Infection Control
in Ambulatory Care

Other Titles of Interest

An Introduction to Epidemiology, Third Edition, *Timmreck*

Infectious Disease Epidemiology: Theory and Practice, *Nelson*

Infection Control in Home Care, *Friedman/Rhinehart*

Epidemiology: Beyond the Basics, *Szklo/Nieto*

Essentials of Epidemiology in Public Health, *Aschengrau/Seage*

Quick Reference to Outbreak Investigation and Control in Health Care Facilities, *Arias*

AN OFFICIAL APIC PUBLICATION

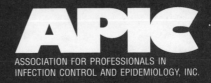

ASSOCIATION FOR PROFESSIONALS IN
INFECTION CONTROL AND EPIDEMIOLOGY, INC.

Infection Control
in Ambulatory Care

Candace Friedman
Manager
Infection Control & Epidemiology
University of Michigan Hospitals and Health Centers
Ann Arbor, Michigan

Kathleen H. Petersen
Staff Specialist
Infection Control & Epidemiology
University of Michigan Hospitals and Health Centers
Ann Arbor, Michigan

JONES AND BARTLETT PUBLISHERS
Sudbury, Massachusetts
BOSTON   TORONTO   LONDON   SINGAPORE

World Headquarters
Jones and Bartlett Publishers
40 Tall Pine Drive
Sudbury, MA 01776
978-443-5000
info@jbpub.com
www.jbpub.com

Jones and Bartlett Publishers Canada
2406 Nikanna Road
Mississauga, ON L5C 2W6
CANADA

Jones and Bartlett Publishers International
Barb House, Barb Mews
London W6 7PA
UK

Library of Congress Cataloging-in-Publication Data

Friedman, Candace.
   Infection control in ambulatory care / Candace Friedman, Kathleen H. Petersen.
     p. cm.
   Includes bibliographical references and index.
   ISBN 0-7637-3190-0
    1. Ambulatory medical care. 2. Infection—Prevention. I. Petersen, Kathleen H. II. Title.

RA974.F75 2003
362.1'2—dc21

                                    2003044700

Acquisitions Editor: Penny M. Glynn
Production Manager: Amy Rose
Editorial Assistant: Amy Sibley
Manufacturing Buyer: Amy Bacus
Composition: Northeast Compositors
Cover Design: Kristin Ohlin
Printing and Binding: Courier Stoughton
Cover Printing: Courier Stoughton

Printed in the United States of America
07 06 05 04 03   10 9 8 7 6 5 4 3 2 1

To our families, especially Robert and Bob and Leah, for their confidence and support over the years.

Table of Contents

Preface

An increasing number of patients with a variety of illnesses are cared for in ambulatory care settings. These patients are often immunocompromised due to underlying illness or treatment practices. In addition, many diagnostic and treatment modalities, including invasive and surgical procedures, are now performed in ambulatory settings. The combination of immunocompromised patients and complexity of care in ambulatory settings results in a need to focus on prevention of infection.

We wrote this book to assist all individuals who practice infection prevention and control and health care epidemiology in ambulatory settings. There are few comprehensive references outlining appropriate practices in these areas. It was our intent to glean information from various resources in order to compile as complete a reference as possible.

Infection prevention and control issues are important across the continuum of care. The basic principles of prevention and control are similar in these areas; however, circumstances may influence specific practice issues. We attempted to provide background information, review basic principles, and describe recommended practices for various ambulatory care settings.

Acknowledgements

This book exists because of the encouragement and support of various colleagues and friends, including Emily Rhinehart, Rochelle Berg, and Barbara Soule. We thank authors Carol Chenoweth, Susan Blitz, and Mary Carol Fromes for their contributions.

Thoughtful and critical review was crucial to the accuracy of this book. Reviewers include Joan Wideman, Marlene Turk, Brian Noonan, Kristi Vander Hyde, Jennifer Arndt, Virginia Walter, Barbara White, Marcia Sojkowski, and Susan Thoms. In addition, we are grateful to Debra Johnson and Eileen Schlather for taking time to review the entire manuscript.

We appreciate the support of co-workers, family, and friends who understood the demands of this project.

CHAPTER 1

Infection Control and Ambulatory Care

HISTORICAL PERSPECTIVE

The first infection prevention and control efforts in the United States began in the 1950s concurrent with the growth of intensive care and increasing staphylococcal infections in hospitals.[1] Formal infection prevention and control (IC) programs then became common in hospitals during the 1970s when IC professionals were hired by many facilities.

There were no governmental or private regulations or standards for IC until 1976 when IC programs became a requirement for accreditation by the Joint Commission on Accreditation of Healthcare Organizations.[1] The Joint Commission's standards are used by many institutions to establish a general framework for infection prevention and control activities. A publication by the Association for Professionals in Infection Control and Epidemiology and the Society for Healthcare Epidemiology of America outlines the structure and function of these programs.[2]

AMBULATORY CARE SETTINGS

Ambulatory care can be defined as health care rendered for acute and chronic diseases and for surgical interventions performed in facilities in which patients reside for less than 24 hours.[3] This type of care is delivered in a variety of settings, such as physician and dental offices, clinics or practices administered by groups of physicians, health maintenance organizations, and facilities attached to hospitals. Other settings include emergency and urgent care centers, diagnostic treatment centers or procedure suites, radiology and imaging centers, dialysis centers, chemotherapy or infusion centers, and short-stay facilities (e.g., 23-hour clinics). Surgical procedures are also performed in surgery centers, whether freestanding, office-based, or part of a traditional healthcare facility.

The risk of infection has traditionally been considered to be low in ambulatory care. This is because most persons seen in these settings have relatively minor illnesses or injuries, or have chronic conditions that have not seriously compromised their host defenses.[4] In addition, ambulatory care visits are typically of limited duration and consist of primarily noninvasive procedures. Few investigators have systematically evaluated the rates of infection in ambulatory care populations. However, because more invasive diagnostic and surgical procedures are being performed in outpatient settings and patients with unrecognized infectious diseases are seen, there is increased focus on infection prevention and control programs.

IC IN AMBULATORY CARE

Infectious diseases account for 20 to 30% of physician office visits, with acute infection of the respiratory tract as the most common reason for consulting a physician.[5] There have been multiple outbreaks of measles,[6–7] tuberculosis,[8] and other infectious diseases[9] traced to physician offices or clinics. Most of these outbreaks were associated with noncompliance with IC procedures.

Medical conditions that were once managed in the acute care hospital are now being treated in ambulatory care settings. These conditions require infusion therapy, dialysis, endoscopy, and other invasive procedures. In addition, an increasing number of surgical procedures have shifted from inpatient to ambulatory settings.[10–11] The range of procedures performed in ambulatory care settings is broadening; surgeons may even have an entire surgical suite incorporated into their office.[12] Immunocompromised and chronically ill patients as well as increasingly invasive procedures pose a risk for the development of infection in these patients. Outbreaks of health care-associated infections have occurred in these various ambulatory care settings.[13]

Thus, transmission of both community- and heath care-associated infections poses a risk to patients in ambulatory care. There is also concern about the potential for occupational transmission of infection in these settings. However, scant published information or recommendations exist regarding the specific risk of infections and prevention strategies in the outpatient setting.

IC PROGRAMS

The Joint Commission's Surveillance, Prevention and Control of Infection Standards for Ambulatory Care[14] are almost identical to those focused on the hospital. In fact, its Shared Visions–New Pathways initiative likely will result in completely identical standards.[15] This seems appropriate, because the basic principles of disease transmission and prevention are the same in ambulatory care service areas as in traditional hospital settings. However, the prevention strategies will vary based on the patient population served and the specific setting,[16] and various practices may need to be adapted for application in some ambulatory care areas.

IC RESOURCES

Infection prevention and control program oversight should come from a group or an individual with infection control expertise and the authority to carry out the components of the program. However, the IC program itself should be the responsibility of one individual. Specific training relevant to IC knowledge and practice will make this individual more effective in managing an IC program.[17] In many facilities this individual may also have other assigned activities; that is, the IC component will be part-time.[2]

As more care is provided in ambulatory care settings, patients and healthcare workers alike are at risk for developing or transmitting infection. The IC community has an opportunity to apply the large body of knowledge related to heath care-associated infections, risk factors, and prevention strategies learned from the hospital setting and to develop programs that meet the needs of ambulatory care.

References

1. McDonald, L. L. Health policy for infection control and epidemiology in critical care. *Crit Care Nurs Clin.* 1995; 7:727–732.

2. Friedman, C., Barnette, M., Buck, A. S., Ham, R., Harris, J., and Hoffman, P., et al. Requirements for infrastructure and essential activities of infection control and epidemiology in out-of-hospital settings: A Consensus Panel report. *Am J Infect Control.* 1999; 27:418–430.

3. Nafzinger, D. A., Lundstrom, T., Chandra, S., and Massanari, R. M. Infection control in ambulatory care. *Infect Dis Clin North Am.* 1997; 11:279–296.

4. Jackson, M. M. Ambulatory Care Facilities. In: Abrutyn, E., Goldmann, D. A., Scheckler, W. E., eds., *Saunders Infection Control Reference Service.* 2nd Ed. Philadelphia: W. B. Saunders Co., 2001: 139.

5. Palmer, S., Giddens, J., and Palmer, D., eds. *Infection Control.* El Paso, TX: Skidmore-Roth Publishing, Inc., 1996: 245.

6. Bloch, A. B., Orenstein, W. A., Ewing, W. M., Spain, W. H., Mallison, G. F., Herrmann, K. L., and Hinman, A. R. Measles outbreak in a pediatric practice: Airborne transmission in an office setting. *Pediatrics.* 1985; 75:676–683.

7. Davis, R. M., Orenstein, W. A., Frank, J. A., Jr., Sacks, J. J., Dales, L. G., and Preblud, S. R., et al. Transmission of measles in medical settings. 1980 through 1984. *JAMA.* 1986; 255:1295–1298.

8. Askew, G. L., Finelli, L., Hutton, M., Laraque, F., Porterfield, D., and Shilkret, K., et al. *Mycobacterium tuberculosis* transmission from a pediatrician to patients. *Pediatrics.* 1997; 100:19–23.

9. Goodman, R. A., and Solomon, S. L. Transmission of infectious diseases in outpatient health care settings. *JAMA.* 1991; 265:2377–2381.

10. Manian, F. A. Surveillance of surgical site infections in alternative settings: Exploring the current options. *Am J Infect Control.* 1997; 25:102–105.

11. Davis, J. E. Ambulatory surgery...how far can we go? *Med Clin North Am.* 1993; 77:365–375.

12. Wade, B. H. Outpatient/Out of Hospital Care Issues. In: Wenzel, R. P., ed., *Prevention and Control of Nosocomial Infections*. 3rd Ed. Baltimore: Williams & Wilkins, 1997: 252.

13. Herwaldt, L. A., Smith, S. D., and Carter, C. D. Infection control in the outpatient setting. *Infect Control Hosp Epidemiol.* 1998; 19:41–74.

14. Joint Commission on Accreditation of Healthcare Organizations. *Standards for Ambulatory Care*. Oakbrook Terrace, IL: JCAHO, 2000: 230.

15. Shared Visions–New Pathways. *Perspectives*. 2002; 22:1–15.

16. Jennings, J., Thibeault, M., Olmsted, R., and Craig, C. Ambulatory. In*: APIC Text of Infection Control and Epidemiology*. Washington, DC: Association for Professionals in Infection Control and Epidemiology; 2000: 38:1–29.

17. Goldrick, B. A., Dingle, D. A., Gilmore, G. K., Curchoe, R. M., Plackner, C. L., Fabrey, L. J., and The Certification Board of Infection Control and Epidemiology, Inc., 2001 Advisory Committee. *Am J Infect Control*. 2002; 30:437–448.

CHAPTER 2

The Infectious Disease Process

Contributing Author:
Carol E. Chenoweth, M.D.
Clinical Associate Professor
Division of Infectious Diseases
Department of Internal Medicine
University of Michigan Health System

AGENT, HOST, ENVIRONMENT

Human beings live in dynamic interaction with their environment and microorganisms. The human body is host to numerous bacteria, fungi, and some viruses that live in a commensal relationship. The term **normal flora** refers to microorganisms that inhabit various parts of the body and may have a protective role in preventing infection. As an example, in most people *Escherichia coli*, *Enterococcus faecalis*, and millions of anaerobic bacteria live in the intestinal tract as normal flora. The presence of these microorganisms is beneficial to the host because they provide nutrients for absorption and competitively inhibit the growth of pathogenic microorganisms. **Colonization** is a term that describes growth of microorganisms in the body without damage to tissues. Normal flora may be described as colonization; however, other microorganisms, which are not usual inhabitants, may colonize the human body as well. Examples of microorganisms not considered to be normal flora that may colonize human beings include methicillin-resistant *Staphylococcus aureus* or vancomycin-resistant enterococci (VRE).

The body has multiple immune defense mechanisms that prevent colonizing microorganisms from causing infection. Infection occurs when a microorganism evades the normal host immune defenses and causes tissue damage and disease. Host factors, including age, underlying illness, or compromised immune defenses such as those occurring with corticosteroid therapy, other immunosuppressive medications, or irradiation, result in increased risk of infection. In addition, medi-cal procedures, including surgical operations, anesthesia, and indwelling catheters, break down the normal first line of defense and make patients more susceptible to infection.

TYPES OF INFECTIONS

An infection occurs when an infective agent establishes itself and multiplies in or on a suitable host. Individuals are susceptible to an infection if they do not have sufficient resistance against a microorganism to prevent the infection if exposed to the microbe. The host immune response to infection results in clinical signs and symptoms of inflammation. These consist of systemic signs and symptoms, including fever, muscle aches, and malaise, or local signs of inflammation, such as pain, redness or erythema, and swelling. Many infections occur with very few recognizable signs and symptoms; these are considered to be subclinical infections. Other infections are associated with obvious signs and symptoms and are recognized as an infection. For example, chicken pox may cause a subclinical infection if the symptoms are mild and there is no observable rash. Alternatively, chicken pox usually presents with fever, malaise, and a characteristic rash.

There are some infectious agents that can cause a chronic infection that does not damage the host tissues and is not associated with any signs or symptoms. This is called a **carrier state**. An example of a carrier state occurs in 10% of patients who are infected with hepatitis B virus. These patients remain asymptomatic and never develop damage to the liver. They are considered to be carriers because even though they lack symptoms and signs of infection, they may act as a reservoir or source of transmission of hepatitis B virus to other people.

TRANSMISSION OF INFECTIOUS AGENTS

The method by which a microorganism spreads from the environment or from person to person is critical for developing infection prevention and control strategies. There are five main methods for spread of microorganisms: contact transmission, droplet transmission, airborne transmission, common vehicle transmission, and vectorborne transmission (see Table 2.1).[1–2] Most pathogenic microorganisms are spread in the ambulatory care setting through contact, droplet, or airborne transmission. Vectorborne transmission occurs when vectors, such as mosquitoes or ticks, spread microorganisms; this is an uncommon method of infectious spread in a healthcare setting and will not be discussed further here.

Contact Transmission

Contact transmission is the most important mode of spread of microorganisms in the healthcare setting. **Direct contact transmission** occurs when person-to-person contact results in the transfer of microorganisms from an infected or colonized person to a susceptible host. Direct contact transmission occurs, for example,

Table 2.1 Examples of Modes of Transmission for Common Pathogenic Agents

Mode of Transmission	Agent
Airborne	Chicken pox
	Measles (rubeola virus)
	Tuberculosis
Contact	Enteric pathogens
	Vancomycin-resistant enterococci
Respiratory droplet	Influenza
	Respiratory syncytial virus
	Rubella (German measles)
Common vehicle	Contaminated multidose vials
Vector	Lyme disease

when a nurse with herpetic whitlow transfers herpes virus to a patient. **Indirect contact transmission** occurs when an intermediate object, such as a contaminated needle, instrument, or hands of a healthcare provider, transfers microorganisms to a susceptible host. A primary example of indirect contact transmission is when a healthcare provider performs a patient care activity and spreads a resistant microorganism, such as VRE, to the patient from unwashed hands, thus acting as an intermediary in patient-to-patient spread.

Droplet Transmission

Droplet transmission occurs primarily from persons infected with upper respiratory viruses. Infectious droplets are generated from the infected person during coughing, sneezing, and talking. Certain medical procedures, including sputum induction and bronchoscopy, may generate droplets as well. These droplets are propelled through the air for a short distance (approximately three feet) and then fall to the floor or other environmental surfaces. Transmission occurs when infectious droplets contact the mucous membranes or conjunctiva of a susceptible host. An example of droplet transmission is when influenza virus is spread from a coughing infected child to a susceptible child while playing in the waiting room of an ambulatory clinic.

Airborne Transmission

Airborne transmission occurs when airborne droplet nuclei are carried through the air from an infected person and inhaled by a susceptible host. Droplet nuclei are tiny evaporated respiratory droplets that can float in the air for long periods of time and can be disseminated in air currents or ventilation systems. Important examples of microorganisms spread via airborne transmission are *Mycobacterium tuberculosis*, chicken pox, and measles virus (rubeola).

Common Vehicle Transmission

Common vehicle transmission occurs when microorganisms are spread from contaminated food, water, medications, or equipment. In the ambulatory setting, this type of transmission may occur from contaminated multi-dose medication vials or from contaminated bronchoscopes.

INFECTION RISKS

Several host factors may increase the risk of acquiring infections in the ambulatory setting. One important factor is age, as the very young and the very old are more susceptible to a variety of infections. Infants, especially in the neonatal period, have not developed an adequate immune response to many common pathogens. The infant immune system may take several months to mature to a fully functioning system. *Listeria monocytogenes* is an example of a pathogenic microorganism that is more likely to infect a neonate than an older person.

Pediatric patients, including infants, toddlers, and preschool children, are also at risk of acquiring infections in the ambulatory setting. At this age, children will begin attending day care and preschool facilities where viruses are spread easily from child to child.[3] These children usually have not learned proper hygienic practices to prevent the spread of enteric and respiratory infections. Symptomatic children in the ambulatory care waiting area may inadvertently spread viruses while playing with other children through direct contact with infectious secretions or indirect contact with contaminated toys.

Unvaccinated children are also susceptible to a number of childhood viruses that cause a rash and can be spread through the airborne route. Chicken pox and measles (rubeola) are examples of childhood infections that can be spread through the air of a clinic.[4] These diseases are seen less frequently with the advent of vaccines. However, sporadic cases, especially chicken pox, still occur. Children are infectious in the early stages of their rash in chicken pox, until their lesions crust. Unfortunately, children may be infectious for up to 24 hours before their chicken pox rash becomes apparent. Measles is contagious from the beginning of prodromal symptoms until about four days after onset of rash. Because these infections are transmittable in ambulatory care settings, procedures for identifying patients with rash and those who are in the incubation period for these diseases and reaching their contagious period must be developed for ambulatory sites that may encounter pediatric patients.

Elderly persons are also at risk of developing infections. As a person ages, the immune system function wanes, increasing the risk of acquiring an infection and increasing the risk of death from infection.[5] In addition to a weaker immune system, elderly patients frequently have more chronic medical illnesses, such as diabetes, chronic lung disease, malignancy, dementia, or malnutrition, which complicate their course of disease and increase the risk of infection. Finally, elderly patients residing in long-term care facilities are at risk of acquiring infections with microorganisms that are endemic to nursing homes (e.g., methicillin-resistant staphylococcus) and infections related to treatments used in nursing homes (e.g., catheter-related urinary tract infections).

Patients with one or more defects in normal human defense mechanisms may be predisposed to common infectious agents and microorganisms that would not normally cause infection in humans (opportunistic pathogens).[6] Patients may have increased risk of infection due to immunosuppressive therapy (including corticosteroid therapy), the absence of a functioning spleen, or breakdown in normal protective mucosal barriers. Underlying diseases, such as infection with human immunodeficiency virus or hematological malignancies, alter the human immune system. Metabolic factors, such as malnutrition, uremia, or hyperglycemia, may also decrease the function of immune cells, putting the patient at increased risk of infection. As noted, a patient may have several factors simultaneously, which work together to increase the risk of infection.

Medical procedures performed in the ambulatory setting may also put patients at risk of infection. Intravascular devices are used to administer intravenous fluids, medications, blood products, and parenteral nutrition. The use of these catheters, however, may put the patient at risk of infectious complications, including catheter site infection, bloodstream infection, septic thrombophlebitis, or endocarditis.[7–8] Long-term intravascular catheters are also used frequently for chronic dialysis in the ambulatory setting. These patients are at high risk for the development of catheter-related bloodstream infection. Other invasive procedures, including surgical procedures, endoscopies, bronchoscopies, and cystoscopies, are associated with an increased risk of infection due to disruption of normal host barriers. All healthcare providers should know the risks of infections associated with medical procedures and the necessary measures for preventing those infections.

REDUCING THE RISK OF INFECTION

Patients and staff in the ambulatory setting have risks for the development of various infections. Many of these infections are preventable through standard infection prevention and control measures. Correction of underlying diseases, such as diabetes or malnutrition, can improve the patient's ability to fight infection. Immunosuppressive medications and antibiotics must be used judiciously. Healthcare providers can improve patient and staff ability to resist infection through effective vaccine use.[9]

Standard infection prevention and control practices are the most effective means for reducing the risk of infection in the ambulatory setting. Handwashing remains the most important intervention for the prevention of infection in any healthcare setting.[10-11] Isolation precautions are necessary to prevent transmission of infection from patient to patient, patient to staff, or staff to patient[1] (see Chapter 6). In addition, procedures for the prevention of infections due to medical procedures are important for the prevention of health care-associated infections.[8-9, 12]

References

1. Garner, J. S. and The Hospital Infection Control Practices Advisory Committee. Guidelines for isolation precautions in hospitals. *Am J Infect Control.* 1996; 24:24–52.

2. Aitken, C., and Jeffries, D. J. Nosocomial spread of viral disease. *Clin Microbiol Rev.* 2001; 14:528–546.

3. Butz, A. M., Larson, E., Fosarelli, P., and Yolken, R. Occurrence of infectious symptoms in children in day care homes. *Am J Infect Control.* 1990; 18:347–353.

4. Chin, J. ed. *Control of Communicable Diseases Manual.* 17th Ed. Washington, DC: American Public Health Association, 2000.

5. Crossley, K. B., and Peterson, P. K. Infections in the elderly. *Clin Infect Dis.* 1996; 22:209–215.

6. Risi, G. F., and Tomascak, V. Prevention of infection in the immunocompromised host. *Am J Infect Control.* 1998; 26:594–606.

7. Mermel, L. A., Barr, B. M., Sheretz, R. J., Raad, I. I., O'Grady, N., Harris, J. S., and Craven, D. E. Guidelines for the management of intravascular catheter-related infections. *Infect Control Hosp Epidemiol.* 2001; 22:222–242.

8. Centers for Disease Control and Prevention. Guidelines for the Prevention of Intravascular Catheter-Related Infections. *MMWR.* 2002; 51(No. RR-10):1–32.

9. Bolyard, E. A., Tablan, O. C., Williams, W. W., Pearson, M. L., Shapiro, C. N., Deitchman, S. D., and The Hospital Infection Control Practices Advisory Committee. Guidelines for infection control in healthcare personnel, 1998. *Am J Infect Control.* 1998; 26:289–354.

10. Larson, E. Skin hygiene and infection prevention: More of the same or different approaches. *Clin Infect Dis.* 1999; 29:1287–1294.

11. Centers for Disease Control and Prevention. Guideline for Hand Hygiene in Health-Care Settings: Recommendations of the Healthcare Infection Control Practices Advisory Committee and the HICPAC/SHEA/APIC/IDSA Hand Hygiene Task Force. *MMWR.* 2002; 51 (No. RR-16):1–44.

12. Mangram, A. J., Horan, T. C., Peason, M. L., Silver, L. C., Jarvis, W. R., and The Hospital Infection Control Practices Advisory Committee. Guideline for prevention of surgical site infection, 1999. *Am J Infect Control.* 1999; 27:97–132.

CHAPTER 3

Cleaning, Disinfecting, and Sterilizing Patient Care Equipment

INTRODUCTION

Effective reprocessing of patient care equipment and devices is one of the most challenging aspects of infection prevention and control in ambulatory care. Numerous occurrences and outbreaks of infections linked to devices have been reported, as described in the background sections of other chapters. Many disinfectants are toxic and require special handling. Developing and following standard protocols will prevent cross-contamination and minimize exposure of staff to chemicals or biohazardous material. Standard practices are also cost-effective, prolong the life of instruments, provide adequate documentation for regulatory agencies or managed care surveyors, provide for consistent reprocessing after each patient use, and can be flexible enough to accommodate the addition of new instruments.

DEFINITION OF TERMS

A precise use of terminology is crucial to informed decision making about reprocessing practices for instruments.[1–3]

Antiseptic. A chemical that either inhibits the growth of microorganisms or destroys them; this term refers to agents used on living tissue. Manufacturers develop germicides for specific uses; therefore, it is not advisable to use antiseptics on inanimate objects or, conversely, to use disinfectants on living tissue.

-cidal, -cide. Suffix meaning "to kill"; thus a germicide is an agent that destroys microorganisms, particularly pathogenic microorganisms ("germs"), and a bacteriocide is an agent that kills bacteria.

Cleaning. The removal of all visible dust, soil, and other foreign material, usually done using water with soaps, detergents, or enzymatic products along with physical action such as brushing. Meticulous cleaning must precede disinfection or sterilization of medical instruments.

Decontamination. The process of removing disease-producing microorganisms and rendering an object safe for handling.

Disinfection. A process that kills or destroys nearly all disease-producing microorganisms. Disinfectants are used on inanimate objects. There are three levels of disinfection, defined by the hardiness of microorganisms that are to be killed or inactivated (see Figure 3.1).

- High-level disinfection kills vegetative bacteria, tubercle bacillus, fungi, lipid, and nonlipid viruses, but not necessarily high numbers of bacterial spores.
- Intermediate-level disinfection kills vegetative bacteria, most fungi, tubercle bacilli, and most viruses; it does not kill resistant bacterial spores.
- Low-level disinfection kills most vegetative bacteria, some fungi, and some viruses, but cannot be relied on to kill mycobacteria or bacterial spores.

Figure 3.1　Descending Order of Resistance of Microorganisms to Disinfectants* [3]

Most Resistant: Bacterial spores
(Examples: *Bacillus subtilis, B. anthracis, B. stearothermophilus, Clostridium botulinum, C. tetani, C. difficile*)

↓

Mycobacteria
(Examples: *Mycobacterium tuberculosis, M. avium,* and other nontuberculous mycobacteria)

↓

Nonlipid or small viruses
(Examples: coxsackievirus, rhinovirus, polio virus)

↓

Fungi
(Examples: Trichophyton, Aspergillus, Candida, Cryptococccus)

↓

Vegetative bacteria
(Examples: *Pseudomonas species, Staphylococcus aureus, Salmonella,* Enterococci)

↓

Least resistant: Lipid or medium-sized viruses
(Examples: herpes simplex, cytomegalovirus, hepatitis B, hepatitis C, human immunodeficiency virus (HIV), respiratory syncytial, hantavirus, ebola virus)

*Adapted with permission from Rutala, W. A. APIC guideline for selection and use of disinfectants. *Am J Infect Control.* 1996; 24:313–342.

Germicide. An agent that destroys microorganisms, particularly pathogenic microorganisms ("germs").

Pasteurization. The process for high-level disinfection using a minimum of 30 minutes of continuous exposure to water heated to at least 160–180°F (60–70°C). Most commonly used for respiratory therapy and anesthesia equipment.[2, 4]

Pathogens. Microorganisms (bacteria, viruses, fungi, molds, yeasts, and parasites) capable of causing infection.

Reprocessing. For the purposes of this book, the method used to render instruments safe for patient contact.

Sanitization. A process that results in a reduction in the microbial population on an inanimate object to a safe or relatively safe level; the term is usually associated with the food, beverage, or dairy industry.[1]

Sterilization. A process by which all forms of microbial life, including bacteria, viruses, spores, and fungi, are destroyed or eliminated, most commonly accomplished in the ambulatory healthcare setting by steam under pressure.

REUSE OF SINGLE-USE DEVICES

In late 2000 the Food and Drug Administration (FDA) passed new federal regulations on reuse of single-use devices. To summarize, the law indicates that when any item labeled as a single-use device (SUD) is reprocessed after use on one patient, the reprocessing hospital becomes a manufacturer and is subject to all the laws that apply to the manufacturing process. Copies of this document can be obtained from *http://www.fda.gov/cdrh/reuse/singleuse.pdf* or by calling CDRH Facts-on-Demand at (800) 899-0381 or (301) 827-0111, specifying document shelf number 2525 at the prompt. The FDA may be contacted directly for additional questions.

The FDA rules apply specifically to hospitals and third-party reprocessing companies, not to ambulatory care. However, due to legal ramifications and potential risks, reprocessing of SUDs is not recommended in the ambulatory care setting. In addition, many physician offices, clinics, and surgery centers maintain reporting relationships or close affiliation with hospitals, and therefore would be expected to comply with the overall hospital policies for reprocessing. Determining whether an item is single use can be done by checking the packaging, inserts, or instruction material, or by contacting the manufacturer. Labels may indicate "single-use device," "disposable," or "one-time use only." The law does not apply specifically to re-sterilization of SUDs opened, but not used; in general, healthcare facilities have been rewrapping and re-sterilizing SUDs that have not become soiled or contaminated with blood or body fluid.

PATIENTS WITH INFECTIOUS DISEASES

Instruments should be managed and reprocessed using the same method regardless of the diagnosis of the patient. To modify procedures for patients suspected or known to have HIV, viral hepatitis (B, C, or other types), antibiotic-resistant microorganisms (e.g., methicillin-resistant *S. aureus*, vancomycin-resistant enterococcus, or vancomycin-resistant *S. aureus*), tuberculosis, or other infections is inconsistent with the concept that all patients are potentially infectious.[2] Therefore, reprocessing procedures must be developed and followed consistently to ensure that all instruments are safe for every patient.

Prion agents, such as Creutzfeld-Jakob Disease (CJD), present an exception regarding decontamination of instruments used directly in the brain, spinal cord, or on nerve tissue. In the rare ambulatory care setting where these tissues may be handled, special procedures must be developed. Consult the CDC Web site at *http://www.cdc.gov/ncidod/diseases/cjd/ cjd_inf_ctrl_qa.htm.*

REPROCESSING PRINCIPLES

In 1968 Spaulding developed a classification system that divides instruments into categories based on the risk of infection according to whether they contact sterile tissue, mucous membrane, or skin (see Table 3.1).[5-6] This is the most widely accepted system used by infection control specialists in the United States. With few exceptions, instruments can be classified into one of three categories: critical (contact with sterile tissue), semi-critical (contact with mucous membrane), or noncritical (contact with skin), as outlined in Table 3.2.

GUIDELINES AND PROCEDURES

Written instructions should be developed for each instrument reprocessed. Written procedures provide references for orientation and training of staff, help ensure that instruments are reprocessed consistently, and can be used to develop competencies and quality improvement activities. Managerial staff and staff who perform the reprocessing should review written procedures on a periodic basis and update as necessary. Copies of procedures should be readily available near the instrument reprocessing area for easy reference. Each procedure should provide detailed information on:

- The responsible person
- Personal protective equipment (PPE) required
- Disassembly instructions, when applicable
- Decontamination/cleaning and rinsing
- Disinfection or sterilization method
- Rinsing and drying, for items disinfected
- Storage location
- Any special instructions from the manufacturer

Sample formats that may be used as templates for procedures are located in Appendix F. Table 3.3 provides a guide for many items that are reprocessed in outpatient settings.

Table 3.1 Classification of Devices[3]

Device Classification	Examples of Devices Common in Ambulatory Care	Spaulding Process Classification	Product Classification or Methods
Critical: Enters sterile tissue or vascular system	Needles, scalpels, biopsy forceps, other surgical instruments	Sterilization	Sterilant/disinfectant.
			Sporicidal chemical—prolonged contact time.
			Steam or ethylene oxide (ETO) gas sterilizer.
Semi-critical: Touches mucous membranes, non-intact skin	Flexible and rigid endoscopes, laryngoscopes, vaginal specula	High-level disinfection	Sterilant/disinfectant.
			Sporicidal chemical—short contact time.
			Pasteurization.
Noncritical: Touches intact skin	Stethoscopes, tabletops, blood pressure cuffs, exam tables	Intermediate-level disinfection	Hospital disinfectant with label claim for tuberculocidal activity.
		Low-level disinfection	Hospital disinfectant without label claim for tuberculocidal activity.

Table 3.2 Methods of Sterilization and Disinfection *

| Object | Sterilization | | Disinfection | | |
| | Critical items | | High-level | Intermediate-level | Low-level |
	Procedure	Exposure Time (hr)	Procedure (exposure time ≥20 min.)	Procedure (exposure time ≤10 min.)	Procedure (exposure time ≤10 min.)
Smooth, hard surface	A	MR	C	H	I
	B	MR	D	I	J
	C	10	E	K	K
	D	6	F	L	L
	E	MR	G	M	
	F	8	H		
Rubber tubing and catheters	A	MR	C		
	B	MR	D		
	C	10	E		
	D	6	F		
	E	MR	G		
	F	8	H		
Polyethylene tubing and catheters	A	MR	C		
	B	MR	D		
	C	10	E		
	D	6	F		
	E	MR	G		
	F	8	H		
Lensed instruments	B	MR	C		
	C	10	D		
	D	6	E		
	E	MR	F		
	F	8	G		
Hinged instruments	A	MR	C		
	B	MR	D		
	C	10	E		
	D	6	F		
	E	MR	G		
	F	8	H		

A: Heat sterilization using steam or hot air

B: Low-temperature sterilization such as ethylene oxide or hydrogen peroxide plasma

C: Glutaraldehyde, 2%

D: Hydrogen peroxide, 7.5%

E: Peracetic acid, 0.2%

F: Hydrogen peroxide/Peracetic acid, 1%/0.08%

G: Wet pasteurization

H: Sodium hypochlorite, 1,000 ppm (1:50 dilution of household bleach)

I: Ethyl or isopropyl alcohol, 70–90%

J: Sodium hypochlorite, 100 ppm (1:500 dilution of household bleach)

K: Phenolic

L: Iodophor

M: Quaternary ammonium compound

MR: Manufacturer's recommendation

*Reprinted by permission from Rutala, W. A., and Weber, D. J. Cleaning, disinfection and sterilization. In: *APIC Text of Infection Control and Epidemiology.* Washington, DC: Association for Professionals in Infection Control and Epidemiology; 2000: 55:1–6.

Table 3.3   Equipment Reprocessing Guidelines for Instruments Reprocessed in Medical Offices and Clinics

Equipment	Processing Procedure	Comments
Acupuncture needles	Sterilize	Or use disposable, single use
Alligator forceps	High-level disinfect	
Auricular (ear) specula	High-level disinfect	
Biopsy forceps or punches	Sterilize	Or use disposable, single use
Colposcopy equipment	Sterilize	
Cryosurgery tips	High-level disinfect	Immerse the tip according to manufacturer instructions
Diaphragm (vaginal or cervical) fitting rings	High-level disinfect	
Ear irrigation syringe	Clean with instrument soap and soak in 70% alcohol for 10 minutes	Disposable syringe preferred
Endocervical curettes	Sterilize	
Exam tables	Fresh table paper for each patient; clean with low-level disinfectant or disinfectant cleaner when visibly soiled (urine, fecal material, blood) and at regular, defined intervals	
External surfaces of equipment and horizontal surfaces	Clean with low-level disinfectant or disinfectant cleaner when visibly soiled (urine, fecal material, blood) and at regular, defined intervals	
Fiberoptic endoscopes	High-level disinfect if touches mucous membrane; sterilize if touches sterile tissue	See Chapter 9
Forceps used for surgical procedures	Sterilize	
Glucometers	Low-level disinfect at regular intervals and when soiled	Follow manufacturer's instructions for safe product use
Hemostats used for surgical procedures	Sterilize	
Hyfrecator tips/needles	Sterilize	Or use disposable, single use
Infant scales	Fresh paper for each child; clean with low-level disinfectant or disinfectant cleaner when visibly soiled (urine, fecal material, blood) and at regular, defined intervals	
Laryngoscope blades	High-level disinfect	
Leep equipment, including tenaculum, speculum, and loops	Follow manufacturer instructions: minimum high-level disinfection for items contacting mucous membrane	If labeled for single-patient use, discard items after each patient, including grounding pad
Liposuction cannula	Clean lumen with brushes; sterilize after each use	
Masks, non-disposable, e.g., for oxygen uptake	High-level disinfect	Or use disposable, single use

(continued)

Table 3.3   (continued)

Equipment	Processing Procedure	Comments
Monofilament	Clean after each use with alcohol or other low-level disinfectant	Or use disposable, single use
Mouthpieces, nondisposable, e.g., for pulmonary function testing	High-level disinfect	Or use disposable, single use; use 1-way valve on pulmonary function testing machine
Nail clippers	High-level disinfect	May cause bleeding or contact non-intact skin
Nasal tongs	High-level disinfect	
Otoscope handles	Clean at regular intervals and when visibly soiled; use low-level disinfectant or disinfectant cleaner	Dispose of tips after each patient
Peak flow meters	Disinfect when visibly soiled	Use with mouthpiece
Punch biopsy	Sterilize	Or use disposable, single use
Scalpels	Disposable	Discard in sharps container
Scissors for surgical procedures	Sterilize	
Scissors for suture removal	High-level disinfect	Discard disposable in sharps container
Sigmoidoscopy biopsy forceps	Sterilize	
Sigmoidoscopes	Follow manufacturer's instructions. High-level disinfect	See Chapter 9
Staple removers	High-level disinfect	Or use disposable, single use
Stethoscope	Wipe with alcohol pad (70–95% isopropyl or ethyl alcohol) at regular intervals and when visibly soiled.	
Surgical instruments/trays	Sterilize	
Suture removal equipment	High-level disinfect	Or use disposable, single use
Thermometers, electronic	Clean at regular intervals and when visibly soiled; use low-level disinfectant or disinfectant cleaner	Dispose of tip covers after each patient
Thermometers, glass	Soak in 70% alcohol for 10 minutes; separate oral and rectal	Historically acceptable, even if not strictly according to Spaulding classification
Tonometer tips, other lenses	Remove and soak in disinfectant	See Chapter 14
Toys	Sanitize at regular intervals and when visibly soiled	See Chapter 7
Tympanogram tips	Clean when visibly soiled; avoid testing when there is ear drainage	Or use disposable, single use
Ultrasound probes (skin contact)	After each use wipe off gel, then disinfect with low-level disinfectant or disinfectant cleaner	
Vaginal specula	High-level disinfect (or sterilize unwrapped if high-level disinfectant is not used)	Sterilize wrapped, if sterile specula are requested
Vaginal ultrasound probes	High-level disinfect, whether or not a probe cover is used	Most references recommend high-level disinfectant because probe covers can break;[3] see Chapter 16

CLEANING

Meticulous cleaning is one of the most important concepts in instrument reprocessing.[4] After use on or in patients, instruments, particularly lumened instruments,[7] are contaminated with bioburden, that is, microorganisms, organic debris, blood, and other body fluids. Presence of soil or organic matter may not allow penetration of the disinfectant or sterilant to the surface of the item.[8] Cleaning removes this debris, reduces the quantity of microorganisms, and renders the item safe to handle.

Before instruments are disinfected or sterilized, they must be cleaned thoroughly. Cleaning includes physical removal of soil, blood, tissue, or other organic matter[3] with instrument detergent, mechanical action, and rinsing.[7] Placing items in a presoak of water or detergent solution immediately after use facilitates cleaning and prevents organic matter from hardening.[2, 8-9] Enzymatic instrument detergent, diluted according to label instructions, should be used for cleaning.[4, 8-9] Enzymatic detergents do not contain germicides, but are formulated to effectively remove organic matter. Hand soap is not recommended, because emollients in the soap may remain on the surface of the item, preventing complete contact with the disinfectant or sterilant.

Delicate instruments should be cleaned by hand using soft brushes or cloths, as needed. Instruments with lumens, crevices, or coils are much harder to clean than smooth or flat surfaces and also need special handling. Brushes, designed for this purpose, must be used to clean the inner surfaces of lumens. Ultrasonic cleaners are recommended for instruments with coils and crevices, such as biopsy forceps.[9] Ultrasonic cleaners should be drained each day of use, dried, and refilled with fresh water to prevent overgrowth of water microorganisms. Water should be changed more often if it becomes heavily soiled during the day. If recommended by the manufacturer, enzymatic or other instrument detergent may be added, diluted according to product label. After removal from ultrasonic cleaners, instruments should be thoroughly rinsed with fresh, running water. Central sterile supply and dentistry departments often use ultrasonic cleaners and washer sterilizers to decontaminate heavily soiled surgical or dental instruments. Until they have been decontaminated, highly contaminated devices, such as dental instruments, should be handled wearing gloves.[8]

DISINFECTION

Types of Disinfectants

Choosing an appropriate disinfectant and reprocessing method depends on a number of factors:

- Where the device fits into the Spaulding Classification
- Device manufacturer's recommendations
- Safety considerations, such as work space and ventilation
- Numbers and types of devices that are in use
- Level of contamination of the device (bioburden)
- Cost
- FDA clearance (510k) for safety and efficacy of liquid chemical disinfectants/sterilants intended for use on critical and semicritical items[3]
- Environmental Protection Agency (EPA) clearance for disinfectants intended for use on noncritical items[3]

As an example, surfactants are soapy-type substances that may form bubbles; for lumened instruments, bubbles inside the lumen will prevent complete contact of all surfaces with the agent. Therefore, a non-surfactant disinfectant should be chosen for devices with lumens. Before purchase of and during training about new devices, information from the manufacturer must be reviewed to ensure that reprocessing is understood thoroughly and that the device can be reprocessed based on the Spaulding Classification. Table 3.4 lists the most common disinfectants used in ambulatory care settings and their applications. Articles by Rutala[3] and Chapter 43 in Block[10] provide details on additional products.

Environmental Surface Disinfection

Noncritical items contacting intact skin include blood pressure cuffs, crutches, exam tables and lights, exam and waiting room chairs and other furniture, external surfaces of machines such as tympanograms, and stethoscopes. Intact skin is an effective microbial barrier and these items may be low-level disinfected. Low-level disinfectants and disinfect cleaners are commonly used for this purpose. Quaternary ammonium compounds and phenols are the most common

Table 3.4 Typical Disinfectants Available for Ambulatory Care Settings

Chemical, Use—Dilution	Level of Disinfection	Typical Application	Exposure Time	Comments
Glutaraldehyde, 2.4–3.4%, alkaline or acidic, with or without surfactant	Sterilant, high-level disinfectant	Devices contacting mucous membranes, such as vaginal specula, fiberoptic endoscopes	20–90 minutes for disinfection, varies by formulation; 10 hours for sterilization	Must never be used as an environmental surface disinfectant due to toxicity; many brands on the market; maximum reuse is product-specific and commonly 14 or 30 days.
Peracetic acid, 0.2%	Sterilant; used to high-level disinfect	Fiberoptic endoscopes	12 minutes	Currently available only as a single-use formulation.
Orthophalaldehyde, 0.55%	High-level disinfection	Vaginal specula, fiberoptic endo-scopes	12 minutes	Maximum reuse of 14 days; minimal health hazards have been associated with its use.
Chlorine, 1,000 parts per million (ppm) available chlorine (1:50 dilution of full-strength bleach)	High-level disinfection	Limited application; may be used on some plastic masks	20 minutes	Damaging to many surfaces; corrosive to metal; check with manufacturer of item to be disinfected; must be made fresh daily; double concentration (1:25) is effective for one month. Store in opaque, closed containers (shielded from sunlight).[2]
Chlorine, 500 ppm (1:100 dilution of full-strength bleach)	Intermediate/low-level disinfection	Surface disinfection	10 minutes; allow to dry on surface	Clean surface first; inactivated by organic material. Must be made fresh daily; double concentration (1:50) is effective for one month. Store in opaque, closed containers (shielded from sunlight).[2]
Alcohol, Isopropyl, 60–95%	Intermediate-level disinfection	Surface decontamination; skin anti-sepsis	Allow to dry on surface	No cleaning properties; concentrations above 95% are not effective.
Quaternary ammonium compounds (QACs), 0.4–1.6% aqueous	Intermediate/low-level disinfection	Surface decontamination; unacceptable for semi-critical or critical items	Generally 10 minutes	Most commonly used as cleaner-disinfectant solutions for environmental surfaces. Available as liquid or wipes.
Hydrogen peroxide, 3–6%	Intermediate-level disinfection	Ophthalmic lenses, tonometer tips	Follow manufacturer directions	
Hydrogen peroxide, 7.5%	High-level disinfection	Items contacting mucous membrane	30 minutes	Corrodes copper, zinc, brass.[3]

(continued)

Table 3.4   (continued)

Chemical, Use— Dilution	Level of Disinfection	Typical Application	Exposure Time	Comments
Phenolics, 0.4–5% aqueous	Intermediate/low-level disinfection	Surface decontamination		May leave film, may depigment skin; do not use on surfaces in contact with infants.[2]
Iodophors, 30–50 ppm free iodine	Intermediate-level disinfection	More commonly used for skin antisepsis	Follow manufacturer directions	May stain objects; make sure formulation specifies environmental surfaces.

active ingredients in these products. Labels should indicate that the product is registered by the EPA.

Neither alcohol nor bleach is recommended as a general environmental cleaner. Alcohol contains no cleaning agent, is flammable, and evaporates rapidly. Bleach is corrosive, harmful to clothing, and easily inactivated by organic material.[2] Disinfectant wipes may be used for small areas or items. Spray containers are commonly used and practical in most settings. Concentrated products may be more cost effective but must be diluted strictly according to product instructions into clean containers. Items should be cleaned on a regular basis and when soiled; see Table 3.3 for some examples. For discussion on cleaning environmental surfaces in specific settings refer to Chapters 7 to 18.

Effective Use of High-Level Disinfectants

Many high-level disinfectants are used in health care, including glutaraldehyde, peracetic acid, orthophalaldehyde, hydrogen peroxide, chlorine compounds (e.g., bleach), and various combinations. Each formulation of ingredients is unique; brands cannot be assumed to be interchangeable and should not be mixed.

To assure efficacious use of disinfectants on medical instruments, the following measures must be taken:

- If applicable, activate or dilute product precisely according to label instructions.
- Label activated (in-use) product with the expiration date and discard according to this expiration date.
- Store activated or diluted product in tightly covered containers to avoid evaporation and excessive staff exposure.
- If the solution is reused (e.g., glutaraldehyde), check with a chemical indicator each day of use to

make sure the active ingredient remains at an effective level, that is, maintains its minimum effective concentration. Chemical indicators, usually easy-to-use dipsticks, are supplied by the disinfectant manufacturer. If the solution fails, it must be discarded. Reusable solutions are formulated to maintain efficacy according to label claims (typically 14 to 30 days) with normal use. Therefore, if indicators show early failure, make sure only clean and dry instruments are placed into the solution, that the solution container is tightly covered, and that it has been properly activated, when applicable. If the disinfectant is used in a high-volume setting, such as in an automatic endoscopic reprocessor in a busy endoscopy unit, the disinfectant may be diluted to ineffective levels before the normal expiration date.

- Store and use product at temperature indicated on the label.
- Pre-clean and tap-water rinse each instrument before immersing into the disinfectant. In many settings the same sink will be used to rinse off detergent and disinfectant. Although there are no studies defining the risk, it may be prudent to wipe the sink with a disinfectant cleaner after the detergent rinse to prevent potential splash contamination during the disinfectant rinse.
- Drip dry or rough dry instruments before immersing into the disinfectant to avoid dilution.
- Completely immerse instruments so that all surfaces are covered, including all lumens or other internal surfaces. For electronic devices, for example, vaginal ultrasound probes or cryosurgery tips, immerse as far as indicated by the manufacturer.
- Soak instruments in the product for the time indicated on the label. Glutaraldehyde soak times

of 20 minutes, after thorough instrument cleaning, have been shown to be effective;[11] product labels of 45 minutes are related to regulatory testing of unwashed instruments. Time the soak with a timer or post the end-time in a clearly visible location.

- After soaking, thoroughly rinse each item to completely remove residual disinfectant. Use potable running tap water or a pan of fresh potable water for each instrument to avoid a buildup of disinfectant in the water. At least 500 ml of fresh water should be used for each instrument.[12]
- Dry and store instruments in a manner to prevent recontamination.

Safe Use of Disinfectants

To avoid toxicity to users, the following additional recommendations are suggested or required by the Occupational Safety and Health Administration, as indicated:

- Do not attempt to pour diluted or activated disinfectants back and forth from the original container to the soaking pan. This activity increases potential for spills, splashes, evaporation, and exposure of staff. After the product is activated and in the soaking container, keep it in the container until the expiration date.
- Use all chemicals with adequate ventilation, as required.[13–14]
- Wear gloves for any hand contact with the disinfectant. If there is potential for splashing, wear other PPE such as gowns and face protection.[13–14] If face protection is worn, it must cover eyes, nose, and mouth to protect all of these mucous membranes from exposure.
- Make available Material Safety Data Sheets (MSDS) for all chemical disinfectants used.[14]
- Label all chemical disinfectants. Labels on secondary containers need to contain the following information: the brand name of the contents of the container and any health (e.g., irritant, corrosive, sensitizer) and/or physical (e.g., flammable) hazards. For example, bleach should be labeled "corrosive" and glutaraldehyde should be labeled "irritant, sensitizer."
- Cover containers of disinfectants at all times.

Glutaraldehyde, one of the most commonly used high-level disinfectants, presents special safety concerns. It is a strong irritant to the nose, eyes, and skin, and exposure can cause sensitization.[13–14] Due to increased safety concerns, in 1998 the American Conference of Governmental Industrial Hygienists lowered its recommended threshold limit value-ceiling from 0.2 ppm to 0.05 ppm.[14] The American Institute of Architects (AIA) recommends 15 air changes per hour (ACH) where glutaraldehyde will be used to provide enough ventilation to maintain safe glutaraldehyde levels.[15] In rooms where ventilation is not sufficient, local exhaust should be provided with a hood or specially designed glutaraldehyde filter system. This guideline should be considered during the design phase for new or renovated facilities.

In addition, the following guidelines should be instituted for use of glutaraldehyde:

- Conduct all glutaraldehyde operations under local exhaust ventilation whenever possible.
- Make sure exhaust fans are functioning at all times and are not blocked off or covered up.
- When disposing of the solution, take extreme care to prevent spilling. If a spill occurs, clean it up immediately with absorbent material.
- If the solution is disposed of in the sink drain, run water to rinse the sink of residual glutaraldehyde. Check local and state ordinances for any laws prohibiting disposal of glutaraldehyde into the sewerage system.
- For prolonged contact, wear gloves made of such substances as butyl rubber or nitrile that have been shown to provide full protection from glutaraldehyde permeation. For short exposures and if changed frequently (that is, every 10 to 15 minutes), latex gloves can be used.[16]
- Check glutaraldehyde air levels in newly opened soiled utility rooms when glutaraldehyde is first used or if there are employee complaints about odors or irritation. Industrial hygienists or environmental safety specialists typically are consulted about this testing.

Pasteurization

Pasteurization is very effective for high-level disinfection. It works by exposing instruments to water at 70 to 75°C (158 to 167°F) continuously for at least

30 minutes.[2] Requiring special equipment that can validate water temperature, pasteurization is not commonly used for high-level disinfection in the outpatient setting. It is useful for devices that can withstand contact with hot water, such as vaginal specula and some types of anesthesia and respiratory care equipment. Prior to pasteurization, items must be thoroughly cleaned, as for other reprocessing methods.

STERILIZATION

Background

Sterilization must be used for items that come into contact with the vascular system or with normally sterile tissue and body cavities. In the outpatient setting, items may be purchased sterile (and disposed of after use, e.g., hypodermics needles, syringes), sterilized by a third party, or sterilized on-site.

The Association for Professionals in Infection Control and Epidemiology,[3, 6] the Association for the Advancement of Medical Instrumentation,[8, 17] the Association of Perioperative Registered Nurses (AORN),[18] and the American Society for Healthcare Central Service Professionals[19] have published guidelines and standards for steam sterilization of medical instruments. For sites surveyed by the Joint Commission on Accreditation of Healthcare Organizations (JCAHO), in general, JCAHO is less prescriptive about the details of sterilization policy and is more interested in determining that every department and location within an institution is sterilizing equipment using standard methods. Standard IC.6 states: "The organization's infection control *process* [author's italics] is designed to lower the risks and improve the rates or trends of epidemiologically significant infections."[20]

Currently, steam autoclaves are the most dependable and cost-effective method of sterilization and are commonly used for heat-resistant items such as suture sets, vaginal specula, surgical instruments, and trays.[2] Carefully maintained, steam autoclaves can be used for decades. Details on their safe and effective use follow.

Parameters

There are four parameters of steam sterilization.[21] All four parameters must be met to ensure that an individual instrument is sterile at the time of use (see Table 3.5).[19, 21]

1. Time: Temperatures must be maintained for specified time periods to kill microorganisms. The greater the temperature, the less time required.
2. Temperature level: Temperatures must reach a specific level to ensure killing of microorganisms.
3. Pressure: Pressure is necessary to raise the temperature above the boiling point of water. Steam is directed into a closed chamber and pressure is applied. The manufacturer of the autoclave presets the pressure.
4. Moisture: Steam must be saturated for effective sterilization. For tabletop models, moisture is supplied by adding water to the autoclave.

Cleaning and Wrapping

If an instrument needs to be sterile at the time of use, it must be wrapped to protect it from touch or environmental contamination. Thus, using chemical sterilization to provide sterile instruments is impractical. Cleaning should be performed as outlined earlier in the

Table 3.5 Sterilization Times for Gravity Steam Autoclaves

Temperature	Minimum Exposure to Steam*
Wrapped: 121–123°C (250–254°F)	15–30 minutes; follow autoclave manufacturer instructions
Wrapped: 132–135°C (270–272°F)	10–25 minutes; follow autoclave manufacturer instructions
Unwrapped: 132–135°C (270–272°F) Nonporous, no lumen, metal (e.g., vaginal specula)	3 minutes (flash)
Unwrapped: 132–135°C (270–272°F) Metal with lumen, porous items (e.g., plastic)	10 minutes (flash)

*Times are for exposure to steam and do not indicate the total time of the cycle.

chapter. Peel pouches and traditional wrap are both acceptable. In many clinics and medical office settings, small instruments are sterilized and peel pouches are most practical. To aid in sterility assurance, choose peel pouches that contain chemical indicators incorporated into the paper or plastic of the pouch and that can be tightly sealed with self-sealing tape or heat sealer.

Preventive Maintenance

Steam autoclaves, including tabletop models, are extremely reliable but depend on preventive maintenance and cleaning to maintain their effectiveness. Records should be kept of any maintenance or repairs. If the instruction manual is not available, contact the sterilizer manufacturer or representative to secure this document. Distilled (or deionized) water must be added to the correct level and drained according to the owner's guide to prevent build-up of minerals inside the autoclave. The gasket must be cleaned and checked for deterioration. Cleaning to prevent build-up of minerals or residue inside the autoclave is best done with a lint-free cloth. Use either the agent recommended by the owner's guide or alcohol that will evaporate, leaving no residue. To prevent a fire, packs must not be allowed to touch the inner wall, which becomes extremely hot during the sterilization cycle. Load the sterilizer according to the owner's guide to avoid overloading or improper orientation of packs that can impede steam penetration.

Sterilization Monitors

To provide assurance of sterilization, the following indicators and records are necessary:

- Internal chemical indicators should be used in each package to be sterilized and should be placed in the area of the package considered to be least accessible to steam penetration. The chemical indicator must be examined before the contents are used. Indicators that are part of the peel pouch itself, inside the plastic or paper, can serve as both the internal and the external indicator.
- External chemical indicators should be on each package to differentiate between processed and unprocessed products. For wrapped items, autoclave tape with hash marks that darken during sterilization is most often used. Peel pouches usu-

ally have indicators incorporated into the pouch material.
- Biological indicators (BI) should be used at least weekly (or with each load if the autoclave is used less than weekly), but preferably daily, and must be used with each load containing implantable devices. In addition, BI should be used after any repair or to establish that a new autoclave is functional. The BI must be placed inside a pack that is representative of the loads autoclaved. Records must be kept for all BI. Appendix F contains an example of a record-keeping log.
- Recording charts are available on some models of tabletop autoclaves. If recording devices are available, the operator must examine the record at the end of the cycle to ensure that all the parameters were met and then maintain this record. If recording devices are unavailable, the operator must monitor the time- and temperature-indicating gauges during the cycle to ensure that parameters were met. Mechanical malfunction can be detected quickly if it is noted during the cycle that the parameters were not met.
- Written records of each load should be kept. To determine how long written logs should be kept, consult legal counsel or, if the site is associated with a larger institution or hospital, the infection control department. It is most efficient to keep all of the sterilizer records together in one file or binder.
- Bowie-Dick tests are used only for pre-vacuum sterilizers and are not applicable to gravity-displacement sterilizers, such as tabletop autoclaves, or to steam-flush pressure-pulse sterilizers. If a pre-vacuum sterilizer is used, the Bowie-Dick test must be run daily.

Failure and Recall Policy

Despite the reliability of sterilizers, it is necessary to have a written plan for a failure. The plan can be a checklist or a flow sheet. Whenever there is a failure, a record must be kept to include what parameter failed, corrective action, and any recall of items performed:

- If the BI was positive, run another BI and do not release any packs from the load during which the potential malfunction occurred. If the repeat BI is negative and there are no other indications of failure, continue to monitor as usual. It is advisable to re-run the load during which the positive BI occurred.

- If the repeat BI is positive, recall all products processed since the most recent negative BI. Contact the supervisor and the autoclave maintenance staff. Complete a sterilizer failure report that includes the time and date, a description of the load(s) and lot control number, the results of mechanical monitoring and chemical indicators, and any other information relevant to the validity of the test or mechanical or human error. Notify the infection control professional to perform follow-up surveillance if any nonrecalled items were used on patients. Notify physicians of patients who had contact with these items. After the corrections have been made, retest the sterilizer with a BI. Do not use the sterilizer until results of the biological test are satisfactory.

Shelf Life and Event-Related Sterility

The shelf life of a packaged sterile item is typically termed "event related"[8] and depends on the quality of the wrapper material, the storage conditions, the conditions during transport, and the amount of handling. Shelf life is not simply a matter of sterility maintenance but is also a function of device degradation and inventory control. There should be written policies and procedures for how shelf life is determined and how it is indicated on the product.

In general, stock rotation according to the "first in, first out" principle should be maintained. Each item should be labeled with the sterilization date to allow for stock rotation. A statement on each package, such as "Product is not sterile if packaging is open, damaged, or wet. Check before using," may be a helpful reminder. Because sterility assurance is generally event-related, expiration dating on sterilized items is needed only when there is a component in the package that will degrade or has an expiration date, such as a chemical.

Sterile supplies should be handled carefully; care should be taken to avoid crushing, bending, compressing, or puncturing the packaging or otherwise compromising the sterility of the contents. Packs should be removed from the autoclave and handled only after complete drying and cooling. Packaging should be given thorough visual inspection for integrity and labeling prior to use. The pack must also be opened using

aseptic technique. Upon opening a sterile pack, the internal indicator also must be checked before using any component.

Flash Sterilization

Except in surgery centers where transport of a flashed item can be controlled, flash sterilization should not be performed in ambulatory care. According to the AORN, flash sterilization "should be carefully selected to meet special clinical situations [and] should be used only when there is insufficient time to sterilize an item by the preferred prepackaged method. . . . When performed correctly, flash sterilization is a safe and effective process. . . . Implants should not be flashed."[18] The major risk for contamination after flash sterilization is during transport of the item from the sterilizer to the sterile field.

Detailed procedures should be written to include what and under what circumstances items can be flashed (e.g., dropped instruments), precleaning methods, the flash sterilization procedure itself (time and temperature), transport methods of the item, and record keeping (e.g., date, time, item flashed, and parameters of sterilization).[23] The printout from the sterilizer can be used for this record and can be stored with the other sterilization records.

OTHER REPROCESSING METHODS

Gas (ethylene oxide or ETO) is not a practical option in ambulatory care due to health and environmental hazards, cost, and lengthy cycle time.[2] Dry heat ovens are used in some settings, such as dentistry;[17] however, the slow rate of microbial killing makes this impractical for most settings.[2]

Periodically, new technologies are introduced, such as low-temperature gas plasma sterilization.[24] A thorough analysis must be performed before considering the purchase of any new sterilization system, including complete review of product literature describing efficacy studies, availability of FDA 510(k) clearance, what items are suitable for sterilizing with the proposed system, limitations of the proposed system, and initial capital outlay and operating expense. Upon installation, the manufacturer must be required to completely train all staff about operating instructions for the specific instruments that will be reprocessed, use of special instrument wrap that may be needed, biological and other monitoring, record keeping, preventive maintenance, safety considerations, and troubleshooting.

Glass bead "sterilizers," microwaves, dishwashing machines, and boilers have been used for reprocessing in the past; however, these methods are not acceptable. In addition, decontaminating machines and washer sterilizers are not adequate for terminal reprocessing. Any method that lacks monitoring capability or scientific research for validation of disinfection or sterilization claims should be viewed with skepticism and probably rejected as inadequate.

SPECIAL SITUATIONS

A steam autoclave may be used in place of a high-level disinfectant soak for heat-resistant instruments that contact mucous membranes. For example, a clinic with an autoclave may choose to autoclave vaginal specula rather than use chemical high-level disinfection. Instruments that contact mucous membranes that are autoclaved need not be wrapped, although chemical indicator tape should be run along with each unwrapped load to indicate that the cycle is completed. The advantage of this method is that staff only need to be knowledgeable about sterilizer operation and monitoring, and concerns for staff exposure to high-level disinfectants are eliminated.

If very few items are sterilized, it may be more cost-effective to eliminate the autoclave and purchase disposable instruments or send instruments to a central processing department in an affiliated hospital. This eliminates the need to ensure that staff are thoroughly knowledgeable and competent to both operate and monitor the autoclave and/or to use high-level disinfectant. High-level disinfectants will sterilize with a prolonged soak; however, because there is no way to ensure sterility during removal from the disinfectant, rinsing, and storing or transporting the instruments to the point of use, this method is not useful for reprocessing critical items.

Policies need to be developed for instruments that clinicians bring in to the facility or that are borrowed from another institution.[22] If reprocessing, transport, and storage conditions are unknown, these items should be cleaned and reprocessed according to the facility procedures upon return. Any questions should be directed to the manufacturer. For more details on instrument handling in areas such as endoscopy, den-

tistry, or ophthalmology, refer to Chapters 9, 12, and 14, respectively, on those topics.

WORKPLACE DESIGN

Optimally, reprocessing activities should occur in a separate soiled utility room.[15] In some states there may be regulatory agency requirements for room separation. Functional work areas should be physically separated by walls, partitions, or space to contain contaminants generated during reprocessing. AIA recommends a minimum of 6 ACH under negative pressure in the soiled/decontamination rooms of central supply departments and a minimum of 10 ACH under negative pressure in the soiled workrooms of diagnostic and treatment areas.[15]

Work flow and traffic patterns should flow from soiled to clean areas. Separating "clean" and "dirty" areas limits the potential for contamination of sterile items or inadvertent use of soiled items. Because there may be a variety of staff coming and going in the work area, it is best to label the intake area as "soiled" and the area where reprocessed items are placed before distribution to storage areas as "clean/patient ready." Soaking and cleaning basins should be positioned to leave ample room in the sink for rinsing instruments under running water. Handwashing sinks must be available and conveniently located in or near the decontamination and clean preparation areas. In surgery centers there will be a decontamination room, as well as more stringent recommendations as described in Chapter 8.

STORAGE

The following guidelines should be observed for storage and handling of clean or sterile items:

- Disinfected and sterile supplies must be stored in a manner that will prevent contamination. Items stored in the utility, treatment, or exam rooms should be stored in closed cupboards or drawers. Small items may be placed in covered bins or containers on open shelves. Supplies must be protected from water damage and dust. If supplies are stored in a dedicated clean storage room, open shelving is acceptable. Clean items must be stored away from the splash zone around a sink and must not be stored under a sink.
- Clean should be separated from sterile to avoid using a nonsterile item when a sterile item is needed.

- Sterile instruments and supplies should be stocked and rotated "first in, first out" so that the oldest items are used first.
- Instruments should not be stored in disinfecting solution, but should be rinsed and dried.
- Supplies and instruments must not be pre-set up or left on counter tops or stands. These items must be set up immediately prior to use. For sterile procedures such as surgery or central line insertions, aseptic technique must be used and a sterile field must be maintained. For clean technique, such as for obtaining pap smears, a sterile field need not be maintained.

STAFF EDUCATION AND QUALITY IMPROVEMENT

Adequate training and continuing education minimize the possibility of operator error during reprocessing and handling of instruments. Negative outcomes have occurred where training has not been adequate. Workup of an outbreak involving 34 of 82 patients after liposuction revealed many deficiences: Surgical technicians had no formal training in infection control practices, glutaraldehyde levels were not monitored, tubing was rinsed but not sterilized, surgical equipment was washed but not sterilized, and the autoclave was not monitored.[25]

Staff training includes orientation, continuing education, and competencies. Initial training should include review of written procedures and return

demonstration of the reprocessing technique. Training should include care of the instruments from the time they are used on one patient through the transport, cleaning, disinfection or sterilization, storage, and set-up for the next patient. It should also include safety precautions for the staff and work flow in the utility room. Records of training and competencies must be documented in the employee files. Examples of competencies are included in Appendix F.

For quality monitoring and improvement, periodic inspections or spot checks should be performed to correct any deficiencies in a timely manner.[26–27]

FURTHER INFORMATION

If a specific ambulatory care setting is affiliated with a hospital, it is important to contact the infection prevention and control department to discuss instrument processing. Each ambulatory care site may be expected to follow similar protocols. The infection control or central sterile supply departments can provide assistance on ordering cost-effective cleaners, disinfectants, and monitoring devices. The goal is to standardize procedures, chemicals, and supplies as much as possible.

Professional reference Web sites include American Society for Healthcare Central Service Professionals (*http://www.ashcsp.org/*) and Association for the Advancement of Medical Instrumentation (*http://www. aami.org/*).

References

1. Block, S. S. Definition of Terms. In: Block, S. S., ed. *Disinfection, Sterilization, and Preservation.* 5th Ed. Malvern, PA: Lea & Febiger, 2001: 19–28.

2. Rutala, W. A. Disinfection, Sterilization and Waste Disposal. In: Wenzel, R. P., ed. *Prevention and Control of Nosocomial Infections.* 3rd Ed. Baltimore, MD: Williams & Wilkins, 1997: 539–593.

3. Rutala, W. A. APIC guideline for selection and use of disinfectants. *Am J Infect Control.* 1996; 24:313–342.

4. AORN. Recommended practices for high-level disinfection. In: *AORN. Standards, Recommended Practices, and Guidelines.* Denver, CO: Association of periOperative Registered Nurses, Inc., 2002: 211–216.

5. Spaulding, E. H. Chemical disinfection of medical & surgical materials. In: Lawrence, C. A., and Block, S. S., eds. *Disinfection, Steriliza-*

tion and Preservation. Philadelphia, PA: Lea & Febiger, 1968: 517–531.

6. Rutala, W. A., and Weber, D. J. Cleaning, disinfection and sterilization. In: *APIC Text of Infection Control and Epidemiology.* Washington, DC: Association for Professionals in Infection Control and Epidemiology, 2000: 55:1–6.

7. Chan-Myers, B. S., McAlister, D., and Antonoplos, P. Natural bioburden levels detected on rigid lumened medical devices before and after cleaning. *Am J Infect Control.* 1997; 25:471–476.

8. Association for the Advancement of Medical Instrumentation (AAMI). Steam sterilization & sterility assurance in office-based, ambulatory-care medical, surgical & dental facilities. *AAMI Standards and Recommended Practices, Volume 1.1: Sterilization, Part 1—Sterilization in Healthcare Facilities.* Arlington, VA: Association for the Advancement of Medical Instrumentation, 2001: 89–132.

9. Alvarado, C. J., and Reichelderfer, M. APIC Guidelines Committee. APIC guideline for infection prevention and control in flexible endoscopy. *Am J Infect Control.* 2000; 28:138–155.

10. Favero, M. S., and Bond, W. W. Chemical disinfection of medical and surgical materials. In: Block, S. S., ed. *Disinfection, Sterilization and Preservation.* 5th Ed. Philadelphia, PA: Lea & Febiger, 2001: 881–917.

11. Rutala, W., and Weber, D. J. FDA labeling requirements for disinfection of endoscopes: A counterpoint. *Infect Control Hosp Epidemiol.* 1995; 16:231–235.

12. Alfa, M. J., Olson, N., DeGagne, P., and Jackson, M. A survey of reprocessing methods, residual viable bioburden, and soil levels in patient-ready endoscopic retrograde choliangiopancreatography duodenoscopes used in Canadian centers. *Infect Control Hosp Epidemiol.* 2002; 23:198–206.

13. Publication #2001-115. *Glutaraldehyde: Occupational hazards in hospitals.* Washington, DC: National Institute for Occupational Safety and Health, 2001. *http://www.cdc.gov/niosh/2001-115.html.*

14. Walker, S. B. *Guideline for the Use of High-Level Disinfectants and Sterilants for Reprocessing of Flexible Gastrointestinal Endoscopes.* Society of Gastroenterology Nurses and Associates, Inc., 2000. *http://www.sgna.org/resources/HLD.html.*

15. American Institute of Architects Academy of Architecture for Health. In: *Guidelines for design and construction of hospital and health care facilities.* Washington, DC: American Institute of Architects Press, 2001: 73,79–80.

16. Miles, J. B. *Standard Interpretation and Compliance Letters. Use of latex surgical exam gloves for protection from glutaraldehyde.* Washington, DC: OSHA; 10/3/1997. *http://www.osha.gov/pls/oshaweb/owadisp.show_document?p_table=INTERPRETATIONS&p_id=224 81&p_text_version=FALSE.*

17. Association for the Advancement of Medical Instrumentation (AAMI). Tabletop dry heat (heated air) sterilization and sterility assurance in dental and medical facilities. *AAMI Standards and Recommended Practices, Volume 1.1: Sterilization, Part 1—Sterilization in Healthcare Facilities.* Arlington, VA: Association for the Advancement of Medical Instrumentation, 2001: 133–168.

18. AORN. Recommended practices for sterilization in the practice setting. In: *AORN. Standards, Recommended Practices, and Guidelines.* Denver, CO: Association of periOperative Registered Nurses, Inc., 2002: 333–342.

19. American Society for Healthcare Central Service Professionals. Sterilization. In: *Training Manual for Central Service Technicians.* 3rd Ed. Chicago: American Hospital Association, 1997: 157–192.

20. JCAHO. *Standards for Ambulatory Care.* Oakbrook Terrace, IL: Joint Commission on Accreditation of Healthcare Organizations, 2000.

21. Rutala, W. A., and Shafer, K. General information on cleaning, disinfection, and sterilization. In: Olmsted, R. N., ed. *Infection Control and Applied Epidemiology Principles and Practice.* Chicago, IL: Mosby Co., 1996: 15–17.

22. Vyhlidal, S. A. Central service. In: *APIC Text of Infection Control and Epidemiology.* Washington, DC: Association for Professionals in Infection Control and Epidemiology, 2000: 54:1–6.

23. Association for the Advancement of Medical Instrumentation (AAMI). Flash Sterilization: Steam sterilization of patient care items for immediate use. *AAMI Standards and Recommended Practices, Volume 1.1: Sterilization, Part 1—Sterilization in Healthcare Facilities.* Arlington, VA: Association for the Advancement of Medical Instrumentation, 2001: 61–88.

24. Jacobs, P. T., and Lin, S. M. Sterilization processes utilizing low-temperature plasma. In: Block, S. S., ed. *Disinfection, Sterilization and Preservation.* 5th Ed. Philadelphia, PA: Lea & Febiger, 2001: 747–763.

25. Meyers, H., Brown-Elliott, B. A., Moore, D., Curry, J., Truong, C., Zhang, Y., and Wallace, Jr., R. J. An outbreak of *Mycobacterium chelonae* infection following liposuction. *Clin Infect Dis.* 2002; 34:1500–1507.

26. Kramer, J., and Shafer, P. Monitoring steam sterilization practices in primary care settings. *J Healthcare Quality.* 2000; 22:4–8.

27. Coulter, W. A., Chew-Graham, C. A., Cheung, S. W., and Burke, F. J. T. Autoclave performance and operator knowledge of autoclave use in primary care: A survey of UK practices. *J Hosp Infect.* 2001; 48:180–185.

CHAPTER 4

Personal Protective Equipment

BACKGROUND

The use of **personal protective equipment (PPE)** is a key element in protecting both patients and healthcare workers from acquiring infections in ambulatory care settings. PPE provides a barrier between a susceptible site (e.g., surgical wound, intravascular site, healthcare workers' [HCW] mucous membranes) and a potential source of microorganisms (e.g., HCW's hands, patient's infected wound) and reduces the likelihood that microbes will reach the site and cause an infection.[1]

PPE can be defined as specialized clothing or equipment worn for protection against a hazard. PPE is intended to prevent the spread of microorganisms from patient to caregiver or caregiver to patient.

Studies have shown that health care-associated infections in patients can be reduced when gloves are used appropriately. In one study, as compliance with gloving increased, patient infection or colonization with marker microorganisms decreased significantly.[2] Studies in pediatric populations indicated that the use of gloves or gowns provided protection for patients.[3–4]

Healthcare workers (HCW) face a well-recognized risk of acquiring bloodborne pathogens in their workplace.[5-10] Although a variety of microorganisms may be spread through blood and body fluids, the pathogens of greatest concern are hepatitis B virus (HBV), hepatitis C virus (HCV), and human immunodeficency virus (HIV). The risk for HCWs varies among job practices within a healthcare setting and depends on several factors, including immunization status and the frequency of exposure to blood and body fluids.[11–12]

It has been shown that blood contact, rather than patient contact, is associated with an increased prevalence of bloodborne pathogens in healthcare personnel. The Occupational Safety and Health Administration (OSHA) rules,[13] the Centers for Disease Control and Prevention's Standard Precautions (see Chapter 6), and other guidelines[14] detail procedures to use to avoid exposure to bloodborne pathogens, including the use of PPE (e.g., gloves, protective clothing, and eye/face protection).

Healthcare workers in ambulatory care settings are at risk of infection whenever they have exposure to blood or other potentially infectious materials (OPIM). OPIM refers to the following human body fluids: semen, vaginal secretions, cerebrospinal fluid, synovial fluid, pleural fluid, pericardial fluid, peritoneal fluid, amniotic fluid, and all body fluids in situations where it is difficult or impossible to differentiate between body fluids.[13] Also of importance are saliva in dental procedures and unfixed tissue.[15]

Microorganisms may be present at all moist body sites and in moist body substances. Ambulatory care facilities need to evaluate the tasks performed by staff and then determine what types of PPE are needed to prevent exposures to patients and staff, and when PPE are to be used.

USE OF PERSONAL PROTECTIVE EQUIPMENT

The type, route, and degree of exposure anticipated to blood and OPIM will determine the selection of appropriate PPE.[16] Thus, if a procedure is performed that routinely exposes staff to blood on their hands, gloves should always be worn for that procedure. If a procedure exposes a patient's mucous membrane, non-intact skin, or sterile body site to a staff member's hands (e.g., wound care), gloves should be worn to protect the patient and caregiver. General requirements for use of PPE in ambulatory care settings are outlined in Table 4.1.

PPE, if used properly, can minimize exposure to pathogens. If blood or OPIM penetrates PPE, it must be removed as soon as possible. Strategies for using PPE are specific for each setting and procedure.

Gloves

The use of gloves is not meant to be a substitute for handwashing, but rather as an additional protective measure. Gloves, whether examination or surgical, are available in many different materials and types. There are natural rubber, latex, powdered, non-powdered, hypoallergenic, non-allergenic, and synthetic rubber materials (e.g., vinyl, neoprene, nitrile). The type used should be based on the specific activity, allergy of the wearer, and personal preference.

Vinyl gloves tear more easily than latex or synthetic gloves and often have a looser fit. Therefore, latex or synthetic gloves may be preferred for lengthy procedures or activities with an increased risk of exposure to blood or body fluids. Sterile gloves are required for procedures where there is contact with sterile tissue in order to protect patients (e.g., surgery and catheter insertion). Heavy-duty reusable rubber gloves should be worn when cleaning instruments.

Gloves should be worn when it can be reasonably anticipated that an employee may have hand contact with blood, OPIM, mucous membranes, or non-intact skin (see Table 4.1). OSHA requires gloves for vascular procedures, including phlebotomy; they are not required for injections. Gloves do not need to be worn for contact with intact skin or during routine care (e.g., wiping a nose).[17] However, when worn, gloves must be changed between tasks, procedures, and patients. Disposable gloves must never be washed and used again.

Table 4.1   Requirements for Personal Protective Equipment in Ambulatory Care Settings

Personal Protective Equipment	Indications for Use	Comments
Gloves	• All vascular access procedures (e.g., phlebotomy, finger sticks) • When handling blood or body-fluid contaminated items • When hands are likely to have contact with blood or body fluids • During equipment reprocessing activities • During invasive procedures	• Use correct size, type • Wash hands after removing gloves • Change gloves between tasks • One hand may remain ungloved, if necessary, to prevent cross-contamination
Protective gown/apron	• When clothes are likely to be splattered with blood or body fluids • During gastrointestinal endoscopic procedures • During minor surgical procedures • During wound irrigations	• Must prevent penetration of blood, body fluids, or other potentially infectious material
Facial protection	• When face is likely to be splattered with blood or body fluids • During endoscopic procedures • During equipment reprocessing activities, if face is likely to be splattered with blood or body fluids	• Ensure that vision is not distorted • Ensure that eyes and mouth are fully protected

Allergic responses to latex materials have been identified as a significant issue for healthcare workers and some patients. The precautions taken by a healthcare worker with latex allergy depend on the manifestation of the allergy. Latex proteins become fastened to the lubricant powder used in some gloves. When workers change gloves, the protein/powder particles become airborne and can be inhaled. Powder-free gloves with reduced protein content can decrease this problem. An additional way to protect employees who are sensitive to latex is to use vinyl gloves, latex-free gloves, or glove liners.[18-19]

Other Garb

Protective attire must be worn when there is a possibility of splashes or sprays of blood or OPIM. It can be reusable or disposable and semipermeable or nonpermeable (moisture repellent). Types of protective attire available are gowns, aprons, lab coats, and jackets that will protect staff clothing from splashes. Clothing is unlikely to play a major role in spread of microorganisms; however, clothing should be covered for aesthetic reasons and to prevent subsequent contamination of hands and surfaces.

General work clothes (e.g., lab coats or uniforms) that are not intended to function as protection against a hazard cannot be considered PPE.[20] PPE must not permit pass through of the potentially infectious substance to skin, eyes, mouth, or clothes.

Staff must wear face and eye protection to prevent splashes, sprays, splatters, or droplets of blood and OPIM.[13, 21-23] These items are intended to protect the mucous membranes of the eyes, nose, and mouth.

Eye protection can consist of goggles, glasses with side shields (add-on plastic adapters), or face shields that protect both eyes and face. Masks should be worn in combination with goggles or glasses to protect facial mucous membranes. These devices should be comfortable, easy to clean or disposable, and not restrict movement or vision.

Masks may be flat or molded in a cone shape. Flimsy tissue paper masks do not provide significant filtration or prevent droplets from soaking through.[1] The type of mask best suited to a particular situation depends on the body substances likely to be encountered and the nature of the activity. For example, a

fluid-repellent mask should be used when aerosolization or splattering of blood or body fluids is probable. Masks may also be worn to protect against airborne spread of microorganisms (e.g., tuberculosis). A particulate mask capable of filtering 1-micron particles and with the best possible fit should be worn when caring for patients with pulmonary tuberculosis (see Chapter 6).

In routine ambulatory care practices, other types of PPE, such as head or shoe covers, are not required. In specific settings (e.g., surgery), disposable head covers, shoe covers, or shoes dedicated for use in the operating room are often worn.[24]

Mouth-to-mask or mouth-to-bag devices should be readily available for resuscitation to prevent mucous membrane contact.

PPE AND CHEMICALS

Anyone who handles chemicals (e.g., cleaners and disinfectants) must be aware of the potential hazards associated with the product and the appropriate PPE to use for protection. At a minimum, gloves should be worn during cleaning activities. The material safety data sheets supplied with the product will outline other PPE to use (see Chapter 3).

EXPOSURE PREVENTION

Ambulatory care settings must take appropriate precautions to protect patients and staff likely to be exposed to blood or OPIM. In addition to using proper PPE, staff hands should be washed immediately or as soon as feasible after removing gloves and other PPE. The hands of the healthcare worker are in contact with patients and their environment, and they are most at risk for contamination during patient care. They may then transfer microorganisms between patients, to staff members, and to environmental surfaces.

Proper care and handling of sharp items is necessary in all settings. There should be no recapping, bending, or breaking of needles; in fact, the use of safety devices is required, when available.[22, 25-26] Impermeable, puncture-resistant sharps containers must be available to discard items appropriately. They should be easily accessible in areas where sharp-item disposal is required (e.g., infusion centers, injection areas, surgical suites, dialysis centers, etc.). The containers should be replaced when approximately three-quarters full. Handle as waste according to state and local regulations.

Potentially infectious agents (e.g., bloodborne pathogens) may be present in all moist body fluids. Therefore, ambulatory care facilities should use Standard Precautions for all patients (see Chapter 6). Under Standard Precautions, all body substances are handled as though potentially infectious.[27] The emphasis is on good hand hygiene practices and proper use of barriers (i.e., PPE).

ACCESS TO AND LOCATION OF PPE

PPE must be supplied at no cost to staff. Employers must provide easy access to PPE and enforce its appropriate use. Appropriate PPE, as determined by the facility, should be placed at the point of use for staff. Important areas for gloves include each examination and treatment room. Infrequently used PPE can be placed in a central location known to all staff. Alternatively, there could be a "PPE kit" stocked with these items placed in a known location. This kit could be easily transported to a site when needed. In addition, resuscitation equipment that eliminates direct mouth-to-mouth contact must be readily available.

TRAINING

Education and training programs have been shown to have a positive impact on reducing exposures to blood and body fluids.[28] However, studies evaluating compliance have been only partially encouraging.

In a 1995 national survey of dentists in Canada,[29] 95% of respondents routinely used gloves in their practice. Only 82% wore face protection when splatter was anticipated. The authors noted that those using appropriate barriers and careful handling/disposing of sharp items reported fewer exposures.[21] A similar study in Australia noted that complete compliance with PPE recommendations by dentists had not been achieved.[30] A survey of family practice physicians also indicated inconsistent compliance with the use of PPE.[31]

Employers must provide instruction and information to all employees who might be exposed to blood or OPIM. There should be a manual of protocols that outlines PPE requirements and appropriate engineering and work practice controls for protection of patients and staff. Employees must be aware of how to avoid exposure and know the area's exposure control plan (see Chapter 22).

EXPOSURES

Staff should be informed that any skin surfaces contaminated with blood or OPIM should be washed immediately and thoroughly. Then they should be directed to policies regarding the management of exposures (see Chapter 19).

References

1. Lynch, P. Barrier Precautions and Personal Protection. In: Soule, B. M., Larson, E. L., Preston, G. A., eds. *Infections and Nursing Practice*. St. Louis: Mosby-Year Book, Inc., 1995: 106–128.

2. Lynch, P., Cummings, M. J., Roberts, P. L., Herriott, M. J., Yates, B., and Stamm, W. E. Implementing and evaluating a system of generic infection precautions: Body substance isolation. *Am J Infect Control.* 1990; 18:1–12.

3. Klein, B. S., Perloff, W. H., and Maki, D. G. Reduction of nosocomial infection during pediatric intensive care by protective isolation. *N Engl J Med.* 1989; 320:1714–1721.

4. Slota, M., Green, M., Farley, A., Janosky, J., and Carcillo, J. The role of gown and glove isolation and strict handwashing in the reduction of nosocomial infections in children with solid organ transplantation. *Crit Care Med.* 2001; 29:405–412.

5. Thomas, D. L., Factor, S. H., Gabor, D., and Kelen, M. D. Viral hepatitis in health care personnel at the Johns Hopkins Hospital. *Arch Intern Med.* 1993; 153:1705–1712.

6. *CDC Hepatitis Surveillance Report No. 56.* Atlanta, GA: Centers for Disease Control and Prevention; 1996: 3–6.

7. Dienstag, J. L., and Ryan, D. M. Occupational exposure to hepatitis B virus in hospital personnel: Infection or immunization. *Am J Epidemiol.* 1982; 115:26–39.

8. White, M. C., and Lynch, P. Blood contact and exposures among ambulatory care personnel. *Amb Surg.* 1994; 2:152–155.

9. Bower, W. A., and Alter, M. J. Risks and prevention of occupational hepatitis B virus and hepatitis C virus infections. *Semin Infect Control.* 2001; 1:19–29.

10. Evans, M. R., Henderson, D. K., and Bennett, J. E. Potential for laboratory exposures to biohazardous agents found in blood. *Am J Public Health.* 1990; 80:423–427.

11. Petrosillo, N., Puro, V., DeCarli, G., and Ippolito, G. Occupational exposure in healthcare workers: An Italian study of occupational risk of HIV and other blood-borne viral infections. *Br J Infect Control.* 2001; 2:15–17.

12. Puro, V., DeCarli, G., Petrosillo, N., and Ippolito, G. Risk of exposure to bloodborne infection for Italian healthcare workers by job category and work area. *Infect Control Hosp Epidemiol.* 2001; 22:206–210.

13. Occupational exposure to bloodborne pathogens: Final rule. *Fed Reg.* 1991; 56:64175–64182.

14. Health Canada. Preventing the Transmission of Bloodborne Pathogens in Health Care and Public Service Settings. *Canada Communicable Disease Report.* 1997; 23S3. *http://www.hc-sc.gc.ca/pphb-dgspsp/publicat/ccdr-rmtc/97vol23/23s3/index.html.*

15. Favero, M. S., and Sadovsky, R. Office infection control, OSHA, and you. *Patient Care.* 1993; 27:117–134.

16. Chiarello, L. A., and Bartley, J. Prevention of blood exposures in healthcare personnel. *Semin Infect Control.* 2001; 1:30–43.

17. American Academy of Pediatrics. Infection control in physicians' offices. *Pediatrics.* 2000; 105:1361–1369.

18. Aldape, T. The material truth: When choosing a glove you should consider the hazards, functions, physical demands, length of exposure, frequency of use, and other conditions found in the workplace. . . choosing the appropriate hand protection. *Occupational Health Safety.* 2000; 69:62.

19. Cuming, R. G. Reducing the hazards of exposure to cornstarch glove powder. *AORN J.* 2002; 76:288–295.

20. American Society for Gastrointestinal Endoscopy. PPE. *Gastrointest Endoscopy.* 1999; 49:854–857.

21. McCarthy, G. M., Kovel, J. J., and MacDonald, J. K. Occupational injuries and exposures among Canadian dentists: The results of a national survey. *Infect Control Hosp Epidemiol.* 1999; 20:331–336.

22. Infection control in the health care setting. *Guidelines for the prevention of transmission of infectious diseases.* Australia, 2000. *http://www.health.gov.au/pubhlth/strateg/communic/review/.*

23. Hansen, M. E. Bloodborne pathogens and procedure safety in interventional radiology. *Semin Ultrasound CT MR.* 1998; 19:209–214.

24. Recommended practices for surgical attire. In: *2002 Standards, Recommended Practices, and Guidelines.* Denver: Association of Operating Room Nurses, Inc., 2002: 199–203.

25. Occupational Exposure to Bloodborne Pathogens: Needlestick and Other Sharps Injuries: Final Rule. *Fed Reg.* 2001; 66:5317–5325. *http://www.osha-slc.gov/pls/oshaweb/owadisp.show_document? p_table=FEDERAL_REGISTER&p_id=16265.*

26. Frank, G., and City, E. Nurses welcome standards provided by new needlestick law. *J Emerg Nurs.* 2001; 27:489–491.

27. Jackson, M. M, and Lynch, P. Ambulatory Care Settings. In: Bennett, J. V., Brachman, P. S., eds. *Hospital Infections.* 4th Ed. Philadelphia: Lippincott-Raven Publishers, 1998: 431–444.

28. Sellick, J. A., Hazamy, P. A., and Mylotte, J. M. Influence of an educational program and mechanical opening needle disposal boxes on occupational needlestick injuries. *Infect Control Hosp Epidemiol.* 1991; 12:725–731.

29. McCarthy, G. M., Koval, J. J., and MacDonald, J. K. Compliance with recommended infection control procedures among Canadian dentists: Results of a national survey. *Am J Infect Control.* 1999; 27:377–384.

30. Lange, P., Savage, N. W., and Walsh, L. J. Utilization of personal protective equipment in general dental practice. *Aust Dent J.* 1996; 41:164–168.

31. Miller, K. E., Krol, R. A., and Losh, D. P. Universal precautions in the family physician's office. *J Fam Practice.* 1992; 35:163–168.

CHAPTER 5

Hand Hygiene

BACKGROUND

Hand hygiene is the general term that applies to washing with plain (non-antimicrobial) soap and water, antiseptic handwash, waterless antiseptic hand rub, and surgical hand antisepsis. It is a key element for prevention of cross-infection in the healthcare setting.[1-3] Inadequate handwashing in outpatient settings has contributed to outbreaks of infection.[4]

Although an essential component of infection prevention and control programs,[5] hand hygiene is performed far too infrequently in health care,[3, 6-7] including ambulatory care settings.[8] Many healthcare professionals complain of chapped and damaged skin[9-10] and/or lack of time for handwashing.[11] The practice of hand hygiene includes the issues of product selection, use of hand lotion, and skin care. Additionally, fingernails, both long and artificial nails, and nail polish play a role in the spread of infection.[3, 12-16] Finally, methods to motivate staff to improve hand hygiene are important considerations in this most basic infection prevention practice.[3]

DEFINITIONS

Alcohol-based hand rub. An alcohol-containing preparation designed for waterless application to the hands to reduce microorganisms, comprised of 60% to 95% ethanol or isopropanol. Products formulated for use in health care usually contain emollients.

Antimicrobial soap. Soap containing an antiseptic agent.

Hand antisepsis. Either antimicrobial handwash or waterless antiseptic hand rub.

Decontaminating hands. Reducing the number of microorganisms on hands by using an alcohol-based hand rub or washing with antimicrobial soap.

Persistent or residual activity. Prolonged antimicrobial activity that prevents or inhibits the proliferation or survival or microorganisms after application of the product.

Plain soap. Handwashing agents with no antimicrobial agents or low concentrations that are effective only as preservatives.

INDICATIONS FOR HANDWASHING AND HAND ANTISEPSIS

When to wash hands depends on the level of soiling of the hands, the activity that follows handwashing, and in some circumstances, the type of microorganism contaminating the hands. To summarize the Centers for Disease Control and Prevention (CDC) Guidelines for Hand Hygiene in Health-Care Settings[3] for ambulatory care settings, wash hands with plain or antimicrobial soap and water or use an alcohol-based hand rub before contact with each patient.

More specifically, wash hands with plain soap or antimicrobial soap and water at these times:

- When hands are visibly soiled or contaminated with proteinaceous material, blood, body fluids, secretions, or excretions

31

- After contact with mucous membranes, non-intact skin, urinals, sputum containers, wound dressings, if hands are visibly soiled
- After glove removal, if hands are visibly soiled
- After changing a dressing or diaper, if hands are visibly soiled
- Before eating, drinking, handling, or serving food
- Following personal hygiene (e.g., use of toilet, blowing nose)
- If exposure to *Bacillus anthracis* is suspected or proven. The physical action of washing and rinsing hands is recommended because alcohols and antiseptic agents have poor activity against spores.[3]

When hands are not visibly soiled, use an alcohol-based hand rub or wash with soap and water at these times:

- Before having direct contact with patients
- Before preparing or handling sterile products or medications
- After contact with a patient's intact skin (e.g., when taking a pulse or blood pressure)
- After contact with a contaminated-body site and before contact with a clean-body site during patient care
- After contact with inanimate objects, including medical equipment in the immediate vicinity of the patient
- After removing gloves

HAND HYGIENE TECHNIQUES

The purpose of basic handwashing is to mechanically remove soil, organic material, and transient microorganisms.[2, 3] The handwashing method is simple:

1. Moisten hands with warm (not hot) water.
2. Apply soap. Use the amount recommended by the manufacturer.
3. Vigorously rub all surfaces for 15 seconds,[3] paying particular attention to areas around fingernails and between the fingers.
4. Rinse hands thoroughly under running water to completely remove soap.
5. Pat hands dry thoroughly with a disposable paper towel.
6. Use the paper towel to turn off the faucet.

The procedure for decontaminating hands with an alcohol-based hand rub is as follows:

1. Apply product to palm of one hand; use the amount recommended by the manufacturer.
2. Rub hands together, covering all surfaces of hands and fingers, until hands are completely dry.

SELECTION OF HAND HYGIENE AGENTS

Plain soap is effective in physically removing soil, dirt, organic substances, and loosely adherent transient microorganisms. However, plain soaps have minimal ability to destroy microorganisms, are often associated with skin irritation and dryness, occasionally have become contaminated, and consistently have failed to remove pathogens from hands of healthcare personnel.[3] Therefore, an antimicrobial product is recommended at these times:

- Before performing minor surgical procedures
- Before placing intravascular devices or urinary catheters
- Before accessing intravascular devices in severely immunocompromised patients (such as in an infusion center)

Historically, many antimicrobial agents have been used in soap products, and many have been found unsafe or ineffective. Therefore, the Food and Drug Administration's (FDA) Division of Over-the-Counter Drug Products now oversees and regulates antiseptic handwash products intended for use by healthcare workers; products are listed in the FDA Tentative Final Monograph for Healthcare Antiseptic Drug Products.[3] In the United States currently, only a handful of agents are considered both safe and effective: alcohol, chlorhexidine, iodophor, chloroxylenol, and triclosan. For overall comparisons of these products, see Table 5.1. For comparisons of antimicrobial properties, see Table 5.2.

Alcohol-Based Hand Rubs

Studies on alcohol-based waterless hand rubs show that they have excellent antimicrobial activity,[2–3, 18] high user acceptability,[3, 19–21] and are time saving.[11]

Table 5.1 Widely Available Antimicrobial Handwashing Agents[2, 17]

Ingredient, Effective Concentrations	Characteristics
Alcohol, usually 60–70%	• Most rapid and effective antimicrobial activity • Nontoxic; stings broken skin • Drying; with addition of emollients is less drying or irritating than other agents or soaps • Not a good cleansing agent • No persistency on skin (increased persistency with addition of 0.5–1.0% CHG) • Flammable; placement of dispensers may be regulated through state fire safety requirements
Chlorhexidine gluconate (CHG), 4%; 2% with 4% alcohol; 0.5–1.0% in 60% alcohol	• Broad-spectrum activity • Nontoxic on skin; allergies uncommon • Damaging to eye, ear, neuro tissue (brain, meninges) • Good persistency on skin • Only minimally affected by organic matter
Iodophor, 7.5–10% povidone-iodine (1% available iodine; 1 part per million free iodine)	• Broad-spectrum activity • Some persistency; inactivated in presence of blood, sputum, other organic substances • More contact dermatitis than other antiseptics • More commonly used as a surgical scrub or patient skin prep
Chloroxylenol (Parachlorometaxylenol, PCMX), 0.3 to 3.75%	• Less active than CHG or iodophors • Broad-spectrum activity • Persistent effect on skin less than CHG • Allergic reactions uncommon
Triclosan, 0.2–2%	• Broad-spectrum, but less potent activity against Gram-negative bacteria (e.g., pseudomonas) • Excellent persistence • Few allergic reactions

Hands have been shown to be less dry and irritated after using alcohol-based hand rubs that contain emollients than after using chlorhexidine,[19] other antimicrobial soaps,[3] or plain soap and water.[20] Although there are no published studies specific to ambulatory care, evidence shows that increased use of these products may lead to increased hand cleansing compliance in the in-patient setting.[22] These products contain alcohol (commonly 60–70% ethanol or isopropyl alcohol) with emollients to mitigate the drying effects of alcohol. Formulations (liquid, gel, foam, or cream) and scents vary. A wide variety of containers, with and without pumps, and dispensers are available. Guidelines[3] for use of alcohol-based hand rubs in ambulatory care include:

• Apply before each patient contact when hands are not visibly soiled (e.g., when performing physical examinations where there is contact with intact patient skin). When hands are visibly soiled, use soap and water. Alcohol is not a good cleaner.
• Use of both alcohol-based hand rub and handwashing with soap and water between patient contacts is unnecessary.
• After several applications of alcohol-based hand rubs, hands may feel sticky or gritty from the build-up of emollients and should be washed with soap and water.
• After glove removal hands may feel gritty from the combination of powder and emollients and may need to be washed with soap and water.

Table 5.2 Antimicrobial Spectrum and Characteristics of Hand-Hygiene Antiseptic Agents[*3]

Group	Gram-Positive Bacteria	Gram-Negative Bacteria	Mycobacteria	Fungi	Viruses	Speed of Action	Comments
Alcohols	+++	+++	+++	+++	+++	Fast	Optimum concentration 60–90%; no persistent activity
Chlorhexidine (2% and 4% aqueous)	+++	++	+	+	+++	Intermediate	Persistent activity; rare allergic reactions
Iodine compounds	+++	+++	+++	++	+++	Intermediate	Causes skin burns; usually too irritating for hand hygiene
Iodophors	+++	+++	+	++	++	Intermediate	Less irritating than iodine; acceptance varies
Phenol derivatives (PCMX)[**]	+++	+	+	+	+	Intermediate	Activity neutralized by nonionic surfactants
Triclosan	+++	++	+	−	+++	Intermediate	Acceptability on hands varies
Quaternary ammonium compounds	+	++	−	−	+	Slow	Used only in combination with alcohols; ecologic concerns

NOTE: +++ = excellent; ++ = good, but does not include the entire bacterial spectrum; + = fair; − = no activity or not sufficient.

[*]Hexachlorophene is not included because it is no longer an accepted ingredient in hand disinfectants.

[**]PCMX = parachlorometaxylenol

- Staff should be reminded that immediately after application there will be an alcohol scent and slight stinging if applied to broken skin; both will dissipate after drying.

Before implementing use of alcohol-based products, evaluate several types and brands for acceptable scent and dispensers. Placement of containers should be in areas where sinks are unavailable (e.g., in ambulances and medical helicopters), in offices where sinks may be inaccessible between patients (e.g., in social or psychiatric workers' offices), or at the check-in station for clerks. Where alcohol hand rubs are offered in addition to soap and water, place the alcohol product away from the soap dispenser/sink so that staff will not confuse the products. For example, alcohol dispensers might be placed near the doorway of an examination room to encourage staff to sanitize hands as they enter the room. Individual pocket-sized containers may also be provided to encourage hand hygiene.[3] Recent concerns about flammability have led some states[23] to prohibit dispenser placement in corridors, so before installing dispensers check with the fire marshal or health department.

Other Products

When selecting antimicrobial soaps, determine the following:

- Know the active ingredient and its concentration. Chlorhexidine (CHG), chloroxylenol (PCMX), and triclosan are the most common active ingredients (see Table 5.1).
- Review product information regarding potential interactions between the proposed antimicrobial soap, types of gloves, and hand lotions in use.
- Evalute products in the clinical setting to evaluate staff acceptance of dispensers, fragrance of the product, and skin irritation.
- Evaluate the containers for criteria such as ease of replacement of product and potential for contamination and/or dripping.

The following products are not recommended for hand hygiene in ambulatory care settings:[2]

- Hexachlorophene: At typical concentrations (3%) this product is slow acting and effective against a narrow range of microorganisms. As a result of neurotoxicity in burn patients and premature infants, its use has been severely curtailed, and it is currently available by prescription only. Use on broken skin or mucous membranes is contraindicated.[2]
- Benzylammonium chloride: This product was widely available historically. However, it is inactivated by cotton and organic material, and there have been reports of its contamination leading to outbreaks of Gram-negative bacterial infection.[24]
- Non–alcohol-based waterless hand rubs have not been studied sufficiently and are not currently recommended.[3]

SURGICAL HAND ANTISEPSIS

Factors that influence the effectiveness of surgical hand antisepsis include the agent used, the duration of the scrub, the technique, the condition of the hands,[25] and implementation of standardized policies and procedures.[26] Ongoing research evaluating the safety and efficacy of surgical scrubs neccssitates regular review of surgical and infection prevention and control literature and recommendations. Surgical hand antisepsis should be performed prior to surgical and some diagnostic procedures.

The most commonly used antimicrobial agents are iodophors (e.g., povidone-iodine), alcohol-containing products, CHG, and PCMX.[25] Although alcohol products are widely used in Europe and alcohol is recognized as an excellent antiseptic, its acceptance for surgical hand antisepsis has been slow in the United States. However, research now supports the use of alcohol for surgical hand antisepsis,[21, 27] and both the CDC[3] and the Association of periOperative Registered Nurses (AORN)[26] endorse its use. AORN states that "vigorous rubbing with enough alcohol-based hand cleanser to wet the hand and forearms completely has been shown to be an effective method for antisepsis." Alcohol-based preparations containing 0.5 to 1.0% CHG have persistency exceeding that of plain alcohol, and in some cases, that of CHG alone.[3]

Because of allergies or skin sensitivities, operating room (OR) staff should be offered a choice of products. Products may be supplied in several forms: impregnated, individually wrapped sponge/brushes; pumps; or other bulk containers. It is important to evaluate any new product, including evaluation of the dispenser, for input from staff.[3] Product should be labeled as a surgical hand antiseptic, and product literature should be reviewed for both efficacy and acceptability studies. Use of sponges or brushes has been considered necessary in the past. However, recent research concludes that sponges or brushes may not be needed[27] and, in fact, may increase skin damage.[28] In studies evaluating alcohol-based products, the alcohol is applied without sponges or brushes following a handwash with plain soap.[3, 21]

Recommendations for duration of a surgical scrub have been controversial and confusing, with times ranging from two to ten minutes. Although optimum scrub time is unknown,[25] more recent research supports times of two to four minutes[26] or two to six minutes[3] as effective, reducing skin irritation and saving water. Product instructions should be followed. AORN recommends that initial and subsequent scrubs be of the same duration.[26]

Standardized protocols should include the following steps:

1. Remove rings, watches, and bracelets.[3]
2. Thoroughly wash hands and forearms with plain soap, under running water, before the first surgery of the day, including use of nail cleaner.
3. When using antimicrobial soap, scrub hands and forearms for the length of time recommended by the manufacturer, usually two to six minutes, followed by rinsing and drying with sterile towels.
4. When using an alcohol-based hand rub, follow the manufacturer's instructions for quantity and application method. Allow hands and forearms to dry completely before donning sterile gloves.
5. Apply sterile gloves in a manner to prevent recontamination.

To help ensure adherence to policies for surgical hand antisepsis, the following guidelines should be implemented:

- Application times for each product and anatomic instructions, when applicable, should be posted at the scrub sink, and a clock should be available.
- Expectations should be reviewed at orientation and annual infection prevention and control in-services.
- Staff, including technicians, nurses, medical students, residents, and new staff physicians, should be thoroughly trained at orientation and when new products are instituted.
- Surgical hand antisepsis protocols should be included in the OR and other diagnostic and treatment area procedure manuals.

ARTIFICIAL FINGERNAILS AND NAIL POLISH

AORN forbids use of artificial nails and limits nail polish to "unchipped, 4 days" of wear.[26] Thus, OR policies routinely forbid staff to wear artificial nails. This restriction should be strictly enforced for anyone in the OR theatre who will have direct (all pre-op, recovery, and OR staff) or indirect (e.g., anesthesia technicians who prepare the anesthesia trays) patient contact. Although there are no firm recommendations forbidding other healthcare professionals from wearing artificial nails, hospitals are beginning to develop policies banning artificial fingernails and requiring short nails with no chipped nail polish for all direct caregivers. Studies have not included the nonsurgical ambulatory care setting.

SKIN CARE

Adverse reactions can develp after use of any hand hygiene product, including alcohol-based hand rubs.[29] Staff who develop dermatitis, allergy, or sensitivity to handwashing products should be assessed. Damaged skin carries many more pathogenic microorganisms than intact skin.[2] Because latex can also cause skin problems, staff should be referred to occupational health for evaluation and treatment (see Chapter 19). Staff with soap allergies or sensitivities can be provided with alternate products; if bar soap solves the skin issue, small bars should be provided and should be maintained in a dry, sanitary environment for use exclusively by affected staff. Detergent in hand soap is often harsh, and hands should be thoroughly rinsed and patted dry after washing.

Hand lotions and moisturizers are recommended for use while off duty and during breaks. Lotion should be supplied in small containers that are more likely to be emptied before becoming contaminated. Lotion should be compatible with any handwashing antiseptic product, such as CHG.[3, 17] Some products contain antibiotics (e.g., bag balm [hydroquinoline]). Although there have been no reports of an increase in antibiotic resistance using these products, if clusters of antibiotic resistant bacteria occur it may be prudent to monitor or investigate their use. Any trial of new products should include evaluation of hand irritation.

SINKS AND DISPENSERS

Sinks should be conveniently located. The American Institute of Architects recommends placement of sinks in examination and treatment rooms.[30] Ideally, sinks should be equipped with foot- or elbow-operated controls. In addition, many local or state public health codes regulate sink location and type. Separate sinks should be maintained for handwashing versus instrument cleaning or disposal of laboratory specimens. Only disposable paper toweling should be used.[3] Before any renovation or construction, plans should be reviewed for placement of sinks and soap and paper towel dispensers. Soap and towel dispensers should be within easy reach of the sink. The soap dispensers should be placed away from countertops where stray drips of soap could fall on patient-care items.

Disposable soap containers are recommended.[2] There have been reports of contamination of and infections related to the "topping off" of pump bottles or the soap in reused containers.[3, 31] If containers must be reused, the container and pump must be thoroughly cleaned before refilling. In most cases it is not practical or cost-effective to clean containers. If individual-sized containers are provided, they must not be placed where the top or pump can become contaminated with water or patient secretions; there is at least one report of extrinsic contamination of containers leading to infection.[3, 32] Except for individual patient use, bar soap may be forbidden in healthcare settings by state health departments and managed care organizations.

EDUCATION AND MOTIVATION

Staff should receive education about the importance of hand hygiene to prevent infection in patients and themselves and instructions in proper products and techniques.[3] Education should occur during orientation,

whenever new products are introduced, and during outbreaks—either community outbreaks such as diarrheal illness or influenza or when healthcare–associated cases are attributable to lack of hand hygiene. Unfortunately, increases in compliance tend to be transitory.[3] Therefore, periodic reminders are needed and can include posters, flyers, newsletters, educational lectures, and verbal reminders during staff meetings. Periodically culturing healthcare worker fingertips on agar plates after brief encounters with patients[33] or using educational resources, such as fluorescing lotions or powders that mimic microbial contamination, can interactively demonstrate the effect of handwashing. One successful intervention increased physician hand hygiene through personal, direct meetings with an infectious disease physician and videotaped in-services, as compared to e-mail newsletters.[34]

Patient teaching should include the importance and methods of handwashing as part of the community effort in decreasing infections. Patient education is especially important during community outbreaks of diarrheal illness, influenza, "cold" season, or when a family or household is experiencing an outbreak of infections that can be spread by lack of handwashing.

PERFORMANCE IMPROVEMENT

As part of performance improvement, the following may be monitored[3] with feedback to staff:

- The volume of hand soap or alcohol-based hand rub used per day of operation, comparing usage over time
- Adherence to policies regarding wearing artificial nails or nail polish

Improved hand hygiene should be an institutional priority as part of an overall culture of patient safety and quality of care. Adherence may increase by providing alcohol-based hand rub to staff who work in areas with high workload and high intensity of patient care. Staff involvement in choosing products and dispensers may also increase compliance.

References

1. Rotter, M. L. Handwashing, hand disinfection, and skin disinfection. In: Wenzel, R. P., ed. *Prevention and Control of Nosocomial Infections*. 3rd Ed. Baltimore, MD: Williams & Wilkins, 1997: 691–709.

2. Larson, E. L. APIC guideline for handwashing and hand antisepsis in health-care settings. *Am J Infect Control*. 1995; 23:251–269.

3. Boyce, J. M., and Pittet, D. Recommendations of the Healthcare Infection Control Practices Advisory Committee. Guideline for hand hygiene in health-care settings. *MMWR*. 2002; 51(RR-16):1–45. *http://www.cdc.gov/mmwr/PDF/rr/rr5116.pdf*.

4. Herwaldt, L. A., Smith, S. D., and Carter, C. D. Infection control in the outpatient setting. *Infect Control Hosp Epidemiol*. 1998; 19:41–74.

5. Boyce, J. M. It is time for action: Improving hand hygiene in hospitals. *Ann Intern Med*. 1999; 130:153–155.

6. Widmer, A. F. Replace handwashing with use of a waterless alcohol hand rub? *Clin Infect Dis*. 2000; 31:136–143.

7. Larson, E., and Kretzer, E. K. Compliance with handwashing and barrier precautions. *J Hosp Infect*. 1995; 30 (Suppl):88–106.

8. Lohr, J. A., Ingram, D. L., Dudley, S. M., Lawton, E. L., and Donowitz, L. G. Handwashing in pediatric ambulatory settings: An inconsistent practice. *Am J Dis Child*. 1991; 145:1198–1199.

9. Larson, E. L., Norton Hughes, C. A., Pyrek, J. D., Sparks, S. M., Cagatay, E. U., and Bartkus, J. M. Changes in bacterial flora associated with skin damage on hands of health care personnel. *Am J Infect Control*. 1998; 26:513–522.

10. Larson, E., Friedman, C., Cohran, J., Treston-Aurand, J., and Green, S. Prevalence and correlates of skin damage on the hands of nurses. *Heart Lung*. 1997; 26:404–412.

11. Voss, A., and Widmer, A. F. No time for handwashing!? Handwashing versus alcoholic rub: Can we afford 100% compliance? *Infect Control Hosp Epidemiol*. 1997; 18:205–208.

12. Edel, E., Houston, S., Kennedy, V., and LaRocco, M. Impact of a 5-minute scrub on the microbial flora found on artificial, polished, or natural fingernails of operating room personnel. *Nursing Research*. 1998; 47:54–59.

13. Wynd, C. A., Samstag, D. E., and Lapp, A. M. Bacterial carriage on the fingernails of OR nurses. *AORN J*. 1994; 60:796, 799–805.

14. Parry, M. F., Grant, B., Yukna, M., Adler-Klein, D., McLeod, G. X., and Taddonio, R., et al. Candida osteomyelitis and diskitis after spinal surgery: An outbreak that implicates artificial nail use. *Clin Infect Dis*. 2001; 32:352–357.

15. Moolenaar, R. L., Crutcher, M., San Joaquin, V. H., Sewell, L. V., Hutwagner, L. C., and Carson, L. A., et al. A prolonged outbreak of *Pseudomonas aeruginosa* in a neonatal intensive care unit: Did staff fingernails play a role in disease transmission? *Infect Control Hosp Epidemiol*. 2000; 21:80–85.

16. McNeil, S. A., Foster, C. L., Hedderwick, S. A., and Kauffman, C. A. Effect of hand cleansing with antimicrobial soap or alcohol-based gel on microbial colonization of artificial fingernails worn by health care workers. *Clin Infect Dis*. 2001; 32:367–372.

17. Rotter, M. L. Handwashing and hand disinfection. In: Mayhall, C. G., ed. *Hospital Epidemiology and Infection Control*. Baltimore, MD: Williams & Wilkins, 1996: 1052–1068.

18. Zaragoza, M., Salles, M., Gomez, J., Bayas, J. M., and Trilla, A. Handwashing with soap or alcoholic solutions? A randomized clinical trial of its effectiveness. *Am J Infect Control*. 1999; 27:258–261.

19. Pereira, L. J., Lee, G. N., and Wade, K. J. An evaluation of five protocols for surgical handwashing in relation to skin condition and microbial counts. *J Hosp Infect*. 1997; 36:49–65.

20. Boyce, J. M., Kelliher, S., and Vallande, N. Skin irritation and dryness associated with two hand-hygiene regimens: Soap-and-water handwashing versus hand antisepsis with an alcoholic hand gel. *Infect Control Hosp Epidemiol*. 2000; 21:442–448.

21. Bryce, E. A., Spence, D., and Roberts, F. J. An in-use evaluation of an alcohol-based pre-surgical hand disinfectant. *Infect Control Hosp Epidemiol*. 2001; 22:635–639.

22. Earl, M. L., Jackson, M. M., and Rickman, L. S. Improved rates of compliance with hand antisepsis guidelines: A three-phase observational study. *Am J Nursing*. 2001; 101:26–33.

23. Office of Fire Safety, Consumer and Industry Services, Michigan Department of Public Health. Policy: 2–25. Alcohol Based Waterless Hand Sanitizing Cleaner. October 10, 2002. *http://www.michigan. gov/cis/0,1607,7-154-10575_17573_19004-55731—,00.html*.

24. Favero, M. S., and Bond, W. W. Chemical disinfection of medical and surgical materials. In: Block, S. S., ed. *Disinfection, Sterilization, and Preservation*. 5th Ed. Philadelphia, PA: Lea & Febiger, 2001: 881–917.

25. Mangram, A. J., Horan, T. C., Pearson, M. L., Silver, L. C., and Jarvis, W. R. Guideline for prevention of surgical site infection. *Am J Infect Control*. 1999; 27:97–134.

26. AORN. Recommended practices for surgical hand scrubs. In: *Standards, Recommended Practices, and Guidelines*. Denver, CO: Association of periOperative Registered Nurses, 2002: 255–260.

27. Jones, R. D., Jampani, H., Mulberry, G., and Rizer, R. L. Moisturizing alcohol hand gels for surgical hand preparation. *AORN J*. 2000; 71:584–592.

28. Kikuchi-Numagami, K., Saishu, T., Fukaya, M., Kanazawa, E., and Tagami, H. Irritancy of scrubbing up for surgery with or without a brush. *Acta Derm Ven*. 1999; 79:230–232.

29. Cimiotti, J. P., Marmur, E. S., Nesin, M., Hamlin-Cook, P., and Larson, E. Adverse reactions associated with an alcohol-based hand antiseptic among nurses in a neonatal intensive care unit. *Am J Infect Control*. 2003; 31:43–48.

30. American Institute of Architects Academy of Architecture for Health. In: *Guidelines for Design and Construction of Hospital and Health Care Facilities*. Washington, DC: American Institute of Architects Press, 2001: 103–127.

31. Sartor, C., Jacomo, V., Duvivier, C., Tissot-Dupont, H., Sambuc, R., and Drancourt, M. Nosocomial *Serratia marcescens* infectious associated with extrinsic contamination of a liquid nonmedicated soap. *Infect Control Hosp Epidemiol*. 2000; 21:196–199.

32. Archibald, L. K., Corl, A., Shah, B., and Schulte, M., et al. *Serratia marcescens* outbreak associated with extrinsic contamination of 1% chlorxylenol soap. *Infect Control Hosp Epidemiol*. 1997; 18:704–709.

33. Ray, A. J., Hoyen, C. K., Eckstein, E. C., and Donskey, C. J. Improving healthcare workers' compliance with hand hygiene: Is a picture worth a thousand words? *Infect Control Hosp Epidemiol*. 2002; 23:418–419.

34. Salemi, C., Canola, T., and Eck, E. K. Handwashing and physicians: How to get them together. *Infect Control Hosp Epidemiol*. 2002; 23:32–35.

CHAPTER 6

Isolation Precautions

BACKGROUND

Several outbreaks have demonstrated that bacterial and viral pathogens can be transmitted within outpatient facilities by airborne or droplet spread to both healthcare workers and patients.[1–9] These diseases include tuberculosis, rubella, and measles (rubeola virus). The following factors enhance spread of infections in ambulatory care facilities:[10]

- Many people congregate in outpatient settings.
- Many patients with infections are in outpatient facilities for evaluation and treatment.
- Rare or unusual infectious diseases may not be recognized.
- The number of air exchanges in ambulatory buildings is often low, and air is recirculated.

Current isolation and precautions (I/P) practices developed out of the concept of physically segregating contagious persons from others. This idea of quarantine included techniques for special handling of food, care of equipment, and handling of body wastes. The theoretical basis of quarantine is to identify a person's communicable disease and direct specific intervention strategies at interrupting the spread of disease.[11] Part of the current I/P approach continues to use this concept.

The Centers for Disease Control and Prevention (CDC) developed guidelines for I/P in 1970.[12] They were revised in 1983 and again in 1996.[13] However, the focus still remains on the hospital. The guidelines are being revised and will include healthcare settings outside of acute care.

The CDC guidelines are based on the rationale that identification of a pathogen, its source, and the mode of transmission will suggest a logical means to prevent spread.[14] The source of infection may be the patient or healthcare worker, staff (through contaminated hands), or contaminated surfaces/equipment. The mode of transmission can be either contact (direct or indirect), droplet, or airborne. The focus of I/P is to interrupt transmission. This same rationale can be used in ambulatory care settings to address diseases that have the potential to cause problems, such as chicken pox, measles, tuberculosis, and vancomycin-resistant enterococcus.[15]

Ambulatory care facilities must develop specific strategies to control the spread of infectious diseases pertinent to the setting. Any I/P system implemented must be epidemiologically sound and user friendly. The CDC guidelines may be used as a guide for developing appropriate strategies. However, because these guidelines are currently focused on hospitals, ambulatory care facilities need to adapt them to each unique situation.

The fundamental components of a facility-specific I/P protocol should include:

- hand hygiene,
- use of barriers (e.g., gloves, gowns and face protection),
- patient placement (i.e., waiting rooms, examination room use, "rash" rooms),
- equipment, and
- cleaning.

GENERAL CATEGORIES

The following information is a summary of the CDC guidelines and other references that are of primary importance in ambulatory care (see Isolation Precautions Table, Appendix D).

Standard Precautions

Rationale

This precaution is designed for the care of all patients regardless of their diagnosis. It includes the concept of universal precautions used with bloodborne pathogens.[16] The concept underlying the precautions is that the source for most potentially infectious microorganisms is the colonized body substances of humans, whether the person is infected or not.[11] The precautions apply to blood, all body fluids, non-intact skin, and mucous membranes.

Other terms used for a similar type of precautions are body substance isolation (BSI) and body substance precautions.[17] The primary purpose of BSI is to reduce risks to patients through cross-transmission of microorganisms via the hands of healthcare workers.[18] BSI focuses on using precautions with all moist and potentially infectious body substances from all patients, regardless of infection status. This type of precautions (BSI or Standard Precautions) is especially valuable in ambulatory care settings because staff members often do not know the identity or even suspect the presence of a pathogen when a patient is seen initially.

Specifics

1. Use with all patients.
2. Hands should be washed before and after each patient contact, if contaminated with blood or body fluids, and after removal of gloves. If hands are not visibly soiled, an alcohol-based hand rub may be used[19] (see Chapter 5).
3. Gloves should be used for contact with blood, all body fluids, non-intact skin, mucous membranes, and contaminated items or surfaces. They must be worn when performing venipuncture and other vascular access procedures.
4. Protective eyewear (masks, goggles, face shields) must be used if the face is likely to be splashed; for example, during procedures likely to generate droplets of blood or body fluids.
5. Fluid-resistant gowns or aprons must be used during procedures likely to splatter clothing with blood or body fluids.
6. Sharp items must be handled safely. Needles should never be recapped, bent, broken, or manipulated by hand. Place sharp items in puncture-resistant containers for disposal. Ensure that disposal containers are out of the reach of children; however, make sure they are available at points of use. Provide safety devices as appropriate.
7. Reusable sharp items should be placed in puncture-resistant containers for transport to a processing area.
8. If an environmental surface or piece of equipment is visibly contaminated with blood or body fluid, it should be cleaned with a low-level disinfectant. After all visible blood or body fluid is removed, disinfectant should by reapplied with a fresh disinfectant cloth or paper towel.
9. There should be easy access to resuscitation equipment so that mouth-to-mouth resuscitation may be avoided.

Contact Precautions

Rationale

Used in addition to Standard Precautions, this precaution focuses on microorganisms that may be spread by routes other than direct contact with body substances. It addresses spread of microbes through droplets or contact with contaminated environmental surfaces; examples are respiratory syncytial virus and vancomycin-resistant enterococcus.

Specifics

1. If the diagnosis is suspected prior to arrival, place the patient in a private room as soon as he or she arrives.
2. Wear gloves for any patient contact and for contact with any item that touched the patient. Remove gloves and wash hands before leaving the room.
3. Wear fluid-resistant gowns when entering the room if clothing will have contact with the patient or if working close to the patient.

4. Wipe down all equipment that had patient contact or that is potentially contaminated with blood or body fluid with a disinfectant cleaner prior to removal from the room.

5. Post a sign on the examination or procedure room door to notify staff of the required precautions (see Appendix D).

Droplet Precautions

Rationale

Used in addition to Standard Precautions, this precaution is designed to reduce risk of spread through respiratory droplets larger than five microns in size (e.g., pertussis or rubella). Droplets are generated during coughing, sneezing, or talking, and during certain procedures such as bronchoscopy. Spread requires relatively close contact because these droplets do not remain suspended in the air and usually only travel about three feet or less from the individual.

Specifics

1. If the diagnosis is suspected prior to arrival, place the patient in a private room as soon as he or she arrives.

2. Post a sign on the examination or procedure room door to notify staff of the required precautions (see Appendix D).

3. Wear a standard mask when working within three feet of the patient.

4. Place a standard mask (e.g., surgical mask) on the patient to minimize droplet dispersal if it is necessary to transport the patient.

Airborne Precautions

Rationale

Used in addition to Standard Precautions, this precaution focuses on diseases spread by respiratory droplet nuclei—small particles less than five microns in size that may remain suspended in the air for long periods of time. Microorganisms spread in this manner can then be inhaled by a susceptible person. Microbes spread this way include *Mycobacterium tuberculosis*, chicken pox (varicella-zoster virus), and measles (rubeola virus).

Specifics

1. Patients with potentially communicable diseases such as chicken pox or measles should be identified upon arrival. Identification may occur through prenotification by phone when making an appointment, observation by a reception or clinical staff person, or via a sign notifying patients of the importance of communicating this information.

2. Place patients known to have a disease spread by the airborne route in a private room (one with a solid door) immediately upon arrival. The door must remain closed except during use by staff members. Ideally, the room should be at negative pressure in relation to the hall. (If practical, a fan may be placed in the window that will pull air out of the room.)

3. Post a sign on the examination or procedure room door to notify staff of the required precautions (see Appendix D).

4. A standard mask should be worn by staff when in the same room as the patient. Persons immune to the specific illness (e.g., measles) do not need to wear a mask.

5. If your facility is classified as being moderate- or high-risk for tuberculosis (TB) (see Chapter 22), a special mask (e.g., a N95 respirator) is to be worn with a potential TB patient. Use of these masks requires education and fit testing.[20] If your facility is classified as being at minimal or low risk for TB, a standard mask may be worn with a potential TB patient.

6. Make tissues available for patients. Instruct the patient to cover his or her mouth when sneezing or coughing.

7. Place a standard mask (e.g., surgical mask) on the patient to minimize droplet nuclei dispersal if it is necessary to transport the patient.

Special TB Issues[20]

1. There should be a comprehensive protocol for identifying and treating patients with possible TB. The most important part of a TB control program is early identification and isolation of patients with suspected or confirmed TB. Triage personnel who perform initial evaluations must

know both the signs and symptoms of TB and the appropriate precautions to use for patients. A screening tool for staff may be helpful in identifying patients who might have TB[10] (see Appendix C).

2. Patients with risk factors and suspicious symptoms for TB should be provided a mask and instructed to cover their mouth and nose with tissues when coughing or sneezing. These patients must be separated as much as possible from other patients and not remain in common waiting areas.

3. If sputum induction, bronchoscopy, aerosolized pentamidine treatments, or pulmonary function testing are performed, the area must have adequate facilities, such as booths or other enclosures meeting ventilation requirements for TB.

4. Isolation can be achieved by use of negative-pressure enclosures such as tents or booths. These can be used to provide patient isolation in areas such as emergency rooms and medical diagnostic and treatment areas that do not have private rooms with solid doors and negative pressure.

5. A TB risk assessment should be conducted periodically, and TB infection-control policies based on results of the risk assessment should be developed (see Chapter 22). The policies should include provisions for identifying patients who may have undiagnosed active TB; managing patients who have active TB; and educating, training, counseling, and screening healthcare workers.

Antibiotic Resistance

Rationale

The selective pressure of antimicrobial therapy has resulted in the evolution of bacteria that are resistant to certain antibiotics. The risk of infection or colonization with antibiotic-resistant microorganisms is higher among sicker, debilitated patients and in settings of high antimicrobial use and invasive technology (e.g., intensive care units). Infections due to antibiotic-resistant microorganisms are difficult to treat and are often associated with high morbidity.

These microbes can be spread from patient to patient through transient hand carriage and environmental contamination. Thus, it is important to adopt procedures that will keep the spread of these microorganisms to a minimum. In general, the microorganisms that might be included in such procedures are:

- Methicillin-resistant *Staphylococcus aureus* (MRSA)
- Vancomycin-resistant *S. aureus* (VRSA)
- Vancomycin-resistant enterococci (VRE)
- Gram-negative bacteria that are β-lactam resistant
- Other microorganisms with antibiotic-resistance profiles considered to be epidemiologically significant

Because enterococci are part of the normal flora of the gastrointestinal and female genital tracts, most infections with these microorganisms have been attributed to the patient's endogenous flora.[21] However, reports of healthcare outbreaks caused by enterococci, including VRE, have indicated that patient-to-patient transmission of the microorganisms can occur either through direct contact or through indirect contact via the hands of personnel or contaminated patient-care equipment or environmental surfaces.[22]

Staphylococci are one of the most common causes of community- and hospital-associated infection. Staphylococci resistant to antimicrobials, especially methicillin, have been of major concern for many years.[23] More recently there has been concern regarding potential resistance to vancomycin, resulting in the development of specific prevention and control guidelines.[24] The first clinical isolate of *S. aureus* fully resistant to vancomycin (VRSA) was reported in a dialysis patient.[25] Preventing the spread of these microorganisms is important to avoid the possibility that prophylaxis against and treatment of infections is not effective because of resistance to antibiotics.

Specifics

1. Use of Contact Precautions is recommended.
2. In addition, the patient's record should be flagged with the resistant microbe status, and educational information should be provided to the patient. See Appendix E for sample education sheets.

SPECIAL APPLICATION OF ISOLATION PRECAUTIONS IN AMBULATORY SETTINGS

Waiting Rooms

Waiting rooms and reception areas offer the opportunity for interaction and the potential for transmission of droplet-borne or airborne-spread communicable diseases due to clustering of individuals.[26] Infectious diseases account for 20 to 30% of physician office visits.[27] Therefore, exposure to communicable diseases (e.g., measles,[3] influenza, and RSV) can occur in waiting areas or other areas where many people congregate. Table 6.1 lists common communicable diseases encountered in ambulatory care settings.[13]

Efforts should be made to avoid crowding, shorter wait times, and minimize the sharing of toys.[26] In addition, patients should be assessed as soon as possible, and potentially communicable patients should enter through a separate entrance and go directly to the examination or procedure room.[10] Ideally, immunocompromised children should not wait in a general waiting area to reduce exposure to communicable diseases.[26]

Table 6.1   Common Communicable Diseases in Ambulatory Settings[†]

Infection/Condition	Type of I/P[*]
Acquired immune deficiency syndrome (AIDS)	S
Adenovirus infection in infants and young children	D, C
Anthrax	S
Antibiotic-resistant microorganisms	C
Chicken pox	A, C
Conjunctivitis	S
Cytomegalovirus infection, neonatal or immunosuppressed	S
Diphtheria	
Cutaneous	C
Pharyngeal	D
Gastroenteritis	
E. coli[**]	S
Giardia lamblia	S
Rotavirus[**]	S
Salmonella	S
Shigella[**]	S
Gonorrhea	S
Hepatitis	
A[**]	S
B	S
Other viral	S
Herpes zoster (shingles)	
Disseminated	A, C
Localized	S
Human immunodeficiency virus (HIV)	S
Influenza	D
Lice	C
Measles (rubeola)	A

(continued)

Table 6.1   (continued)

Infection/Condition	Type of I/P*
Meningitis	
Viral	S
H. influenzae	D
N. meningiditis	D
Mumps	D
Parvovirus B19 (Fifth disease)	D
Respiratory disease, infants and young children	C
Rubella	D
Scabies	C
Streptococcus, Group A (e.g., strep throat)	
Adults	S
Infants and children	D
Syphilis	S
Tuberculosis, pulmonary	A
West Nile Virus	S
Whooping cough (pertussis)	D
Wound	
No dressing/dressing does not contain drainage	C
Dressing covers and contains drainage	S

*Isolation Precautions: C—Contact precautions; D—Droplet precautions; A—Airborne precautions; S—Standard precautions

**C if diapered or incontinent

†Adapted from Garner, J. S. The Hospital Infection Control Practices Advisory Committee. Guidelines for isolation precautions in hospitals. *Am J Infect Control.* 1996; 24:24–52.

Scheduling Patients

If a patient has a fever or rash, schedule the appointment at the end of the day or during times of the day when few patients are present.[10]

Triaging Patients

It is important to promptly triage patients who have febrile exanthems. Patients should be triaged by phone whenever possible. Educate reception staff to alert a clinical staff member if a patient presents with a severe cough or a rash. Take the patient promptly into an examination room to minimize spread in the waiting area.

Patients with coughs or respiratory symptoms should be provided tissues and instructed to cover coughs and sneezes with a tissue. Symptom-based evaluation can allow for appropriate triage and application of precautions. Patients with known disease or a high index of suspicion for TB, chicken pox, measles, mumps, rubella, or bacterial meningitis should wear a mask and be placed in a separate room with the door closed and an Airborne Precautions sign posted.[28]

Immunization

The transmission of many infectious diseases can be minimized, if not prevented, by ensuring that patients and staff are appropriately vaccinated. There should be appropriate immunization protocols for children and adults.[29]

The most important preventive measure for control of communicable diseases is to have all staff and patients immune. It is recommended that all susceptible healthcare workers be immunized with varicella, hepatitis B, influenza, measles, mumps, and rubella vaccines.[30]

Design of Area

Many outpatient facilities are not designed for I/P practices. Rarely are rooms designed with negative pressure capabilities. Often the air is recirculated without any filtration, the number of air exchanges is low, and the buildings are airtight. Proper ventilation for I/P may be difficult to achieve.

The duration of time that airborne microbes remain suspended in a room depends on air exchange rates.[20, 31] The current recommended air exchange rate for a medical office examination room is six air changes per hour with two outside air exchanges per hour.[26]

An understanding of airflow patterns and general space requirements in the facility can assist in the development of appropriate I/P protocols. Protocols should include: 1) making efforts to see potentially communicable patients at the end of the day, 2) quickly triaging these patients out of common waiting areas, 3) closing the door of the examination room, and 4) limiting access to the patient by staff members who are not immune to the suspected disease.[26]

INFORMING OTHERS OF ISOLATION PRECAUTIONS

It is important that information regarding the patient's illness be kept as confidential as possible. However, there must be a method to inform staff of appropriate precautions, such as a door sign. In addition, some communicable diseases must be reported to a local health department. See the list of health departments at *http://www.cdc.gov/other.htm.*

TRANSFER OF PATIENTS

When transporting patients to another facility (e.g., a hospital) it is important that the patient wear appropriate garb to protect staff members. The type of garb, such as a mask, will depend on the type of I/P used. In addition, the facility to which the patient is being sent must be informed of the potential infectious disease so they may take appropriate precautions.

PATIENT AND FAMILY EDUCATION

Education of patients and family regarding the use of I/P is important to ensure their compliance and answer any questions. There are many resources available on the CDC Web site at *http://www.cdc.gov/health/default.htm* that may be shared with patients and family members.

In many instances the infectious potential of a patient may not be known until a probable or definitive diagnosis can be determined. Obviously, precautions based on that diagnosis cannot be implemented in advance of a diagnosis. The routine use of Standard Precautions for all patients should greatly reduce the risk of transmission for conditions other than those required for airborne-spread diseases.

References

1. Couldwell, D. L., Dore, G. J., Harkness, J. L., Marriott, D. J., Cooper, D. A., and Edwards, R., et al. Nosocomial outbreak of tuberculosis in an outpatient HIV treatment room. *AIDS.* 1996; 10:521–525.

2. Haley, C. E., McDonald, R. C., Rossi, L., Jones, W. D., Haley, R. W., and Luby, J. P. Tuberculosis epidemic among hospital personnel. *Infect Control Hosp Epidemiol.* 1989; 10:204–210.

3. Istre, G. R., McKee, P. A., West, G. R., O'Mara, D. J., Rettig, P. J., Stuemky, J., and Dwyer, D. M. Measles spread in medical settings: An important focus of disease transmission? *Pediatrics.* 1987; 79:356–358.

4. Bloch, A. B., Orenstein, W. A., Ewing, W. M., Spain, W. H., Mallison, G. F., and Herrmann, K. L., et al. Measles outbreak in a pediatric practice: Airborne transmission in an office setting. *Pediatrics.* 1985; 75:676–683.

5. Remington, P. L., Hall, W. N., Davis, I. H., Herald, A., and Gunn, R. A. Airborne transmission of measles in a physician's office. *JAMA.* 1985; 253:1574–1577.

6. Davis, R. M., Orenstein, W. A., Frank, J. A., Jr., Sacks, J. J., Dales, L. G., and Preblud, S. R., et al. Transmission of measles in medical settings: 1980–1984. *JAMA.* 1986; 255:1295–1298.

7. Sienko, D. G., Friedman, C., McGee, H. B., Allen, M. J., Simonsen, W. F., Wentworth, B. B., Shope, T. C., and Orenstein, W. A. A measles outbreak at university medical settings involving health care providers. *Am J Public Health.* 1987; 77:1222–1224.

8. Gladstone, J. L., and Millian, S. J. Rubella exposure in an obstetric clinic. *Obstet Gynecol.* 1981; 57:182–186.

9. Fliegel, P. E., and Weinstein, W. M. Rubella outbreak in a prenatal clinic: Management and prevention. *Am J Infect Control.* 1982; 10:29–33.

10. Herwaldt, L. A., Smith, S. D., and Carter, C. D. Infection control in the outpatient setting. *Infect Control Hosp Epidemiol.* 1998; 19:41–74.

11. Jackson, M. M., and Lynch, P. Isolation practices: A historical perspective. *Am J Infect Control.* 1985; 13:21–31.

12. CDC. *Isolation Techniques Used in Hospitals.* Atlanta, GA: Centers for Disease Control, 1970.

13. Garner, J. S. The Hospital Infection Control Practices Advisory Committee. Guidelines for isolation precautions in hospitals. *Am J Infect Control.* 1996; 24:24–52.

14. O'Rourke, E. New isolation strategies: Is there a need? *Infect Control Hosp Epidemiol.* 1994; 15:300–302.

15. Willy, M. E. The Epidemiology and Control of Communicable Diseases (in the Outpatient Setting). *Lippincott's Primary Care Practice.* 1999; 3:82–92.

16. Occupational exposure to bloodborne pathogens: Final rule. *Fed Reg.* 1991; 56:64175–64182.

17. Lynch, P., Cummings, M. J., Roberts, P. L., Herriott, M. J., Yates, B., and Stamm, W. E. Implementing and evaluating a system of generic infection precautions: Body substance isolation. *Am J Infect Control.* 1990; 18:1–12.

18. Jackson, M. M., and Lynch, P. An attempt to make an issue less murky: A comparison of four systems for infection precautions. *Infect Control Hosp Epidemiol.* 1991; 12:448–450.

19. Centers for Disease Control and Prevention. Guideline for Hand Hygiene in Health-Care Settings: Recommendations of the Healthcare Infection Control Practices Advisory Committee and the HICPAC/SHEA/APIC/IDSA Hand Hygiene Task Force. *MMWR.* 2002; 51 (No. RR-16):1–44.

20. Centers for Disease Control and Prevention. Guidelines for preventing the transmission of *Mycobacterium tuberculosis* in health-care facilities, 1994. *MMWR.* 1994; 43(RR13):1–132.

21. Murray, B. E. The life and times of the enterococcus. *Clin Microbiol Rev.* 1990; 3:46–65.

22. Recommendations for Preventing the Spread of Vancomycin Resistance Recommendations of the Hospital Infection Control Practices Advisory Committee (HICPAC). *MMWR.* 1995; 44(RR12):1–13.

23. Boyce, J. M. Methicillin-Resistant *Staphyloccocus aureus* Infections. In: Abrutyn, E., Goldmann, D. A., Schlecker, W. E., eds., *Saunders Infection Control Reference Service.* 2nd Ed. Philadelphia: W.B. Saunders Co., 2001: 775–779.

24. Interim Guidelines for Prevention and Control of Staphylococcal Infection Associated with Reduced Susceptibility to Vancomycin. *MMWR.* 1997; 46(27):626–628, 635.

25. *Staphylococcus aureus* Resistant to Vancomycin—United States, 2002. *MMWR.* 2002; 51:565–567.

26. American Academy of Pediatrics. Infection control in physicians' offices. *Pediatrics.* 2000; 105:1361–1369.

27. Palmer, S., Giddens, J., and Palmer, D. *Infection Control.* El Paso, TX: Skidmore-Roth Publishing, Inc., 1996: 245.

28. Jennings, J., and Wideman, J. *APIC Handbook of Infection Control.* 3rd Ed. Washington, DC: Association for Professionals in Infection Control and Epidemiology, Inc., 2002: 354.

29. Pickering, L. K., ed. *2000 Red Book: Report of the Committee on Infectious Diseases.* 25th Ed. Elk Grove Village, IL: American Academy of Pediatrics, 2000.

30. Bolyard, E. A., Tablan, O. C., Williams, W. W., Pearson, M. L., Shapiro, C. N., and Deitchman, S. D., et al. Guideline for infection control in health care personnel, 1998. *Am J Infect Control.* 1998; 26:289–354.

31. AIA. *Guidelines for Design and Construction of Hospital and Health Care Facilities.* Washington, DC: The American Institute of Architects and the Facilities Guidelines Institute, 2001.

CHAPTER 7

Physician Offices and Clinics

BACKGROUND

Risk of infection transmission in primary care offices and clinics is generally considered lower than for hospitalized patients (see Chapter 1). However, infection prevention strategies need to be in place for both patient-care practices and the environment in order to ensure a low risk. Management of infectious patients and the ability to offer patient education may differ significantly from an in-patient setting due to the high number of patients seen in a short time and the brief encounter. Many environmental issues in these areas have overlapping infection control, safety, and aesthetic concerns. The expectation from the Joint Commission on Accreditation of Healthcare Organizations (JCAHO) is for a "safe, functional, and effective environment for patients, staff members, and other individuals in the ambulatory care organization."[1] This section will review infection prevention and control, and environmental and general patient care considerations to help meet this expectation.

ENVIRONMENTAL ISSUES

Housecleaning

A clean environment theoretically may contribute to prevention of infection both to staff and patients; however, there are few references linking the spread of infection from common surfaces in any healthcare setting.[2] Various microorganisms can survive for extended periods on environmental surfaces; however,

the importance of environmental contamination with health care-associated pathogens (e.g., methicillin-resistant *S. aureus*, vancomycin-resistant enterococcus, *C. difficile*) in ambulatory care has not been well defined.[3] During outbreaks in specific settings (e.g., ophthalmology [see Chapter 14]), the environment may contribute to the spread of microorganisms. However, for routine cleaning the following recommendations are based on common sense and aesthetics.

Frequency of Cleaning

Surfaces such as examination tables, countertops, floors, and public areas of the facility, such as waiting rooms and rest rooms need to be cleaned immediately after soiling with blood or body fluids.[4] In addition, these surfaces need to be cleaned at regular intervals, depending on use and function. Occupational Safety and Health Administration standards[4] state that: "Cleaning schedules and methods will vary . . . routine cleaning and removal of soil are required."

General cleaning of examination, waiting, and rest rooms should be performed daily; however, if patient load is heavy, several times a day may be necessary. Treatment or procedure rooms are subject to increased soiling potential, and surfaces visibly soiled should be cleaned after each patient.

Surfaces in contact with intact skin of the patient or a staff member, such as examination tables, baby scales, blood pressure cuffs, stethoscopes, tympanogram equipment, glucometers, and examination lights, should be cleaned when soiled and on a routine basis. If clean paper is used on the examination tables and baby scales between each patient, these surfaces can be cleaned daily and when visibly soiled. If the provider adjusts the exam light during pelvic or other examinations where there is potential of touching mucous membrane or non-intact skin, it should be cleaned after each such exam.

Cleaning Agents

Products used for surface cleaner-disinfectants should be evaluated for and exhibit as many ideal characteristics as outlined in Table 7.1 as possible.[5] Low-level disinfectants (see Chapter 3) are adequate for environmental surface cleaning. Among the most commonly used and best cleaners are quaternary ammonium compounds. Phenolics are sometimes used, but they may leave a film or residue and are not recommended for surfaces in contact with newborns.[5] Neither alcohol nor bleach is recommended as a general environmental cleaner. Alcohol (usually 70–90% isopropyl) is effective in decontaminating blood but contains no cleaning agent, is flammable, and evaporates rapidly. Alcohol as supplied in sealed, small pads contains enough to disinfect a very small area. Bleach is corrosive, harmful to clothing, and easily inactivated by organic material.[5]

Because of the importance of mechanical cleaning, a product containing detergents or surfactants should be selected. Most importantly, the cleaner-disinfectant must be diluted, used, and stored precisely according to the label instructions. If diluted into secondary containers, these containers must be labeled with the brand name of the product and any health or physical hazards as listed on the Material Safety Data Sheet (MSDS). Although convenient, aerosol products usually are more costly and may elicit complaints about odor.

Method of Cleaning

As a practical matter, cleaning should be performed going from the cleanest to the most soiled area. Usually this means that cleaning will start at the highest point in the room (e.g., any spot cleaning on the walls) and then proceed to counters, sinks, examination tables, and so on. Although contact time is usually less than or equal to 10 minutes[5] for cleaner-disinfectants, from a practical, in-use point of view, surfaces are usually wiped and product allowed to dry with no rinsing, so that actual contact time is quite variable. Cleaning solution for general daily cleaning is often made up in a bucket. Cloths soaked with solution are used for mechanical cleaning. Most solutions will not need to be rinsed off. Cloths and buckets of cleaner-disinfectant should be changed often to prevent overloading with soil and microorganisms.

If light soiling is encountered most often, dispensing product from a spray bottle directly on the surface and wiping with clean cloth is practical. If blood or body fluids are being cleaned up, the spill initially should be

Table 7.1 Properties of Cleaner-Disinfectants to Consider

Broad antimicrobial spectrum	Review product specifications and microbiological testing data.
Stability	Review shelf life information for concentrate and in-use dilution.
Toxicity	Review Material Safety Data Sheets for health hazards associated with product use.
Absent or mild odor	To reduce possible sensitivity, allergic, or asthmatic reactions.
Cost	Review cost of pre-diluted, ready-to-use product versus concentrate.
Water solubility	Important if concentrate is under consideration.
Cleaning ability	Evaluate for surfactants or other cleaners that are important for mechanical removal of soil and organic material.
Rinsing	If rinsing is needed, the entire cleaning procedure will take longer.
Contact time	Usually less than or equal to 10 minutes.

absorbed with a moistened cloth or paper towel, the area sprayed with cleaner-disinfectant, and then cleaned again with cloth or paper towel. Follow the product label instructions regarding the length of time the product should remain moist on the surface.[4] Disinfectant-impregnated wipes in "pop-up" containers may be useful for cleaning small areas; for blood, one should be used to clean up the spot and then another one used to disinfect the area.

For floors, cleaning should start with a clean mop head and fresh bucket of cleaner-disinfectant solution. A single bucket and mop head will be sufficient to clean all of the noncarpeted areas in most physician offices and smaller clinics. Used mop heads and buckets of cleaning solution should never be stored overnight or for use at a later time due to the growth potential of microorganisms. Physical removal of soil with friction and scrubbing is as important as the product used and should not be overlooked in maintaining a clean environment. Damp dusting is preferred; dry dusting can cause fungal spore-laden dust particles to become airborne and should be discouraged.[6]

Written Procedures

Written procedures are needed and should describe in detail:

- what and how to clean, the cleaning products, and any instructions for dilution;
- who is responsible (including direct patient care providers for immediate clean-up of a blood or body fluid spill);
- where the cleaning products are stored; and
- when and how often to clean.

All areas need to be included specifically in the written protocols: waiting room, patient examination and treatment/procedure rooms, laboratory, employee lounges, and restrooms. All surfaces should be included, from floors to walls to medical equipment to examination tables to countertops to doorknobs. Frequency of changing cleaning cloths, mop heads, and buckets of cleaner-disinfectant should be specified. Written protocols are important to avoid confusion about house-

cleaning expectations and should be used for training new staff and for verification that tasks are performed. If janitorial services are contracted, performance should be monitored and accountability established in the contract. Products used by the contract service should be reviewed for active ingredients and the other properties listed in Table 7.1, and they should be approved by administration and infection control staff.

Carpet

Carpet has not been shown to increase infection rates[7–9] in hospitals and is widely used in physician offices and clinics. Carpeting should be vacuumed and shampooed regularly.[10] Except during construction, high-efficiency particulate air filter (HEPA) vacuums have not been shown to be necessary.[10] As with other surfaces, blood and body fluid spills should be cleaned up immediately with a disinfectant; carpet choice should be based in part on the manufacturer providing adequate cleaning and disinfecting protocols. In areas where blood or body fluid spills may occur routinely (e.g., laboratories, procedure rooms, and soiled utility rooms), carpeting is not recommended because of aesthetics and odor control.

Supplies

Lack of storage space is chronic in many ambulatory settings. The ideal is to have clean storage and handling of soiled items done in separate rooms. However, because space and design may not permit this complete separation, there are flexible ways to organize the available space to keep supplies clean. However, it is important to review state or local regulations for requirements related to storage and separation of supplies. Codes may specify room function based on whether the facility is located in a hospital, medical professional building, or business occupancy. The American Institute of Architects (AIA) recommends that for outpatient centers a separate room or closet be provided for clean storage. For small, primary outpatient facilities, clean supplies may be stored in a separate room or in an isolated area of a room used for another purpose.[11]

Clean Storage

Guidelines for clean storage are as follows:

- Coordination should be made with delivery services so that clean supplies, such as linen, are not placed on the floor or on soiled shelving. If services also pick up soiled supplies, separate containers must be used for clean versus soiled supplies.
- Open shelves are acceptable in designated clean storage rooms, including linen storage. However, if mesh-type shelving is used, the bottom shelf should be covered or items stored in clean bins on the shelf to protect items from damage or soiling during cleaning of the floor under the shelves.
- Clean storage areas should have limited access and should not be located in a throughway.
- Cleaning should be performed on a regular schedule to remove dust from floors and shelves. It should be performed carefully to avoid damage to or contamination of supplies.
- Supplies should be rotated "first in, first out" so that the oldest supplies are used first.
- In examination and treatment rooms, drawers and closed cabinets should be used for storage.
- To prevent water damage, no patient items should be placed under sinks, the ice machine, or other areas with water pipes.
- Cleaning supplies and disinfectants may be placed under sinks; however, unless the cabinet is locked, they should be kept only in rooms inaccessible to children or developmentally disabled individuals. Cleaner-disinfectant may be kept in treatment and procedure rooms for easy access for surface cleaning after procedures. It can be stored on an upper shelf or cabinet. It is common and generally acceptable for cleaning supplies to be stored under the sink in the soiled utility room.
- Items should be removed from shipping boxes before storage to prevent contamination with soil/debris that might be on the packing container.
- Although it is preferable to store linen in a clean room or in drawers or closed cabinets in exam rooms, it is acceptable to store linen on shelves in designated alcoves or other open areas. In these areas, the linen must be covered at all times to prevent potential soiling from traffic and to reduce the possibility of linen falling on the floor.

- In general, clean linen should not be stored in restrooms. However, in areas where the patient restroom adjoining a procedure room doubles as a locker room, it may be practical to keep a limited supply of patient gowns as long as they are covered and away from water contamination from the sink or toilet.
- Paper products (e.g., paper towels) stored in the janitor closet must not be stored on the floor.
- Clean items, including examination gloves, should be stored away from the "splash zone" around the sink to avoid contamination from microorganisms found in tap water. The precise distance will depend on the size and shape of the sink and water pressure. These items should also not be stored under the soap dispenser to prevent damage from dripping soap.
- It is safe to store clean items in closed cabinets, covered shelves, or drawers in a soiled utility room, but specific state health department regulations should be checked before implementing this practice. The area for storage of clean supplies should be labeled. If there is an autoclave in the utility room, supplies such as autoclave wrap, tape, peel pouches, and towels to be included in sterile packs may be stored in this room.
- If clean supplies will be held in the utility room after reprocessing until they can be delivered to a storage room or patient care areas, the holding space should be labeled to indicate that these items are "clean, patient ready."

Soiled Supplies and Linen

The underlying principle for managing soiled supplies, linen, and trash is to prevent contamination of clean items and to avoid exposure of patients or staff. After use, reusable medical devices should be taken directly to a soiled utility room. If this is not practical, they may be placed in a labeled, covered container in the examination or treatment room so that there is no chance of confusion with clean supplies. However, if there is opportunity for patients to unwittingly touch soiled items, they must be removed before another patient enters the room.

Soiled linen containers should be well defined and obvious, such as closed hampers in examination rooms or large hampers in the utility room. If drawers for soiled linen are provided in the examination table, they should be clearly labeled to avoid confusion with clean linen also found in examination table drawers. Drawers used for soiled linen should be decontaminated on a regular basis with an approved cleaner-disinfectant. Soiled linen should be collected at the point of use and handled minimally to prevent aerosolization of microorganisms. Linen should not be handled differently based on patient diagnosis. If linen is contaminated with blood or body fluid, wear barriers during handling of the items according to Standard Precautions[4, 12] (see Chapter 6). Either plastic or cloth laundry bags are acceptable for managing soiled linen. Blood-saturated linen should be placed in plastic bags to prevent leakage.[12] Soiled and clean linen must be transported and stored separately.

Laundering patient linen on-site is uncommon. To maintain the highest quality and for cost efficiencies, it is rarely recommended that linen be washed on-site.[12] Although linen can harbor many micrcoorganisms, risk of disease spread has been shown to be negligible and linen in these settings is rarely heavily soiled.[2, 12] However, if washing machines are in use for cleaning patient sheets, towels, gowns, and so forth, state regulations must be consulted for proper water temperature, monitoring and record keeping, location of washing machines, and storage of soiled linen prior to washing. Recent guidelines indicate that ≥160°F (71°C) for 25 minutes or a lower temperature (71.6–122°F, i.e., 22–50°C) when bleach is added are effective.[12] The soiled laundry processing area should be physically separated from clean linen storage, patient care areas, food preparation areas, and clean supply and equipment storage areas.[13]

Trash Handling

Regulated medical (infectious) waste and regular trash must be separated for disposal; each state has specific definitions for regulated/medical/infectious waste (see Chapter 22). Approved sharps containers must be located at the point of use;[4] they should be placed in all examination, treatment, and procedure rooms, phlebotomy stations and utility rooms, at heights convenient for all staff (not so high that staff will have difficulty reaching them). Special safety considerations need to be addressed for their placement in pediatrics areas to avoid potential accidental patient injury and access. In these areas they should be placed high enough from the floor to be inaccessible. If there is great concern or history of injury, portable sharps containers may be taken into the room as needed and stored in an inaccessible area between uses.

Space constraints, infrequency of generating regulated medical waste, lack of understanding about items that are classified as regulated medical waste, and ineffective separation of trash and regulated waste often hamper efforts at efficient waste disposal. Red bags, biohazard buckets, or other containers as required by specific state regulations should be placed judiciously. It is often practical and sufficient to place one container for regulated waste in the lab area or utility room and one in each procedure or treatment room that generates regulated waste on a regular basis. Regular reminders to staff via in-service education and posted lists or posters may also help ensure adequate separation.

If there is an unplanned generation of regulated waste, a plastic bag can be used to collect the waste. Then it can carefully be transported to where the regulated waste container is located, or the regulated container can be taken where needed. Accurate sorting of trash and regulated waste is cost-effective due to the expense of disposing of regulated waste.

Refrigerators

Refrigerators should be clean and well maintained. There have been no outbreaks or reports of cross-infection due to refrigeration failure in ambulatory care. However, there have been recalls of immunization products, specifically hepatitis B vaccine in early 2001, due to storage temperatures not being maintained.[14] During the 1970s, articles were published on the impotency of vaccines as a result of improper handling.[15]

State regulations should be consulted for any specific temperature monitoring and record-keeping requirements of refrigerators and freezers. General guidelines include:

- Store patient food, medications, and specimens in separate, labeled refrigerators. Glucose beverages may be stored in the medication or the patient food refrigerator, but never in the specimen refrigerator.
- Store all medications at the temperatures indicated by the product labels or package inserts.

- Label the specimen refrigerator with a biohazard label to comply with OSHA regulations.[4]
- Comply with safe temperature ranges for specimen,[16] food,[17] and medication[18] refrigerators and freezers (see Table 7.2).
- Use a thermometer inside each refrigerator and freezer.
- Monitor and chart temperatures at regular intervals, such as each day the clinic is open. Note on the chart the acceptable temperature range. (See Appendix F for sample temperature recording charts.) If the clinic is part of the Vaccines for Children Program administered through state health departments, there may be additional monitoring requirements (*http://www.cdc.gov/nip/vfc/ default.htm*).
- Develop a procedure to follow should the temperature fall outside the acceptable range. Describe steps to take and who to contact on the temperature log. Consult with drug manufacturing companies or an affiliated pharmacy for how long medications will be safe if outside the acceptable temperature range. Develop alternative storage methods during power or refrigerator failure and post the written procedure for easy access.
- Clean and defrost refrigerators, including staff refrigerators, at regular, defined intervals and when soiled or if a spill occurs. The procedure should be written and include the responsible staff and the cleaning product to use.
- Date patient food and beverages and discard at reasonable time intervals, such as 48 hours after opening. Check for state or local regulations.
- A full refrigerator will retain a constant temperature better than an empty one. Therefore, it may be helpful to place containers of water in refrigerators with extra space. For infection control purposes, label containers with "Water. Not for drinking. Do not remove from the refrigerator. The water needs to stay in the refrigerator to help maintain a constant temperature."

Because many ambulatory sites are not open every day and it may be impractical and cost-prohibitive to install refrigerators with alarms, questions often arise about how to identify power failures. One method is to place a small, water-filled container, such as a paper cup, in the freezer. After the water has frozen, place a coin on the ice. If the refrigerator fails while the clinic is closed, the ice will melt and the coin will sink. Someone must be assigned the duty of checking on the coin the morning after a weekend or holiday closure.

There are no regulations or specific JCAHO standards on staff refrigerators, so common sense should prevail for their cleaning and maintenance.

Toys and Computers

There are many concerns about the risk of cross-infection from toys. Although actual incidence of disease transmission directly linked to toys has been rare, it is known that microorganisms can survive for extended periods of time on environmental surfaces. After a busy morning in a physician's office, one study found that toys appeared unclean, that 10% were contaminated with potential pathogens, and that bacteria were cultured more frequently from soft toys than from hard toys.[19] Another study found higher contamination levels on soft toys, that neither machine washing and drying nor autoclaving were adequate to totally reduce microorganisms on soft toys, and that soft toys in waiting rooms became contaminated much more quickly than hard toys. This study also found that in waiting rooms hard toys that were cleaned weekly or every other week had low total bacterial counts compared with toys cleaned infrequently or not at all.[20]

Professional organizations and publications have made various recommendations; however, there are no definitive standards for toy cleaning. The American Academy of Pediatrics recommends that toys used in day-care settings that are mouthed or contaminated with body secretions should be cleaned, disinfected,

Table 7.2 Recommended Storage Temperatures for Refrigerators/Freezers

Type	Refrigerator	Freezer
Specimen	36 to 46°F (2 to 8°C)	−4 to 14°F (−20 to −0°C)
Food	≤ 41°F (≤ 5°C)	≤ 0°F (≤ −17.8°C)
Medication	36 to 46°F (2 to 8°C)	−4 to 14°F (−20 to −10°C)
		≤ 5°F (≤ −15°C)

and rinsed. Toys frequently touched by infants or toddlers should be cleaned and disinfected daily, and toys used by nondiapered children should be cleaned at least weekly. Soft, nonwashable toys should be discouraged.[21] The Association for Professionals in Infection Control and Epidemiology (APIC) states that in day-care centers only washable toys should be shared, and they should be washed as frequently as possible and at the end of the day.[22] The value of disinfection for toy cleaning has not been proven. Thorough washing with detergent or in a dishwasher will clean and adequately decrease the microbial load on items.[23]

The procedure and frequency for cleaning toys should be practical and based on the patient population. Toys in a very active pediatric practice with many toddlers will need more frequent cleaning than in practices with fewer young children. Safe disinfectants include dilute bleach (1:100), quaternary ammonium hospital-grade disinfectants, and 70% isopropyl alcohol. Phenolics should never be used (see Chapter 3). Small toys should be thoroughly rinsed; if alcohol is used, toys can air dry and need not be rinsed with water. Alternately, small toys can be placed in a mesh bag and run through a dishwasher with standard dishwashing detergent. Large items, such as wall-mounted toys, tables, or playhouses, can be wiped with a disinfectant cleaner on a regular basis.

Written toy-cleaning policies should be developed and include:

- Frequency of routine toy cleaning: May be daily to weekly, depending on intensity of use.
- Types of toys: Soft toys should not be provided; toys should be restricted to those easily cleaned. New soft toys may be given to patients to take home. Books and puzzles are generally seen to pose very little risk and need not be cleaned unless visibly soiled.
- Toy circulation: Mouthed and visibly soiled toys should be removed from circulation until cleaned.
- Training: Staff training should be clearly documented.
- Toy cleaning procedure: Should include washing, disinfection or sanitization, and rinsing.
- Cleaning agent to be used: Substance(s) must be nontoxic for children.

Computers are now common in exam rooms and in some waiting rooms. Computer surfaces cultured in intensive care units in hospitals have harbored bacteria that can cause outbreaks, and some types of bacteria can survive for many days on plastic.[24] The risk for actual disease transmission from computers in ambulatory care is presumed to be very low. However, protocols should be developed to include cleaning the keyboard or keyboard cover and mouse with disinfectant cleaner on a regular basis and when soiled. The computer should be located away from potential splashing from the sink. The computer manufacturer should supply information on types of disinfectants that are safe to use on the hardware. Handwashing by staff before and after patient contact can reduce risk further.[25]

Construction

Plans for a new building or renovation of existing areas should be reviewed for infection prevention and control issues. The AIA's "Guidelines for Design and Construction of Hospital and Health Care Facilities" contains broadly applicable standards;[11] however, local and state health department ordinances should also be consulted. Infection control professionals should identify who in the institution is responsible for construction and renovation and should request to review all building plans for ambulatory care sites. Plans need to be reviewed early enough to effect change.

Whether planning for a new building or renovating an existing site, plans should be reviewed to ensure that the following infection control questions are addressed:

1. Are clean storage and soiled utility rooms large enough to accommodate expansion?
2. Will the utility room be close to treatment/procedure rooms for safe, expedient transport of contaminated, used equipment?
3. Are instrument reprocessing activities planned for a separate room rather than in a clean room or in a patient care room?
4. Are soiled utility rooms and instrument reprocessing rooms fitted with adequate ventilation? Do they have a negative pressure relationship to the adjacent corridor? If glutaraldehyde disinfectant will be used, does the room have 15 air changes per hour with negative pressure?[11]
5. Do instrument processing rooms have adequate counter space to accommodate containers of disinfectant and/or a table-top autoclave? Are sinks large enough to accommodate rinsing of instruments?

6. Are handwashing sinks located in each examination/treatment/procedure room, all restrooms, the laboratory area, the medication preparation area, and all soiled utility/workrooms?
7. Will hand soap and paper towel dispensers be conveniently located?
8. Will sharps disposal containers be conveniently located?
9. What areas will be carpeted? Carpet is not recommended in laboratory areas or procedure/treatment rooms because it cannot be cleaned effectively.
10. Are environmental surfaces, such as walls, cabinetry, and horizontal surfaces, easy to clean?
11. Is there a lounge area so that staff will not be tempted to eat in patient-care, laboratory, utility, or clean areas?
12. Is there a housekeeping room supplied with a service sink and storage for housekeeping supplies and equipment?
13. If bronchoscopies or other aerosol generating procedures are expected to be performed or if a tuberculosis (TB) patient is likely to be seen (e.g., a pulmonary clinic), are there plans for a negative pressure room? (See Chapter 9.)
14. Are doors and windows secured to prevent entrance of insects, rodents, or other pests?

Renovation

For renovation projects, dust abatement[11, 26] must be addressed to prevent exposure to airborne mold spores such as *Aspergillus* and *Penicillium*. Infection prevention and control activities during renovation are outlined by APIC.[26] Regardless of the size of the project, overall planning should include at least the following:

- Evaluate whether and how much dust is likely to be generated.
- Arrange for the area undergoing renovation to be contained within plastic sheeting.
- Arrange for air flow and/or filtration to prevent dust from blowing into adjacent areas.
- Arrange for monitoring the area under construction to determine that barriers are in use.
- Arrange for thorough damp mopping or HEPA-vacuuming daily, or as needed.

- Outline traffic flow and worksite garb for contractors.
- Determine whether there are any immunocompromised patients who will need to be rerouted away from the area to avoid potential exposure.

Construction companies accustomed to working with healthcare facilities are often aware of these special needs and include costs for dust abatement.

Remediation

Water damage requires drastic action if not handled expediently.[26] It can occur following heavy rains, plumbing leaks, or excessive condensation. If water is not swiftly removed and damaged items completely dried, microorganisms, especially mold such as *Stachybotrys*, *Aspergillus*, and *Penicillium*, can quickly multiply. Spore numbers increase exponentially and are released into the air. Inhaling these spores in high quantities can cause allergic reactions, dubbed "sick building syndrome," and/or respiratory infections.

As soon as water damage is detected, intervention should begin. Porous materials must be dried within 48 hours to prevent an exponential increase in fungal spores. If this is not possible, often the only way to mitigate the problem is to completely remove all of the flooring, carpeting, wall covering, ceiling tiles, plaster, or wallboard affected. Any paper, such as medical records or office products, must also be inspected for water damage. Because intervention must begin immediately, it is best to develop a plan, including a list of remediation contractors with emergency, non-business-hour contact numbers, before any such occurrence. After water damage, the immediate (within 24 to 48 hours) response should be to:

- Remove wet carpeting, ceiling tiles, dry wall, baseboard, or vinyl wall covering;
- Remove contents and furniture;
- Damp-wipe books and papers exposed to water with sanitizer;
- Damp-wipe smooth surfaces with sanitizer, such as diluted bleach; and
- Provide dehumidification to maintain relative humidity between 30 and 60%. Use dehumidifiers rather than fans, which can aerosolize any fungal spores to an even greater extent.

The type and extent of protective barriers remediation workers will need to wear during the clean-up will depend on whether the water is from rain, clean water lines, or sanitary sewerage lines.

PATIENT CARE ISSUES

Examination of the Patient

- Before physical examination of the patient, the healthcare provider should wash hands[27] or use alcohol-based hand rubs if hands are not visibly soiled. (Review Chapter 5 for additional details.) During a physical examination, Standard Precautions should be followed: Gloves should be worn for contact with mucous membranes or non-intact skin, and hands should be washed immediately after glove removal. Gloves must also be worn for vascular access and phlebotomy procedures[4] (see Chapter 4).
- Depending on symptoms, the patient should be assessed for risk of contagious disease, travel history, or occupational exposure. Clear procedures should be in place to report any suspected outbreaks or reportable diseases to the health department. Unusual and rare infections should also be reported (see Chapter 22).
- Depending on age, underlying illness, or occupation, immunization status should be assessed and immunizations advised when necessary.
- If the patient presents with an infection of a recent surgical site, the surgeon and infection control department where the surgery was performed should be notified and the site cultured for causative microorganism and antibiotic susceptibility. Reporting will assist in surgical site infection surveillance and control.
- If multidose vials (MDVs), such as local anesthetics, are used, the access diaphragm should be wiped with alcohol prior to puncture. A new sterile device should be used for any access to the medication vial. MDVs should be stored at the temperature recommended by the manufacturer. MDVs must be discarded by the manufacturer's expiration date or according to the policies of the institution.
- Medication should be drawn up into syringes immediately before use on individual patients and not batched. Syringes must be labeled with the contents. Medications and immunizations should be prepared in a designated clean area, away from the splash zone around the sink.

There are no published studies linking stethoscopes or other devices, such as otoscope handles or thermometer cassettes, to cross-infection in the ambulatory care setting. However, there is enough evidence to show that stethoscopes become contaminated in use.[28–30] Thus the American Medical Association passed a resolution recommending cleaning of stethoscopes and other handheld instruments, such as otoscopes, between each patient in all healthcare settings[31] or minimally on a "regular basis."[28–30] In a clinic setting, one study showed that 100% of stethoscopes (and 90% of otoscope handles) were contaminated by skin bacteria in a pediatric clinic and that alcohol swabs were effective in reducing bacterial counts.[30] Prepackaged alcohol wipes or pads were determined to be economical and convenient, as well as effective, to wipe these small areas.[28–30]

Infectious Patients

Triage

To prevent spread of airborne infections (e.g., chicken pox, measles, and TB) the clinic or office needs to develop a triage system to assist in recognizing these diseases and then in managing the patients. Information to consider includes:

- How patients make appointments with the clinic: phone calls versus urgent care walk-ins
- Initial encounter with the clinic: where, how, and who assesses the patient
- The most common types of airborne infection (e.g., chicken pox) in a pediatric practice
- Maintaining an up-to-date list of staff who are immune to childhood diseases, such as chicken pox, measles, mumps, and rubella
- The risk of seeing a patient with TB; for example, it is higher at clinics caring for the medically underserved, low-income populations, alcoholics, foreign-born, and intravenous drug abusers[32]
- Maintaining confidentiality of the patient's diagnosis

- Whether the practice sees patients where there is a likelihood of children accompanying the patient who might be contagious
- How the information will be communicated to facilitate immediate placement of the patient into isolation precautions

Using the previous criteria, a triage procedure should be developed that can be posted for use by admitting clerks, nurses, or other assigned staff who have initial patient contact. Staff with direct responsibility for administering the procedure should be involved in its development. The triage procedure:

- Should begin at the time the office visit is scheduled.[22] If possible, the office visit should be postponed.
- Should be simple enough to administer quickly and unobtrusively to patients.
- Should be posted for easy referral at both intake areas and by phones used to make the appointments.
- Should include key symptoms indicative of airborne infection (rather than diagnoses).
- Should include where to access information on noncontagious rashes (e.g., poison ivy).
- For an exclusively pediatric population, may include whether the patient (or any child accompanying the patient) has had exposure to chicken pox during the past three weeks.
- Should be reviewed periodically to ensure procedure is applied consistently and continues to contain relevant information.
- Should be reviewed with clerical intake staff on a regular basis.
- To aid clerical staff, it may be useful to have tissue available at the intake or check-out desks for patients who are coughing and sneezing.

Examples of triage procedure formats include flow sheets, scripts with questions to ask the patients (or their parents or guardians), or information directly on the patient intake form as part of the patient record (see examples in Appendix C).

After a patient is recognized to potentially have an airborne infection, the patient will need to be isolated promptly.[33] The patient should be admitted directly to an examination room through an alternate entrance, if available, and placed into Airborne Precautions (see Chapter 6).

Some general pediatric clinics maintain a separate waiting room for "infectious" cases. Although there has been spread of airborne disease (measles and TB) in ambulatory care settings[34], there has been no published information on the efficacy in preventing spread by this method.

Diseases that are spread by direct contact (including scabies, lice, impetigo, and diarrheal infections) pose less of a threat for cross-infection in the clinic setting. In most cases, using Standard Precautions and cleaning the environment will be effective in preventing spread.

Development of antibiotic-resistant bacteria poses another threat facing health care across the continuum. Vancomycin-resistant enterococci (VRE) have been shown to survive in the environment for an extended time.[35] In the hospital setting, there are recommendations from the Centers for Disease Control and Prevention (CDC) to prevent nosocomial spread.[36] In physician office and clinic settings, spread has not been shown to be an issue; short length of exposure times, lack of invasive procedures, and generally healthier status probably explain why transmission has not been observed. The first case of vancomycin-resistant *Staphylococcus aureus* (VRSA) was confirmed in 2002 in a dialysis patient with a complicated medical history and many healthcare encounters.[37] The consequences of spread of this microorganism are great; the CDC recommends that "in the health-care setting, a patient with VRSA should be placed in a private room and have dedicated patient-care items. Health-care workers providing care should wear gowns, masks, and gloves and use antibacterial soap for handwashing."[37]

Minor Surgery in Examination Rooms

This topic is covered in Chapter 8, including types of procedures, hand antisepsis, and patient preparation. Any equipment or medications should be prepared immediately before the procedure to avoid contamination of the sterile field.

Patient Education

Overall goals of patient education in infection prevention and control are to promote personal health and improve overall public health. As ambulatory care settings provide increasingly complex services, more patient education is needed.[38] Patients should be encouraged to ask health professionals questions about protecting themselves from infections.

There are many passive and interactive means of patient education for general and specific topics, including:

- Handwashing: reminder signs or posters placed in public rest rooms, phlebotomy stations, laboratories, examination, procedure, and soiled utility rooms
- Immunizations for children and adults: posters, brochures
- Influenza: posters, brochures
- Antibiotic resistance: brochures explaining judicious use of antimicrobials and for what conditions antibiotics are ineffective.[23, 39–40] A number of organizations publish handouts on this topic; the CDC has extensive information available online, both for the public and for healthcare providers.[41] Antibiotic resistance is increasingly a problem, so it is important to provide pertinent information to patients.
- Human immunodeficiency virus/Acquired immunodeficiency syndrome (HIV/AIDS), hepatitis, TB, *Burkholderia cepacia*, sexually transmitted diseases, urinary tract infections, Lyme disease and other infections depending on the demographics of the population served
- Food poisoning: brochures on safe food handling and storage
- Infection potential in popular travel destinations
- Prevention of infection in specific at-risk populations (e.g., diabetics, HIV/AIDS patients, asplenic individuals, and individuals with cystic fibrosis)
- Infection during pregnancy

For specific infections, it is important to assess the overall patient population to determine the most common infectious diseases so that educational resources can be acquired. When patients are diagnosed with an infectious disease or have a procedure that involves post-discharge care, printed information should be reviewed with the patient and phone numbers or Web site addresses provided for concerns that may arise after the patient has left. Many infectious diseases require work restrictions; information provided for healthcare professionals can often be applied to the general population (see Chapter 19).

Resources are published by various public health and private agencies. Web sites as well as printed and audiovisual material from the CDC and from local and state health departments have been reviewed for accuracy and readability. When consulted, infection control professionals can provide expertise in reviewing educational materials.

Resources for patient education include:

- CDC (*http://www.cdc.gov/health/*)
- State and local Departments of Health
- Infection control departments of hospitals or affiliated medical care facilities
- Food and Drug Administration (*http://www.fda.gov/oc/opacom/hottopics/anti_resist.html*)—for antibiotic resistance
- Food and Drug Administration (*http://www.nal.usda.gov/foodborne/index.html*)—for foodborne infections
- Association for Professionals in Infection Control and Epidemiology (*http://www.apic.org/cons/*)

References

1. JCAHO. *Standards for Ambulatory Care.* Oakbrook Terrace, IL: Joint Commission on Accreditation of Healthcare Organizations, 2000–2001.

2. Rhame, F. The inanimate environment. Bennett, J. V., and Brachman, P. S., eds. In: *Hospital Infections.* 4th Ed. Philadelphia, PA: Lippincott-Raven Publishers, 1998: 299–324.

3. Weber, D. J., and Rutala, W. Environmental issues and nosocomial infections. Wenzel, R. P., ed. In: *Prevention and Control of Nosocomial Infections.* 3rd Ed. Baltimore, MD: Williams & Wilkins, 1997: 491–514.

4. Occupational Exposure to Bloodborne Pathogens: Needlestick and Other Sharps Injuries: Final Rule. *Fed Reg.* 2001; 66:5317–5325.

http://www.osha-slc.gov/pls/oshaweb/owadisp.show_document?p_table=FEDERAL_REGISTER&p_id=16265.

5. Rutala, W. Disinfection, sterilization, and waste disposal. Wenzel, R. P., ed. In: *Prevention and Control of Nosocomial Infections.* 3rd Ed. Baltimore, MD: Williams & Wilkins, 1997: 539–593.

6. Chou, T. Environmental Services. In: *APIC Text of Infection Control and Epidemiology.* Washington, DC: Association for Professionals in Infection Control and Epidemiology, 2000: 73:1–8.

7. Fauerbach, L. L., and Janelle, J. W. Practical applications in infection control. Block, S. S., ed. In: *Sterilization, Disinfection and Preservation.* 5th Ed. Malvern, PA: Lea & Febiger, 2001: 935–944.

8. Anderson, R. L., Mackel, D. C., Stoler, B. S., and Mallison, G. F. Carpeting in hospitals: An epidemiological evaluation. *J Clin Microbiol.* 1982; 15:408–415.

9. Lumish, R. M. Carpeting in hospitals: An infection control problem? *JAMA.* 1989; 261:2422.

10. Bartley, J. Construction and Renovation. In: *APIC Text of Infection Control and Epidemiology.* Washington, DC: Association for Professionals in Infection Control and Epidemiology, 2000: 72:1–11.

11. AIA. Guidelines for Design and Construction of Hospital and Health Care Facilities. Washington, DC: The American Institute of Architects and the Facilities Guidelines Institute, 2001: 73, 103–127.

12. Pugliese, G., and Hubbard, C. A. Central services, linens and laundry. Bennett, J. V., and Brachman, P. S., eds. In: *Hospital Infections.* 4th Ed. Philadelphia, PA: Lippincott-Raven, 1998: 325–332.

13. McDonald, L. L., Linen Services. In: *APIC Text of Infection Control and Epidemiology.* Washington, DC: Association for Professionals in Infection Control and Epidemiology, 2000: 75:1–4.

14. U.S. Food and Drug Administration. Recalls / Withdrawals *http:// www.fda.gov/cber/recalls.htm;* U.S. Food and Drug Administration. Voluntary Recall of Hepatitis B Vaccine (Recombinant), Engerix-B 2/22/01. *http://www.fda.gov/cber/recalls/glahepb022201. htm.*

15. Krugman, R. D., Meyer, B. C., Enterline, J. C., Parkman, P. D., Witte, J. J., and Meyer, H. M. Impotency of live virus vaccines as a result of improper handling in clinical practice. *J Pediatr.* 1974; 85:512–514.

16. Miller, J. M., and Holmes, H. T. Specimen Collection, Transport and Storage. In: Murray, P. R., ed. *Manual of Clinical Microbiology.* 7th Ed. Washington, DC: ASM Press, 1999: 33–63.

17. Recommendations of the United States Public Health Service Food and Drug Administration. *Food Code.* Section 3-501.16. Springfield, VA: National Technical Information Service, 2001. *http://www.cfsan.fda. gov/~dms/fc01-3.html#3-5.*

18. Committee on Infectious Diseases. In: *2000 Red Book.* Elk Grove Village, IL: American Academy of Pediatrics, 2000: 9–16.

19. McKay, I., and Gillespie, T. A. Bacterial contamination of children's toys used in a general practitioner's surgery. *Scottish Med J.* 2000; 45:12–13.

20. Merriman, E., Corwin, P., and Ikram, R. Toys are a potential source of cross-infection in general practitioners' waiting rooms. *Brit J Gen Practice.* 2002; 52:138–140.

21. Committee on Infectious Diseases. In: *2000 Red Book.* Elk Grove Village, IL: American Academy of Pediatrics, 2000: 116–119.

22. McFarland, L., and Kelso, K. Y. Child Care. In: *APIC Text of Infection Control and Epidemiology.* Washington, DC: Association for Professionals in Infection Control and Epidemiology, 2000: 40–47.

23. Committee on Infectious Diseases and Committee on Practice and Ambulatory Medicine, American Academy of Pediatrics. Infection control in physicians' offices. *Pediatrics.* 2000; 1361–1369.

24. Neely, A. N., and Sittig, D. F. Basic microbiology and infection control information to reduce the potential transmission of pathogens to patients via computer hardware. *J Am Med Informatics Assoc.* 2002; 9:500–508.

25. Devine, J., Cooke, R. P. D., and Wright, E. P. Is methicillin-resistant *Staphylococcus aureus* (MRSA) contamination of ward-based computer terminals a surrogate marker for nosocomial MRSA transmission and handwashing compliance? *J Hosp Infect.* 2001; 48:72–75.

26. Bartley, J. APIC State of the art report: The role of infection control during construction in health care facilities. *Am J Infect Control.* 2000; 28:156–169.

27. Boyce, J. M., and Pittet, D. Recommendations of the Healthcare Infection Control Practices Advisory Committee. Guideline for hand hygiene in health-care settings. *MMWR.* 2002; 51(RR-16):1–45. *http://www.cdc. gov/mmwr/PDF/rr/rr5116.pdf.*

28. Smith, M., Mathewson, J. J., Ulert, I. A., Scerpella, E. G., and Ericsson, C. D. Contaminated stethoscopes revisited. *Arch Int Med.* 1996; 156:82–84.

29. Marinella, M., Pierson, C., and Chenoweth, C. The stethoscope: A potential source of nosocomial infection? *Arch Int Med.* 1997; 157:786–790.

30. Wurtz, R., and Weinstein, R. Microbiologic contamination and cleaning personal medical equipment. *JAMA.* 1998; 280:519–520.

31. Cohen, H. A., Amir, J., Matalon, A., Mayan, R., Beni, S., and Barzilai, A. Stethoscopes and otoscopes—a potential vector of infection? *Family Practice.* 1997; 14:446–449.

32. Division of Tuberculosis Elimination, Center for Prevention Services, Centers for Disease Control and Prevention. *National Tuberculosis Training Initiative Core Curriculum on Tuberculosis.* Washington, DC: U.S. Department of Health and Human Services, 1991: 7–8.

33. Committee on Infectious Diseases. In: *2000 Red Book.* Elk Grove Village, IL: American Academy of Pediatrics, 2000: 137.

34. Arias, K. M. Outbreaks Reported in the Ambulatory Care Setting. In: Arias, K. M., ed. *Quick Reference to Outbreak Investigation and Control in Health Care Facilities.* Gaithersburg, MD: Aspen Publishers, Inc., 2000: 105–118.

35. Noskin, G. A., Stosor, V., Cooper, I., and Peterson, L. R. Recovery of vancomycin-resistant enterococci on fingertips and environmental surfaces. *Infect Control Hosp Epidemiol.* 1995; 16:577–581.

36. Recommendations for preventing the spread of vancomycin resistance: Recommendations of the Hospital Infection Control Practices Advisory Committee (HICPAC). *Am J Infect Control.* 1995; 23:87–94.

37. *Staphylococcus aureus* resistant to vancomycin—United States, 2002. *MMWR.* 2002; 51:565–567.

38. Friedman, C., Barnette, M., Buck, A. S., Ham, R., Harris, J., and Hoffman, P., et al. Requirements for infrastructure and essential activities of infection control and epidemiology in out-of-hospital settings: A consensus panel report. *Am J Infect Control.* 1999; 27:418–430.

39. Gonzales, R., Bartlett, J. G., Besser, R. E., and Cooper, R. J. Principles of appropriate antibiotic use for treatment of acute respiratory tract infections in adults: Background, specific aims, and methods. *Ann Intern Med.* 2001; 134:479–486.

40. Gonzales, R., Steiner, J. G., Lum, A., and Barrett, P. H. Decreasing antibiotic use in ambulatory practice: Impact of a multidimensional intervention on the treatment of uncomplicated acute bronchitis in adults. *JAMA.* 1999; 281:1512–1519.

41. Centers for Disease Control and Prevention (CDC). Promoting appropriate antibiotic use in the community. *http://www.cdc.gov/drugresistance/community/.*

CHAPTER 8

Ambulatory Surgery

BACKGROUND

The first surgicenter was opened in 1970. The number of centers and the number of procedures routinely performed in an ambulatory setting have risen dramatically since then.[1] In 1996, 31.5 million ambulatory surgery procedures were performed in the United States.[2] The types of ambulatory surgery sites include laser surgery clinics, plastic surgery centers, surgicenters, physician offices, and oral surgery centers.

An increasing number of "not-so-minor" surgical procedures have shifted from inpatient to ambulatory care settings. Along with the provision of more intensive ambulatory surgery procedures has come an increase in the risk of health care-associated infections. Types of surgical procedures often performed in the ambulatory setting include ophthalmology procedures, excision of lesions or tissue, muscle/tendon procedures, reduction of fractures, cholecystectomy, and minor procedures in offices.[3]

Adverse infectious events following surgery (for example, surgical site infections (SSI), bacteremia, and pneumonia) result in increased morbidity and increased use of antibiotics. Various studies have been published outlining the risk of site infection associated with ambulatory surgery. These studies focused on various procedures and used different techniques to determine which patients developed SSIs. Infection rates from these studies are summarized in Table 8.1.

Most SSIs result from microbial contamination of the wound during surgery. The microorganisms typically come from endogenous sites, that is, within the patient. Exogenous contamination can result from the operating room environment or surgical personnel. Prevention techniques are aimed at both endogenous and exogenous microbes.

It is suggested that SSI rates for ambulatory procedures are lower than those conducted in hospitals because:[1]

1. Most procedures are either clean or clean-contaminated.[11] These procedures have the lowest risk of infection.
2. Exposure to multidrug-resistant microorganisms is reduced. Patients are not exposed to microbes of other patients as in hospitals.
3. Patients undergoing contaminated or dirty procedures as outpatients are generally at lower risk. Patients who have more risk factors are generally hospitalized.

Reports of outbreaks related to ambulatory surgery procedures are rare (see Table 8.2).

Staff members involved in ambulatory surgery procedures are also at risk for infection due to the potential for blood and body fluid contamination and injuries from sharp items. In one study[16] at least one person was contaminated with blood in half of the procedures. Cuts or needlestick injuries occurred in 15% of the operations. It was noted that longer operations and use of more needles in an operation lead to increased risk for staff.

There are various requirements for practices in ambulatory surgery centers. The Joint Commission on Accreditation of Healthcare Organizations has special standards for ambulatory surgery.[17] The standards focus on patient care, quality, and safety, and they

Table 8.1   Studies Evaluating Surgical Site Infection Risk after Ambulatory Surgery

Study	Population	Infection Rate*	Comments
Garvey, 1986[4]	Gynecology	0.9% (11 / 1,241)	Infections self-reported by surgeons
Flanders, 1990[5]	All patients	0.7% (15 / 2,060)	Infections self-reported by surgeons
Hugar, 1990[6]	Clean foot surgery	1.4% (2 / 495)	Healthy, compliant patients
Manian, 1990[7]	All patients	0.13% (14 / 10,952)	
Zoutman, 1990[8]	30% orthopedic procedures (half of them arthroscopy)	5.1% (26 / 515) Arthroscopy—6.5% (3 / 48) Laparoscopy—3.6% (5 / 136)	Patients questioned by phone
Audry, 1994[9]	Pediatric inguinal procedures	1% (18 / 1,816)	
Vilar-Compte, 2001[10]	All patients	2.8% (38 / 1,350)	

*Percentage (number of surgical site infections/number of procedures)

require monitoring, analyzing, and improving practice performance. These activities include data collection for infection prevention and control practices, patient outcomes, and adverse events. Medicare rules state that ambulatory surgery centers must establish a program for identifying and preventing infections, maintaining a sanitary environment, and reporting the results to appropriate authorities.[18] States may also have laws or regulations pertaining to office-based surgery.

The same aseptic surgical technique and environmental standards apply to all surgical settings as outlined next. Any differences in practice are slight and should only occur in minor procedures performed in physician or dental offices.

SURGICAL ASEPSIS

Hand Hygiene

A surgical scrub is intended to reduce the number of microbes on the surgical team's hands and reduce contamination of the operative site due to potential breaks in surgical gloves. The ideal duration of a surgical scrub is unknown. Studies have shown that two minutes are as effective as ten minutes—with less irritation.[19–21] Various antimicrobial agents (e.g., an iodophor, chlorhexidine, or parachlorometaxylenol product) may be used. Alcohol-based handrubs with persistent activity are also available. A nail cleaner should be used to clean under the nails.[22]

Table 8.2   Outbreaks of Infection Related to Ambulatory Surgery Procedures

Study	Type of Infection	Comments
Rutala, 1987[12]	Surgical site infection due to *Proteus mirabilis*	Due to contaminated bone drills
Hlday, 1993[13]	Hepatitis B virus	Failure to apply standard precautions and sterile surgical technique
Fridkin, 1996[14]	Endophthalmitis	Environmental source—water in the ventilation system
Weems, 1995[15]	Infections post prostate biopsy	Due to contaminated water

Staff should have clean, healthy nails. Artificial nails should not be worn.[23–24] Jewelry should be confined within scrub attire or removed.[22, 25] Individuals who have exudative lesions or weeping dermatitis should not care for patients directly and should not handle medical devices used for invasive procedures. See Chapter 5 for more information on hand hygiene.

Patient Preparation

- Do not remove hair preoperatively unless the hair at or around the incision site will interfere with the operation. If necessary, remove hair with clippers.[23, 26]
- Thoroughly wash and clean at and around the incision site to remove superficial debris before performing antiseptic skin preparation. Then use an appropriate antiseptic agent (e.g., iodophor [combined alcohol-iodophor solutions], or chlorhexidine) for skin preparation to reduce numbers of microbes on intact skin. Apply the agent per manufacturer's directions.
- Use moisture-impermeable drapes to prevent the patient's microorganisms from transferring to the wound.
- Use aseptic technique before inserting catheters.
- The issue of what type of attire patients should wear is controversial. However, 54% of respondents to a survey noted that patients are allowed to wear their own clothing for certain procedures, especially eye procedures.[27]

Surgical Attire

- All surgical personnel must wear suitable attire, such as scrub suits, hair covering, masks, and protective eyewear.[28] Scrub suits (pants and top) are worn to reduce microbial shedding. Fluid-resistant masks are preferable.
- Wear a sterile gown in procedures that require a sterile field.
- If staff perform procedures at more than one location during the day, any expectation about changing scrubs at each location needs to be addressed and a consistent policy adopted and enforced.[28] Change scrub suits that are visibly soiled, contam-

inated, and/or penetrated by blood or other body fluids.[23]
- Wear a surgical mask that fully covers the mouth and nose when entering the operating room if an operation is about to begin or already underway, or if sterile instruments are exposed. Wear the mask throughout the operation.[23] In 1991, a study[29] found no difference in numbers of surgical-site infections among patients undergoing operations by surgeons who did or did not wear masks. An important role today is to prevent contamination of mucous membranes of the surgical team.
- Wear a cap or hood to fully cover hair on the head and face when entering the operating room during a procedure.
- Scrubbed surgical team members must wear sterile gloves. Put on gloves after donning a sterile gown.
- Double gloving should be practiced if the operator has a break in skin integrity. Double gloving may also be helpful in reducing chances of a puncture.[30–31]
- Use surgical gowns that are effective barriers when wet, that is, materials that resist liquid penetration.
- Many operating suites allow parents of pediatric surgery patients to wear street clothes and cover gowns so that they can stay in the room until their child is anesthetized. These operating suites have not noted higher infection rates related to this practice.[32]
- Shoe covers are rarely required except as described under personal protective equipment.[23]
- Visitors may wear a cover (bunny) suit in place of a scrub suit.

Sterile Field

- Items within the sterile field must be sterile.
- Assemble sterile equipment and solutions immediately prior to use.[23]
- Dispense items and deliver instruments in a manner that will maintain sterility and integrity of the field.
- Unfold packs in a manner that allows the sterile inner surface of the pack to cover the surface of the table or stand. Otherwise a sterile sheet with a moisture barrier must be placed over the table.

- Move around the field in a manner that will maintain sterility.
- Maintain control of the sterile field.

Personal Protective Equipment

All procedures must be conducted as though there is a risk of infection, and Standard Precautions (see Chapter 6) must be used routinely with all patients. Staff must be trained in surgical asepsis,[28] general aseptic technique, and methods for preventing exposure to blood and body fluids.[33] Also see Chapter 4 for information on personal protective equipment.

Gloves must be used for all cases where there is potential for exposure to blood or body fluids. Remove gloves before touching uncovered equipment control panels or other items.

Masks, impervious or fluid-resistant gowns, eye/face protection, and protective caps are important for preventing exposure to the patient's blood that might splatter onto the operator during invasive procedures. Keep a resuscitation device in each examination and procedure room or crash cart.

When there is a reasonable risk of exposure to blood or body fluid during any procedure, additional protective clothing are recommended: shoes worn only for performing procedures, fluid-impermeable gowns, and shoe covers or gaiters to cover lower legs and feet. Any barrier that becomes saturated with blood must be removed and replaced as soon as patient safety permits. All personal protective items must be removed upon exiting the operating area.

Traffic Patterns and Control

- Limit those entering the operating room to necessary personnel.[23]
- Keep patients and supplies separated; allow only authorized staff in the operative area; segregate sterile, clean, and soiled areas.
- Keep doors closed during procedures, and limit unnecessary movement during a procedure.
- Maintain separation of clean and dirty areas.
- Generally, there are three designated areas in operating room suites: (1) unrestricted—e.g., staff change area, (2) semirestricted—e.g., clean areas, and (3) restricted—e.g., the operating room itself. The unrestricted, semirestricted, and restricted areas of the operating suite are not as clearly delineated in some new operating suites as they were in older suites. For example, in the past, operating rooms had higher air pressure than did other areas in the operating suite. In many modern suites the air pressure is higher in the sterile core than in the operating rooms and higher in the operating rooms than in the outer corridor. Thus when staff define the restricted and semi-restricted zones, they must consider the air pressure gradients.[32] Areas in ambulatory surgery facilities may not have a clear demarcation. Therefore, it is important to clearly outline areas and practices in written protocols.
- Family members may be allowed into the preoperative preparation and postoperative recovery areas.

Newer operating suites may have sterilizers with two doors, one through which the nonsterile items are placed into the machine and one through which the sterile items are removed into a sterile corridor. In an operating suite that has this design, healthcare workers may not need to wear masks when near the entry door of a sterilizer but must wear them when near the exit door of the sterilizer, which is in the sterile core.[32]

Equipment and Supplies

- There should be a protocol for transporting clean, sterile and soiled equipment and supplies to/from the operating room.
- Segregate clean and sterile supplies.
- See Chapter 7 for additional information on storage.

Medications and Multiple-Dose Vials (MDV)

- Use single-dose vials of parenteral additives or medications whenever possible.
- The access diaphragm of MDVs should be wiped with 70% alcohol prior to puncture.[34]
- Use a new sterile device for each access into the medication vial.[34]

ANTIMICROBIAL PROPHYLAXIS

Antibiotics may be provided to patients to decrease the potential for infection developing after certain procedures. Surgical antimicrobial prophylaxis refers to a very brief course of an antimicrobial agent initiated just before an operation begins. The antibiotic is administered so that a bactericidal concentration of the drug is established in serum and tissues when the incision is made. Therapeutic levels of the agent are maintained in serum and tissues throughout the operation and until, at most, a few hours after the incision is closed in the operating room.[23]

GENERAL REQUIREMENTS

Sharps

There must be procedures to safely handle contaminated sharp items and minimize percutaneous and skin or mucosal exposure.[35-36] These procedures may include:

- No recapping of needles.
- Conveniently located sharps disposal containers.
- Evaluate and use, as appropriate, devices to prevent exposures, such as blunt suture needles, disposable safety scalpels, closed flush systems, self-sheathing needles, and needle-holding devices.[37]
- Use a container to hold reusable sharp instruments.
- Use a device to hold needles that might be reused during a procedure.
- When needles must be removed from syringes or exchanged, use a clamp, forceps, or other mechanical device.
- Use a no-touch method to pass sharp instruments between individuals by placing instruments on the table and avoiding hand-to-hand transfer.

Instruments

There must be policies and procedures for instruments that describe cleaning and decontamination practices, preparation and assembly of items, loading and unloading methods for sterilizers, matching the container system and the sterilization cycle, transportation practices for the containers to maintain sterility, and quality assurance programs. For more specific information on reprocessing, see Chapter 3.

- Remove all debris from instruments as soon as possible. Instruments can be placed in a basin of water and detergent upon removal from the operating area to prevent drying of organic matter.

Scrub instruments or use an ultrasonic cleaner to remove organic debris.
- Sterilize all surgical instruments according to published guidelines.[23, 38-43]
- Steam sterilization is recommended for heat and moisture-stable items. Wrapped or containerized items should be sterilized for a full steam cycle followed by a drying cycle.[44-46]
- Sterilization of instruments for immediate use is known as flash sterilization. Perform flash sterilization only for patient-care items that will be used immediately, such as to reprocess an inadvertently dropped instrument. Do not use flash sterilization for reasons of convenience, as an alternative to purchasing additional instrument sets, or to save time. Items to be flash sterilized should be unwrapped or placed in containers or wrappers designed specifically for flash sterilization.[23, 45]
- Staff must be trained in use and monitoring of autoclaves (see Chapter 3).
- Store instruments properly to avoid accidental contamination.
- Any reprocessed single-use device must meet the requirements of the Food and Drug Administration (FDA).[47] The FDA rules apply specifically to hospitals and third-party reprocessing companies and not to ambulatory care. However, due to legal ramifications and risks, reprocessing of these devices is not recommended in the ambulatory care setting (see Chapter 3).

Lasers

Airborne contaminants may be a concern when using lasers.[48] There should be policies outlining ventilation requirements and use of respiratory and eye protection by staff. Airborne contaminants should be captured as close as practical to the point of evolution and then vented outdoors. This task can be accomplished by localized exhaust ventilation or by portable smoke extractors with charcoal and/or high-efficiency particulate air-type filters.[32]

The generation of airborne particulate matter and blood spray during laser procedures requires that each staff member working in or near the target area wear face protection. Usual surgical masks filter 5 μm particles with 99% efficiency. However, particles in a laser plume may be as small as 0.3 μm. Masks are available that can filter 0.3 μm particles with an efficiency of 99%; however, they make breathing more difficult.[49] There are masks available specifically for laser procedures. Eye protection should also be worn.

Waste

Follow state regulations for the disposal of medical or biohazard waste.

ENVIRONMENTAL CONTROLS

Cleaning

- When visible soiling or contamination with blood or other body fluids of surfaces or equipment occurs during an operation, use a disinfectant cleaner to clean the affected areas before the next operation.
- Wet vacuum the operating room floor after the last operation of the day or night with an Environmental Protection Agency-registered disinfectant.[23] If a wet vacuum is not available, use a clean mop head and cleaning solution.[25]
- Clean and disinfect surgical lights, floors, equipment, and horizontal surfaces in the operating room on a daily basis.[50]
- Clean patient transport vehicles, including straps, after each case.

Ventilation

- Maintain positive-pressure ventilation in the operating room with respect to the corridors and adjacent areas.[23]
- Maintain a minimum of 15 air changes per hour, of which at least three should be fresh air.[23]
- Filter all air, recirculated and fresh, through appropriate filters per the American Institute of Architects' recommendations.[23, 51]
- Introduce all air at the ceiling and exhaust near the floor.

SURVEILLANCE

It is important to collect data on infections in order to evaluate any change in infection trends. This activity may be difficult because ambulatory surgery facilities may not provide aftercare treatment of patients. Thus, a system for follow-up needs to be designed.

- Develop a process for case finding. One method to assist in this process is to include signs and symptoms of infection in aftercare instructions for patients. Emphasize infection prevention techniques and provide contact information if problems arise. If contacted, the surgery center can then keep track of patients who might have a SSI.
- For each patient undergoing an operation chosen for surveillance, record those variables shown to be associated with increased SSI risk (e.g., surgical wound class, American Society of Anesthesiologists' classification, and duration of operation).[23]
- Report surgical site infection information to the surgical team members on a routine basis, e.g., quarterly.[23]
- See Chapter 20 for additional information on surveillance.

COMMUNICABLE DISEASES IN PATIENTS

Provisions should be made for the use of isolation precautions or for transfer, when indicated, of patients known or suspected of having communicable diseases.[28] Patients should be screened prior to the procedure for any potential exposure to or presence of communicable diseases.

Antibiotic-Resistant Microbes

There are no specific practices required for controlling the spread of these microbes in the operating suite because appropriate garb and environmental cleaning is already part of routine protocol. When caring for patients with a resistant microorganism, preoperative and postoperative areas should follow the precautions outlined in Chapter 6.

Tuberculosis

Elective operative procedures on patients who have tuberculosis (TB) should be delayed until the patient is no longer infectious. TB precautions in the ambulatory-care setting should include placing these patients in a separate area apart from other patients, and not in open waiting areas (ideally, in a room or enclosure meeting Airborne Precautions requirements); giving the patients surgical masks to wear and instructing them to keep their masks on; and giving them tissues and instructing them to cover their mouths and noses with the tissues when coughing or sneezing.[52]

- If operative procedures must be performed, they should be managed, if possible, in operating rooms that have anterooms. For operating rooms without anterooms, the doors to the operating room should be closed, and traffic into and out of the room should be minimal to reduce the frequency of opening and closing the door. Attempts should be made to perform the procedure when other patients are not present in the operative suite and when a minimum number of personnel are present, for example, at the end of day.
- Placing a bacterial filter on the patient's endotracheal tube (or at the expiratory side of the breathing circuit of a ventilator or anesthesia machine if these are used) when operating on a patient who has confirmed or suspected TB may help reduce the risk for contaminating anesthesia equipment or discharging tubercle bacilli into the air.
- During postoperative recovery the patient should be monitored and should be placed in a private room that meets recommended standards for ventilating TB isolation rooms.
- When operative procedures are performed on patients who may have infectious TB, respiratory protection worn by the staff must protect the field

from the respiratory secretions of the healthcare workers and protect the staff from the infectious droplet nuclei generated by the patient. A suitable mask is a N95 mask.

MINOR OFFICE PROCEDURES

It is important to outline which procedures can be performed in examination or treatment rooms. There may be state requirements outlining which procedures are authorized to be performed in office settings.

General areas of consideration include:[53]

- One room should be reserved specifically for procedures involving incisional surgery.
- The room must be easy to clean.
- Masks are unnecessary for brief, minor procedures. However, for long procedures with open defects (e.g., Mohs surgery), masks must be worn.
- Masks, goggles or face shields, and surgical gowns are always required if there is a potential for splattering of blood or body fluids.

Alterations in practice from that of a surgical suite:[54]

- No hat is required. Protect clothing with a disposable plastic apron or gown.
- There is no need to formally scrub; wash with chlorhexidine or povidone iodine soap preparations or alcohol-based products. Dry with paper towels.
- Special drapes are unnecessary. The sterile paper towels included in dressing packs are adequate.
- Patients may not need to change out of street clothes.

References

1. Nafzinger, D. A., Lundstrom, T., Chandra, S., and Massanari, R. M. Infection control in ambulatory care. *Infect Dis Clin North Am.* 1997; 11:279–296.
2. National Center for Health Statistics, *http://www.cdc.gov/nchs/fastats/outsurg.htm.*
3. *Ambulatory and Inpatient Procedures in the United States, 1996.* Washington, DC: National Center for Health Statistics, DHHS Publication No. (PHS) 99-1710, 1998.
4. Garvey, J. M., Buffenmyer, C., Rycheck, R. R., Yee, R., McVay, J., and Harger, J. H. Surveillance for postoperative infections in outpatient gynecologic surgery. *Infect Control.* 1986; 7:54–58.

5. Flanders, E., and Hinnant, J. R. Ambulatory surgery postoperative wound surveillance. *Am J Infect Control.* 1990; 18:336–339.
6. Hugar, D. W., Newman, P. S., Hugar, R. W., Spencer, R. B., and Salvino, K. Incidence of postoperative infection in free-standing ambulatory surgery center. *J Foot Surg.* 1990; 29:265–267.
7. Manian, F. A., and Meyer, L. Comprehensive surveillance of surgical wound infections in outpatient and inpatient surgery. *Infect Control Hosp Epidemiol.* 1990; 11:515–520.
8. Zoutman, D., Pearce, P., McKenzie, M., and Taylor, G. Surgical wound infections occurring in day surgery patients. *Am J Infect Control.* 1990; 18:277–282.

9. Audry, G., Johanet, S., Achrafi, H., Lupold, M., and Gruner, M. The risk of wound infection after inguinal incision in pediatric outpatient surgery. *Europ J Ped Surg.* 1994; 4:87–89.

10. Vilar-Compte, D., Roldan, R., Sandoval, S., Corominas, R., De-LaRosa, M., and Gordillo, P., et al. Surgical site infections in ambulatory surgery: A 5-year experience. *Am J Infect Control.* 2001; 29:99–103.

11. Altemeier, W. A., Burke, J. F., Pruitt, B. A., and Sandusky, W. R. *Manual on Control of Infection in Surgical Patients.* 2nd Ed. Philadelphia: J.B. Lippincott Co., 1984: 28.

12. Rutala, W. A., Weber, D. J., and Thomann, C. A. Outbreak of wound infections following outpatient podiatric surgery due to contaminated bone drills. *Foot Ankle.* 1987; 7:350–354.

13. Hlday, W. G., Hopkins, R. S., Ogilby, T. E., and Allen, S. T. Patient-to-patient transmission of hepatitis B in a dermatology practice. *Am J Public Health.* 1993; 83:1689–1693.

14. Fridkin, S. K., Kremer, F. B., Bland, L. A., Padhye, A., McNeil, M. M., and Jarvis, W. R. *Acremonium kiliense* endophthalmitis that occurred after cataract extraction in an ambulatory surgical center and was traced to an environmental reservoir. *Clin Infect Dis.* 1996; 22:222–227.

15. Weems, J. J., Jr. Usry, G., and Schwab, U. Infection due to rapidly-growing mycobacteria associated with ultrasound directed prostate biopsy. *Infect Control Hosp Epidemiol.* 1996; 17(S):P50. Abstract M67.

16. Quebbeman, E. J., Telford, G. L., Hubbard, S., Wadsworth, K., Hardman, B., and Goodman, H., et al. Risk of blood contamination and injury to operating room personnel. *Ann Surg.* 1991; 214:614–620.

17. *Accreditation Manual for Office-Based Surgery Practices.* Oakbrook, IL: Joint Commission on Accreditation of Healthcare Organizations, 2001.

18. *Code of Federal Regulations* [Title 42, Volume 2] [PART 416—Ambulatory Surgical Services] [Revised as of October 1, 2001]. From the U.S. Government Printing Office via GPO Access. *http://www.access.gpo. gov/nara/cfr/waisidx_01/42cfr416_01.html.*

19. Hingst, V., Juditzki, I., Heeg, P., and Sonntag, H. G. Evaluation of the efficacy of surgical hand disinfection following a reduced application time of 3 instead of 5 minutes. *J Hosp Infect.* 1992; 20:79–86.

20. Wheelock, S. M., and Lookinland, S. Effect of surgical hand scrub time on subsequent bacterial growth. *AORN J.* 1997; 65:1087–92, 1094–1098.

21. Deshmukh, N., Kramer, J. W., and Kjellberg, S. I. A comparison of 5-minute povidone-iodine scrub and 1-minute povidone-iodine scrub followed by alcohol foam. *Mil Med.* 1998; 163:145–147.

22. Centers for Disease Control and Prevention. Guideline for Hand Hygiene in Health-Care Settings: Recommendations of the Healthcare Infection Control Practices Advisory Committee and the HICPAC/SHEA/APIC/IDSA Hand Hygiene Task Force. *MMWR.* 2002; 51 (No. RR-16):1–44.

23. Mangram, A. J., Horan, T. C., Pearson, M. L., Silver, L. C., and Jarvis, W. R. Guideline for Prevention of Surgical Site Infection, 1999. Centers for Disease Control and Prevention (CDC) Hospital Infection Control Practices Advisory Committee. *Am J Infect Control.* 1999; 27(2):97–132.

24. AORN: Recommended practices for surgical hand scrubs. In: *2002 Standards, Recommended Practices, and Guidelines.* Denver: Association of Perioperative Registered Nurses, Inc., 2002: 237–242.

25. Allen-Bridson, K., and Olmsted, R. N. Surgical Services. In: *APIC Text of Infection Control and Epidemiology.* Washington, DC: Association for Professionals in Infection Control and Epidemiology, 2000: 53:1–11.

26. Sebben, J. E. Sterile technique and the prevention of wound infection in office surgery—Part II. *J Dermatol Surg Oncol.* 1989; 15:38–48.

27. Hoffman, K. K., Clontz, E. P., Rutala, W. A., and Weber, D. J. Patient attire in ambulatory surgery. *Am J Infect Control.* 2001; 29:345–346.

28. *ACS Guidelines for Optimal Ambulatory Surgical Care and Office-based Surgery.* 3rd Ed. Chicago, IL: American College of Surgeons, 2000.

29. Tunevall, T. G. Postoperative wound infections and surgical face masks: A controlled study. *World J Surg.* 1991; 15:383–387.

30. Laine, T., and Aarnio, P. How often does glove perforation occur in surgery? Comparison between single gloves and a double-gloving system. *Am J Surg.* 2001; 181:564–566.

31. Thomas, S., Agarwal, M., and Mehta, G. Intraoperative glove perforation—single *versus* double gloving in protection against skin contamination. *Postgrad Med J.* 2001; 77:458–460.

32. Lane, T. W., Herwaldt, L. A., Pottinger, J. M., Perl, T. M., and Steelman, V. M. Infection Control Guidelines for the Operating Suite. In: Abrutyn, E., Goldmann, D. A., Scheckler, W. E., ed. *Saunders Infection Control Reference Service.* 2nd Ed. Philadelphia: W.B. Saunders Co., 2001: 675–704.

33. Occupational exposure to bloodborne pathogens: Final rule. *Fed Reg.* 1991; 56 (Dec. 6):64175–64182.

34. Centers for Disease Control and Prevention. Guidelines for the Prevention of Intravascular Catheter-Related Infections. *MMWR.* 2002; 51(No. RR-10):1–32.

35. Gerberding, J. L. Procedure-specific infection control for preventing intraoperative blood exposures. *Am J Infect Control.* 1993; 21:364–367.

36. AORN: Standard and Transmission-Based Precautions. In: *2002 Standards, Recommended Practices, and Guidelines.* Denver: Association of Perioperative Registered Nurses, Inc., 2002: 321–326.

37. Occupational Exposure to Bloodborne Pathogens; Needlestick and Other Sharps Injuries; Final Rule. *Fed Reg.* 2001; 66:5317–5325.

38. ANSI/AAMI: Guidelines for the selection and use of reusable rigid container systems for ethylene oxide sterilization and steam sterilization in heath care facilities. *AAMI Standards and Recommended Practices.* Vol. 1: Sterilization. ST33. Arlington, VA: Association for the Advancement of Medical Instrumentation. Steam Sterilization Hospital Practices Working Group of the Thermal Sterilization Subcommittee, AAMI Sterilization Standards Committee, 1996.

39. ANSI/AAMI: Biological Indicators for Moist Heat Sterilization. ST19. *AAMI Standards and Recommended Practices.* Arlington, VA: Association for the Advancement of Medical Instrumentation. AAMI Sterilization Standards Committee, 1999.

40. ANSI/ AAMI: Steam sterilization and sterility assurance using table-top sterilizers in office-based, ambulatory-care, medical, surgical, and dental facilities. ST42. *AAMI Standards and Recommended Practices.* Arlington, VA: Association for the Advancement of Medical Instrumentation. AAMI Sterilization Standards Committee, 1998.

41. AAMI: Chemical indicators—Guidance for the selection, use, and interpretation of results. TIR25. *AAMI Standards and Recommended Practices.* Arlington, VA: Association for the Advancement of Medical Instrumentation. AAMI Sterilization Standards Committee, 1999.

42. ANSI/AAMI: Table-Top Dry Heat (Heated Air) Sterilization and Sterility Assurance in Dental and Medical Facilities. ST40. *AAMI Standards and Recommended Practices.* Arlington, VA: Association for the Advancement of Medical Instrumentation. AAMI Sterilization Standards Committee, 1992/(R) 1998.

43. ANSI/AAMI: Safe Handling and Biological Decontamination of Medical Devices in Health Care Facilities and in Non-Clinical Settings. ST35. *AAMI Standards and Recommended Practices.* Arlington, VA: Association for the Advancement of Medical Instrumentation. AAMI Sterilization Standards Committee, 1996.

44. AORN: Recommended practices for Sterilization in the Practice Setting. In: *2001 Standards, Recommended Practices, and Guidelines.* Denver: Association of Perioperative Registered Nurses, Inc., 2001: 309–318.

45. ANSI/AAMI: Flash Sterilization: Steam Sterilization of Patient Care Items for Immediate Use. ST37. *AAMI Standards and Recommended Practices.* Arlington, VA: Association for the Advancement of Medical Instrumentation. Steam Sterilization Hospital Practices Working Group, AAMI Sterilization Standards Committee, 1996.

46. ANSI/AAMI: Steam Sterilization and Sterility Assurance. ST46. *AAMI Standards and Recommended Practices.* Arlington, VA: Association for the Advancement of Medical Instrumentation, 2002.

47. Food and Drug Administration. Center for Devices and Radiological Health. Reuse of Single Use Devices. *http://www.fda.gov/cdrh/reuse/singleuse.pdf.*

48. McKinley, I. B., and Ludlow, M. O. Hazards of laser smoke during endodontic therapy. *J Endodontics.* 1994; 20:558–559.

49. ANSI: *American National Standard for the Safe Use of Lasers in Health Care Facilities.* Z136.3. New York: American National Standards Institute, Inc., 1996.

50. AORN: Recommended practices for environmental cleaning in the surgical practice setting. In: *2001 Standards, Recommended Practices, and Guidelines.* Denver: Association of Perioperative Registered Nurses, Inc., 2001: 221–226.

51. AIA. *Guidelines for Design and Construction of Hospital and Health Care Facilities.* Washington, DC: The American Institute of Architects and the Facilities Guidelines Institute, 2001.

52. Centers for Disease Control and Prevention: Guidelines for preventing the transmission of *Mycobacterium tuberculosis* in health-care facilities. *MMWR.* 1994; 43(RR-13):i–v, 1–132.

53. Sebben, J. E. Sterile technique and the prevention of wound infection in office surgery—Part I. *J Dermatol Surg Oncol.* 1988; 14:1364–1370.

54. Sodera, V. K. *Minor Surgery in Practice.* Cambridge, England: Cambridge University Press, 1994: 41–52.

CHAPTER 9

Endoscopy

BACKGROUND

Flexible endoscopic procedures are increasingly common. Over 10 million gastrointestinal endoscopies are performed each year[1] and almost 500,000 bronchoscopies were performed in 1996.[2] Endoscopes are also used to perform surgery (laparoscopy, arthroscopy) for examination of nasal passages and sinuses, and in urologic procedures.

Although endoscopy poses minimal risk for infection, the Technology Assessment Committee of the American Society for Gastrointestinal Endoscopy identified 28 reported cases of endoscopy-related transmission of infections between 1988 and 1992.[3] Most endoscopy-related infections have been attributed to insufficient reprocessing of the endoscopes, as summarized in Table 9.1. Other microorganisms associated with inadequate gastrointestinal endoscope reprocessing include *Helicobacter pylori* and hepatitis B virus.[4]

Insufficient practices have included inadequate cleaning, improper selection of cleaning and disinfecting agents, failure to follow details of cleaning and disinfection guidelines, and failure to follow automatic endoscopic reprocessor (AER) manufacturer's recommendations for disinfection and maintenance. Endoscopy accessories have also been linked with infection, such as arthroscopy cannulae,[13] biopsy forceps,[14] and devices used to apply lidocaine to the pharynx and nasal passages.[15] Recalls have increased public awareness and concern; specifically, a large multi-state outbreak of *Pseudomonas aeruginosa* in 2001 was attributed to a bronchoscope defect and delay in recall by the manufacturer.[16]

In addition, there are numerous reports of post-endoscopy mucous membrane damage (i.e., colitis) attributed to inadequate final rinsing of disinfectant, specifically glutaraldehyde.[17–20]

Endoscopes by their design are inherently heat-sensitive, structurally complex, fragile, and easily damaged. However, to prevent infection only designated high-level disinfectants or liquid sterilants must be used to ensure effective microbial killing. Glutaraldehyde (2%), despite safety concerns, remains the most commonly used high-level disinfectant, has a proven cost-efficacy, and is approved for use by the manufacturers of all brands of endoscopes. Other disinfectants[21–22] shown to be safe and effective for certain applications include hydrogen peroxide (7.5%), peracetic acid (≤1%), hydrogen peroxide/peracetic acid (1%/0.08%), and orthophthalaldehyde (0.55%). These products must be used according to the labels for soak time, and endoscope manufacturers must be contacted to make sure the product has been approved for use on their endoscopes. Periodically, new disinfectants are marketed; each new product must be tested for safety, efficacy, and nondamage to endoscopes before it can be endorsed.

AERs are increasingly popular in endoscopy units, while manual reprocessing is mostly performed in low-volume physician offices or small clinics. A 1993 study[23] compared manual and automated disinfection. Although there was not a significant difference between the two methods, there were more water bacteria isolated from the AER-disinfected endoscopes. Since then, AERs have undergone numerous improvements; however, the quality of the rinse water in AERs contin-

Table 9.1   Examples of Infections Related to Contamination of Endoscopes

Year Reported	Endoscope Type	Number of patients	Microorganisms	Factors
2001 and 1999	Bronchoscope[5, 6]	18	*Pseudomonas aeruginosa*	Improper connection of endoscope to AER*
2000	Bronchoscope[7]	8	*Pseudomonas aeruginosa*	Improper maintenance of AER; improper storage of bronchoscopes
1999	Bronchoscope[6]	5	*Mycobacterium tuberculosis*	Improper connection of endoscope to AER
1997	Colonoscope[8]	2	Hepatitis C	Inadequate soak time in disinfectant; biopsy channel not mechanically cleaned; biopsy forceps not sterilized
1997	Bronchoscope[9]	2	*Mycobacterium tuberculosis*	Enzymatic cleaner not used; bronchoscope partially immersed; biopsy forceps not always sterilized
1997	Bronchoscope[10]	3	*Mycobacterium tuberculosis*	Inadequate cleaning; only endoscope tips submerged in disinfectant; efficacy of disinfectant and leak testing not performed; alcohol not used for final rinse; endoscope stored coiled
1994	Arthroscope[11]	5	*Staphylococcus aureus*, Coagulase-negative staphylococci	Inadequate soak time in disinfectant; arthroscope sterilized only at end of day
1993	Endoscopic retrograde cholangiopancreatogrphy (ERCP)[12]	53 (3.6% of patients undergoing ERCP)	Post-ERCP bacteremia *Pseudomonas aeruginosa*, *Enterobacteriaceae*	Cleaning and disinfection of blind channel omitted by AER; AER contaminated with bacteria

*AER: Automated endoscope reprocessor

ues to be an important and controversial issue. There are many descriptions of pseudo-outbreaks (where bronchial washing or lavage cultures were contaminated but no illness resulted) of water bacteria such as nontuberculous mycobacteria[6, 24–30] and pseudomonads[29] related to bronchoscopy reprocessing in AERs. With increased culturing of the water, pipes and tubing, manifolds, reservoirs, and other pieces of the AERs, water microorganisms are increasingly recovered; this is related to biofilm build-up and the inability to thoroughly clean the insides of many machines.[31] Although microorganisms can be recovered from the AERs and pseudo-outbreaks have been directly related to AERs, few cases of true infection have been reported.

Water quality poses the biggest issue for bronchoscopes, especially as more at-risk patients undergo bronchoscopy—patients with lung transplants, bone marrow transplants, human immunodeficiency virus/acquired immunodeficiency syndrome, and those receiving other immunosuppressive treatments. Questions about either the necessity or ability to supply "sterile" or "bacteria-free" water remain unanswered at this time. Regardless of the water source, the importance of a final alcohol rinse of the internal channels has been established; a 70% alcohol rinse followed by forced air to dry the endoscope before storage is well documented as a means to prevent infection caused by contaminated rinse water.[32]

Endoscopy staff are at risk of exposure to body fluids, especially by splashing, during procedures. This risk is estimated to occur in over 13% of procedures.[33] During reprocessing of endoscopes, staff are at risk of respiratory tract or skin irritation from exposure to disinfectants, especially to glutaraldehyde, the most widely used chemical for disinfecting endoscopes.[34]

Flexible endoscopes with lumens are particularly difficult to reprocess. The following issues need to be addressed by dedicated endoscopy units as well as by physician offices or clinics that perform occasional endoscopies:

- Reprocessing procedures, including accessories
- If AERs are used, maintenance of water quality
- Storage
- Protection from exposure to disinfectant
- Standard Precautions and use of personal protective equipment by staff
- Protection from exposure to tuberculosis (TB) if bronchoscopy is performed
- Education and competency
- Quality assurance and improvement program

REPROCESSING PROCEDURES

Sufficient and consistent reprocessing of endoscopes is essential to prevent infection. Endoscopes must be reprocessed in the same manner for each patient, regardless of the diagnosis of the patient. The endoscope manufacturer should provide written, detailed instructions and hands-on training for each type of endoscope purchased and when new equipment is introduced. All staff responsible for the reprocessing must be included in the training sessions. Staff should be oriented and be able to demonstrate competency on a periodic basis (refer to sample competency in Appendix F). Ideally, written instructions, preferably illustrated, should be posted in the endoscope reprocessing area. These instructions are available from major endoscope manufacturers.

The following steps must be included in the protocol for manual reprocessing:

- Flush channels with water or enzymatic detergent solution immediately after each procedure to prevent drying of organic material.
- Leak test after the initial flushing according to manufacturer's specifications. If the test indicates a leak, avoid exposure to cleaning brushes and disinfectant to prevent further damage. If the endoscope needs to be returned for repair before completing the disinfection cycle, it should be labeled as biohazardous according to the Occupational Safety and Health Administration's Bloodborne Pathogen Standards (see Chapter 22).
- Remove, clean, and high-level disinfect all caps and valves. Store these separately from the endoscope in a clean, dry location until use to prevent water from trapping between the cap and the channel.
- Immerse endoscope into enzymatic detergent solution and manually clean each internal channel with cleaning brushes and enzymatic detergent, whether or not it was used during the procedure. Continue brushing until all visible debris is removed. Manual cleaning must precede use of an AER and has been demonstrated to reduce bacterial counts by an average of 10^4. The maximum contamination of endoscopes has been reported at 10^8; therefore, cleaning will significantly reduce the amount of bioburden.[35]
- Thoroughly rinse in at least 500 ml[36] of fresh water to remove the detergent. Purge with air to remove the water and wipe the exterior surfaces to prevent dilution of the disinfectant.
- Choose a disinfectant specified by the endoscope manufacturer as compatible with the endoscope. If glutaraldehyde is used it should contain no surfactant; surfactant can cause air bubbles that prevent the solution from completely contacting the entire surface of the endoscope. Monitor to ensure the minimal effective concentration of disinfectant solution is reused (see Chapter 3 for details).
- Completely immerse the endoscope in the disinfectant and ensure that disinfectant is inside each channel, whether or not it was used during the procedure. Pay particular attention to the lumens of the endoscopic retrograde cholangiopancreatography (ERCP) endoscopes; these lumens are very narrow and difficult to access. Non-immersible endoscopes should be phased out of use because they are more difficult to clean.[1]

- Appropriately time the soak in the disinfectant (e.g., at least 20 minutes for 2% alkaline glutaraldehyde).[35]
- Thoroughly rinse each channel with at least 500 ml[36] of fresh tap, filtered, or sterile water to completely remove all traces of disinfectant. If basins are used, the water must be fresh for each endoscope processed. Air purge the water from the lumens.
- Flush all lumens with alcohol (e.g., 70% isopropyl alcohol) followed by forced air to completely dry each channel and prevent overgrowth of water microorganisms. Flush each channel with enough alcohol so that it can be seen exiting the opposite end of the channel in a steady stream. A syringe of 30 to 60 ml may be needed to ensure that the alcohol contacts the entire interior surface of each channel. Alcohol should be used even when sterile or filtered water is used for rinsing.[1] Store alcohol in covered containers to prevent evaporation.
- Store the endoscope hanging vertically in a well-protected area to allow complete drying and to prevent damage or contamination. The endoscope should not be stored in its case because cleanliness cannot be ensured, and there is no air circulation to assist in drying.

If endoscopes are removed from the endoscopy unit for use at other institutions or on inpatient units, there must be a method to ensure that they are reprocessed before being returned for use in the endoscopy unit. Recent concerns about contamination of endoscope cases prompted reminder recommendations that endoscopes not be stored in their cases.[37] Endoscope case interiors cannot be cleaned or disinfected adequately. For transport, small endoscopes should be placed in a closed container, such as a hard plastic, tackle-type box. Upon return to the endoscopy unit, the box can be cleaned with a disinfectant cleaner. If endoscopes are sent for repair in the carrying case, they must be high-level disinfected upon return, before use on a patient.

Accessories such as reusable biopsy forceps must be cleaned with enzymatic detergent in an ultrasonic cleaner and then wrapped and sterilized by steam or gas according to the manufacturer's instructions. Any device that cuts into or incises tissue must be cleaned and sterilized after each use. Reprocessing of labeled single-use devices (SUD) should only be undertaken in strict accordance with Food and Drug Administration regulations. For further discussion, see Chapter 3. The

Society for Gastroenterology Nurses and Associates (SGNA) recommends that cleaning brushes also be soaked in disinfectant and rinsed after each use.[1]

Supplies used pre-procedure for delivery of airway anesthetic should be assessed to make sure there will be no cross-contamination during use. A new tube or nozzle on spray containers should be used for each patient. To avoid inadvertent reuse, it is suggested that the spray nozzle be removed and discarded immediately after each use. If local anesthetic is supplied in multi-dose tubes it should be dispensed individually for each patient, such as on clean gauze, to avoid touch contamination of the tube contents. Irrigation fluid should be sterile regardless of the type of endoscopy; large containers of sterile fluid may be used for a maximum of 24 hours. The container should be dated and timed when opened or discarded at the end of the day.

Suction canisters can be disposed of at regular intervals or when full; the canisters may need to be discarded as regulated medical waste depending on state regulations. Reusable suction units should be emptied using appropriate barriers according to Standard Precautions, and then cleaned and high-level disinfected. Tubing from the patient to the suction unit should be changed for each patient.

Ideally, endoscopes that penetrate sterile tissue, such as arthroscopes, should be sterilized after each patient. Adequate numbers of endoscopes must be purchased to allow for the lengthy ethylene oxide gas sterilization cycle. If sterilization is not feasible, high-level disinfection with a sterile water rinse is required.[38]

Automatic endoscope reprocessors (AER) are very expensive to purchase and maintain. Except for high-volume endoscopy units, they may not be cost-effective. At the present time, manual cleaning of each channel must be performed prior to machine disinfection, somewhat reducing expected time savings. Many AERs require special water filtration systems. Before purchasing an AER, a thorough cost-benefit analysis should be undertaken in conjunction with the infection prevention and control staff.

- It is essential to include installation of the required water filtration system and maintenance of the system in terms of filter costs and personnel time.
- The final filter should eliminate bacteria (i.e., 0.1 or 0.2 micron).

- Upstream water treatment must be considered, based on the local quality of water (i.e., size and quantity of particulate matter, such as mineral content). Water should be analyzed before installation of the filter system to make sure that the particulate filters (from 5 to 20 microns) installed above the final filter will work.
- Routine maintenance of the filtration system is essential; filter housing and tubing from the final filter to the entrance to the machine must be removed, cleaned with enzymatic detergent, and preferably sterilized whenever the final filter is changed, to remove any bio-film.
- In addition, according to the AER specification, all the inner tubing and parts of the machine must be backflushed or exposed to the disinfectant on a regular basis.
- Pressure gauges should be installed and monitored to determine when to change the filters.
- Water supply to AERs is an automatic mixture of hot and cold; therefore, the temperature must be monitored to make sure it remains within manufacturer's specifications to prevent damage to endoscopes or lessen the effectiveness of the disinfectant.

If AERs are in use, bronchoscopy specimens, such as bronchealveolar lavages or bronchial washings, that are positive for water microorganisms (e.g., nontuberculous mycobacteria or pseudomonads) should be monitored to establish a baseline. Any increase over baseline should be investigated as a possible outbreak or pseudo-outbreak. Water specimens should be analyzed for the implicated microorganism; collect water from the intake upstream of the filter, downstream of the smallest filter and from within the water bath of the machine.

Currently, routine culturing of AERs is not recommended by organizations in the United States;[39] however, it is recommended in the United Kingdom.[39] Endotoxin has not been an issue for reprocessing endoscopes.[40]

SGNA[1] recommends the following features in an AER for adequate disinfection and to prevent contamination by water microorganisms:

1. Fluids (i.e., water, detergent, disinfectant) must circulate through all channels without trapping air.
2. Detergent and disinfection cycles must be followed by thorough water rinsing and forced air to remove all fluid.
3. Disinfectant must not be diluted with water or detergent.
4. Machine should be self-disinfecting, that is, disinfectant should circulate through tubing to prevent overgrowth of water microorganisms and build-up of biofilm.
5. No water should remain in hoses or reservoirs for the same reason.
6. Cycles for alcohol flushing and forced air drying are desirable.

In addition to lumened endoscopes there are many non-lumened flexible endoscopes, rhinoscopes and sinuscopes for example. The presence of fiberoptics makes these endoscopes delicate; therefore, they need to be handled with care. They should be disinfected as just described; however, final rinsing with alcohol or sterile water is not needed. Non-lumened endoscopes must also be stored in a clean, dry area to prevent damage or contamination.

PROTECTION FROM EXPOSURE TO DISINFECTANT

Reprocessing of endoscopes should be performed in a dedicated utility room and not in the procedure room.[1] If glutaraldehyde is used, air circulation in the utility room should be adequate to dissipate fumes or special disinfectant utilization stations or hoods should be installed.[40] Vapor levels of disinfectant should be monitored when the endoscopy unit opens and endoscope disinfection first begins, as well as whenever a change is made in type of disinfectant or volume of endoscope reprocessing. Staff must wear protective gloves whenever placing instruments into or removing instruments from the disinfectant. Face shields or goggles/masks are needed if there is splash potential.[41] For further details on appropriate workflow and staff protection, see Chapter 3.

STANDARD PRECAUTIONS

During the endoscopy procedure the operator must wear gloves. Because there are documented reports of splash exposure to staff, face shields or goggles/mask and disposable gowns should also be worn. See Chapter 4 for further discussion of personal protective equipment.

PROTECTION FROM EXPOSURE TO TUBERCULOSIS

The Centers for Disease Control and Prevention (CDC) recommends that special provisions to prevent TB be implemented for cough-inducing procedures, including bronchoscopy.[42] Where bronchoscopies are performed, provisions for Airborne Precautions are needed. Negative pressure rooms or rooms with air circulated through high-efficiency particulate air (HEPA) filters are recommended. Staff performing bronchoscopy and assistants during the procedure must be fit-tested for the required masks (e.g., N95 masks) and must wear them during bronchoscopy procedures where there is any suspicion of TB. Airborne Precautions should also be carried out during the recovery of these patients (see Chapter 6).

QUALITY ASSURANCE AND IMPROVEMENT PROGRAM

Written procedures for every aspect of endoscope care and prevention of adverse events must be developed and reviewed on a regular basis. Each person responsible for reprocessing endoscopes must be trained and shown to be competent on a periodic basis, preferably annually, according to SGNA guidelines.[1] See Appendix F for a sample competency. Each person responsible for performing endoscopy must follow Standard Precautions and Airborne Precautions where applicable, and annual staff training on these policies must be provided. Corrective action should be taken for any lapse in performance.

Procedures for reporting infections and follow-up for any suspected cross infection or outbreak must be developed. Consultation with an infection prevention and control professional is recommended for policy development and review.

Resources

Professional endoscopy organizations can provide additional resources via their Web sites, e.g., American Society for Gastrointestinal Endoscopy, www.asge.org. The Society for Gastroenterology Nurses and Associates, http://www.sgna.org/, publishes guidelines online for endoscope reprocessing at http://www.sgna.org/resources/guideline3.cfm and use of disinfectants at http://www.sgna.org/resources/guideline6.cfm. Articles by Rutala[21] and Alfa[36] provide reviews of chemical disinfectants and reprocessing recommendations, respectively.

References

1. Walker, S. B. *Standards of Infection Control in Reprocessing of Flexible Gastrointestinal Endoscopes.* Chicago: Society of Gastroenterology Nurses and Associates, Inc., 2000. http://www.sgna.org/resources/Infection.html.

2. Weber, D. J., and Rutala, W. A. Lessons from outbreaks associated with bronchoscopy. *Infect Control Hosp Epidemiol.* 2001; 22:403–408.

3. Ostrowsky, B. Endoscopes—Current practices and controversies in infection control. *Semin Infect Control.* 2001; 1:267–279.

4. Alvarado, C. J., Reichelderfer, M., and APIC Guidelines Committee. APIC guideline for infection prevention and control in flexible endoscopy. *Am J Infect Control.* 2000; 28:138–155.

5. Sorin, M., Segal-Maurer, S., Mariano, N., Urban, C., Combest, A., and Rahal, J. J. Nosocomial transmission of imipenem-resistant *Pseudomonas aeruginosa* following bronchoscopy associated with improper connection to the Steris System 1 Processor. *Infect Control Hosp Epidemiol.* 2001; 22:409–413.

6. Bronchoscopy-related infections and pseudoinfections—New York, 1996 and 1998. *MMWR.* 1999; 48:557–560.

7. Schelenz, S., and French, G. An outbreak of multidrug-resistant *Pseudomonas aeruginosa* associated with contamination of bronchoscopes and an endoscope washer-disinfector. *J Hosp Infect.* 2000; 46:23–30.

8. Bronowicki, J. P., Venard, V., Botte, C., Monhoven, N., Gastin, I., and Chone, L., et al. Patient-to-patient transmission of hepatitis C virus during colonoscopy. *N Eng J Med.* 1997; 337:237–240.

9. Michele, T. M., Cronin, W. A., Graham, N. M., Dwyer, D. M., Pope, D. S., and Harrington, S., et al. Transmission of *Mycobacterium tuberculosis* by a fiberoptic bronchoscope. Identification by DNA fingerprinting. *JAMA.* 1997; 278:1093–1095.

10. Agerton, T., Valway, S., Gore, B., Pozsik, C., Plikaytis, B., and Woodley, C., et al. Transmission of a highly drug-resistant strain (strain W1) of *Mycobacterium tuberculosis.* *JAMA.* 1997; 278:1073–1077.

11. Armstrong, R. W., and Bolding, F. Septic arthritis after arthrsocopy: The contributing roles of intraarticular steroids and environmental factors. *Am J Infect Control.* 1994; 22:16–18.

12. Struelens, M. J., Rost, F., Deplano, A., Maas, A., Schwam, V., and Serruys, E., et al. *Pseudomonas aeruginosa* and *Enterobacteriaceae*

bacteremia after biliary endoscopy: An outbreak investigation using DNA macrorestriction analysis. *Am J Med.* 1993; 95:489–498.

13. Blevins, F. T., Salgado, J., Wascher, D. C., and Koster, F. Septic arthritis following arthroscopic meniscus repair: A cluster of three cases. *Arthroscopy.* 1999; 15:35–40.

14. LoPasso, C., Pernice, I., Celeste, A., Perdichizze, G., and Todaro-Luck, F. Transmission of *Trichosporon asahii* esophagitis by a contaminated endoscope. *Mycoses.* 2001; 44:13–21.

15. Southwick, K. L., Hoffmann, K., Ferree, K., Matthews, J., and Salfinger, M. Cluster of tuberculosis cases in North Carolina: Possible association with atomizer reuse. *Am J Infect Control.* 2001; 29:1–6.

16. Notice to readers: *Pseudomonas aeruginosa* infections associated with defective bronchoscopes. *MMWR.* 2002; 51:190.

17. Dolce, P., Gourdeau, M., April, N., and Bernard, P. M. Outbreak of glutaraldehyde-induced proctocolitis. *Am J Infect Control.* 1995; 23:34–39.

18. Hanson, J. M., Plusa, S. M., Bennett, M. K., Browell, D. A., and Cunliffe, W. J. Glutaraldehyde as a possible cause of diarrhea after sigmoidoscopy. *Brit J Surgery.* 1998; 85:1385–1387.

19. West, A. B., Kuan, S. F., Bennick, M., and Lagarde, S. Glutaraldehyde colitis following endoscopy: Clinical and pathological features and investigation of an outbreak. *Gastroenterology.* 1995; 108:1250–1255.

20. Rozen, P., Somjen, G. J., Baratz, M., Kimel, R., Arber, N., and Gilat, T. Endoscope-induced colitis: Description, probable cause by glutaraldehyde, and prevention. *Gastrointestinal Endoscopy.* 1994; 40:547–553.

21. Rutala, W. A., and Weber, D. J. Disinfection of endoscopes: Review of new chemical sterilants used for high-level disinfection. *Infect Control Hosp Epidemiol.* 1999; 20:69–76.

22. Ruddy, M., and Kibbler, C. C. Endoscopic decontamination: An audit and practical review. *J Hosp Infect.* 2002; 50:261–268.

23. Fraser, V. J., Zuckerman, G., Clouse, R. E., O'Rourke, S., Jones, M., and Klasner, J., et al. A prospective randomized trial comparing manual and automated endoscope disinfection methods. *Infect Control Hosp Epidemiol.* 1993; 14:383–389.

24. Maloney, S., Welbel, S., Daves, B., Adams, K., Becker, S., and Bland, L., et al. *Mycobacterium abscessus* pseudoinfection traced to an automated endoscope washer: Utility of epidemiologic and laboratory investigation. *J Infect Dis.* 1994; 169:1166–1169.

25. Fraser, V. J., Jones, M., Murray, P. R., Medoff, G., Zhang, Y., and Wallace, R. J., Jr. Contamination of flexible fiberoptic bronchoscopes with *Mycobacterium chelonae* linked to an automated bronchoscope disinfection machine. *Am Rev Respir Dis.* 1992; 145:853–855.

26. Kressel, A. B., and Kidd, F. Pseudo-outbreak of *Mycobacterium chelonae* and *Methylobacterium mesophilicum* caused by contamination of an automated endoscopy washer. *Infect Control Hosp Epidemiol.* 2001; 22:414–418.

27. Gillespie, T. G., Hogg, L., Budge, E., Duncan, A., and Coia, J. E. *Mycobacterium chelonae* isolated from rinse water within an endoscope washer-disinfector. *J Hosp Infect.* 2000; 45:332–334.

28. Wallace, R. J., Brown, B. A., and Griffith, D. E. Nosocomial outbreaks/pseudo-outbreaks caused by nontuberculous mycobacteria. *Ann Review Microbiol.* 1998; 52:453–490.

29. Nosocomial infection and pseudoinfection from contaminated endoscopes and bronchoscopes—Wisconsin and Missouri. *MMWR.* 1991; 40:675–678.

30. Petersen, K., Bus, N., Walter, V., and Chenoweth, C. Pseudoepidemic of *Mycobacterium abscessus* associated with bronchoscopy. *Am J Infect Control.* 1994; 22:123 (abstract).

31. MacKay, W. G., Leanord, A. T., and Williams, C. L. Water, water everywhere nor any a sterile drop to rinse your endoscope. *J Hosp Infect.* 2002; 51:256–261.

32. Muscarella, L. F. Deja vu . . . all over again? The importance of instrument drying. *Infect Control Hosp Epidemiol.* 2000; 21:628–629.

33. Mohandas, K. M., and Gopalakrishnan, G. Mucocutaneous exposure to body fluids during digestive endoscopy: The need for universal precautions. *Indian J Gastroenterology.* 1999; 18:109–111.

34. Vyas, A., Pickering, C. A., Oldham, L. A., Francis, H. C., Fletcher, A. M., and Merret, T., et al. Survey of symptoms, respiratory function, and immunology and their relation to glutaraldehyde and other occupational exposures among endoscopy nursing staff. *Occupational Environ Med.* 2000; 57:752–759.

35. Rutala, W. A., and Weber, D. J. FDA labeling requirements for disinfection of endoscopes: A counterpoint. *Infect Control Hosp Epidemiol.* 1995; 16:231–235.

36. Alfa, M. J., Olson, N., DeGagne, P., and Jackson, M. A survey of reprocessing methods, residual viable bioburden, and soil levels in patient-ready endoscopic retrograde choliangiopancreatography duodenoscopes used in Canadian centers. *Infect Control Hosp Epidemiol.* 2002; 23:198–206.

37. Olympus Corporation. Proper use of carrying case for flexible endoscopes. Melville, NY: Olympus America, Inc.; 2002. *http://www.olympus.com/msg_section/endo_pr.pdf.*

38. Rutala, W. A. APIC guideline for selection and use of disinfectants. *Am J Infect Control.* 1996; 24:313–342.

39. Muscarella, L. F. Application of environmental sampling to flexible endoscope reprocessing: The importance of monitoring the rinse water. *Infect Control Hosp Epidemiol.* 2002; 23:285–289.

40. Working Party Report. Rinse water for heat labile endoscopy equipment. *J Hosp Infect.* 2002; 51:7–16.

41. Walker, S. B. *Guideline for the Use of High-Level Disinfectants and Sterilants for Reprocessing of Flexible Gastrointestinal Endoscopes.* Chicago, IL: Society of Gastroenterology Nurses and Associates, Inc.; 2000. *http://www.sgna.org/resources/HLD.html.*

42. Guidelines for Preventing the Transmission of *Mycobacterium tuberculosis* in Health-Care Facilities, 1994. *MMWR.* 1994; 43(RR13):1–132.

CHAPTER 10

Infusion Therapy

BACKGROUND

The provision of parenteral infusion therapies in ambulatory settings has expanded dramatically in recent years. General specialized services may include catheter care; implanted port access and removal; blood component administration; antimicrobial, antifungal, and antiviral therapy; continuous or intermittent chemotherapy; intravenous gamma globulin; hydration therapy; pain control; and total parenteral nutrition.[1] Some programs provide only on-site administration of medications, teach patients to self-administer, or may send nurses into patients' homes. Some programs also prepare and dispense drugs. Settings include hospital-based clinics, group practice clinics, physician offices, emergency departments, or free-standing infusion centers.

Outpatient infusion therapy can require the use of sophisticated vascular access devices (VADs) and medication delivery systems.[2] Complications associated with VADs include phlebitis, infiltration, occlusion, clotting, breakage, leakage at the site, and infection.

CAUSES OF INFECTION

Generally, VADs can facilitate transfer of microorganisms from one part of the body to another or from caregivers' hands to the patient. Once inserted, intravascular (IV) catheters become coated with fibrin and other plasma proteins that may promote colonization with microorganisms. The insertion site and the catheter hub are important sources of these colonizing microorganisms and serve as the main reservoirs of microbes causing catheter-related infections. Migration of skin microorganisms at the insertion site into the cutaneous catheter tract with colonization of the catheter tip is the most common route of bloodstream infection for peripherally inserted short-term and central venous catheters. Contamination of the catheter hub is an important contributor to intraluminal colonization of long-term catheters.[3] Contaminated infusate may also cause infections.[4] Important determinants of catheter-related infection are the material of the device and the virulence of the infecting microorganism.[3]

DEVICES

Vascular access types include:

- Short peripheral venous catheters
- Midline catheters
- Nontunneled, noncuffed central venous catheters
- Peripherally inserted central catheters (PICC)
- Skin-tunneled cuffed central venous catheters
- Totally implantable intravascular devices

RISKS

The risks of infection directly related to outpatient infusion therapy have not been quantified. However, it is assumed to be far less than the risk of infection when hospitalized.[1] The following characteristics have been found to be associated with increased risk of VAD-associated infection:[4, 5]

- Duration of catheterization
- Heavy colonization of the catheter hub
- Heavy colonization of the insertion site
- Neutropenia
- Improper catheter care and insertion practices

There have also been instances of infections occurring with flush solutions.[6] The risk of bloodstream infection associated with VADs in hospitals has been reported as:[7]

- Peripheral intravenous catheters: 0.2 per 100 devices
- Nontunneled central venous catheters (multilumen): 3.0 per 100 devices
- PICC: 0.2 per 100 devices
- Skin-tunneled central venous catheters: 0.2 per 100 devices
- Totally implantable intravascular devices: 0.04 per 100 devices

Home infusion-related infection data might be more comparable to outpatient infusion centers. A prospective study of patients receiving home infusion therapy through central or midline catheters found the range of bloodstream infections as 0.16 to 6.8 infections per 1000 catheter-days. The rate was affected by various risk factors, including recent bone marrow transplantation, previous bloodstream infection, receipt of total parenteral nutrition, administration of therapy in an outpatient facility, and use of a multilumen catheter.[8]

PREVENTION

Successful prevention strategies reduce colonization at the insertion site and hub of catheters or minimize microbial spread extraluminally from the skin or intraluminally from hub toward the catheter tip lying in the bloodstream.[9] Factors to focus on include:[3]

- Hand hygiene and aseptic technique
- Skin antisepsis
- Device site care and dressing regimen
- Infusion systems and fluids
- Antimicrobial/antiseptic impregnated catheter and cuffs
- Multidose parenteral medication vials

The Centers for Disease Control and Prevention (CDC) guidelines for the prevention of intravascular catheter-related infections[3] are appropriate for use in ambulatory care settings. Special practices are required for antineoplastic agents.[10] The American Society of Health-System Pharmacists' Best Practices for Health-System Pharmacy may also be used as a resource: *http://www.ashp.org/bestpractices/index.cfm.*

Physical Space

- There should be a clean, well-ventilated area for each patient.[11]
- There should be an isolation room to separate patients who have a communicable disease.[1]
- Surfaces should be easy to clean.
- There should be a dedicated space for staging and compounding drugs. Parenteral solutions must be compounded in a laminar flow hood using aseptic technique.[11] The traffic in this area should be minimized.
- The pharmacy should have an anteroom in which to change into appropriate clothing.[1]

Catheter Insertion

- Short peripheral catheters
  - Use safety catheters whenever possible.
  - Use upper extremities, if possible, for adults; use scalp, hand, or foot for children.[3]
  - Anchor securely.
- Central venous catheters
  - Use a minimum number of lumens or ports.[3]
  - Use an antiseptic or antimicrobial-impregnated catheter in adult patients whose catheter is to remain in place longer than five days if bloodstream infection rates are above benchmark data.[3]
  - Use maximal barrier precautions during insertion. This includes sterile long-sleeved gown, gloves, mask, cap, and large sterile drape.[3]
- Full barrier precautions should be considered for midline catheters.[9]
- Use 2% chlorhexidine for skin preparation before catheter insertion. Secondary choices are tincture of iodine or an iodophor.[9] Do not palpate the insertion site after cleansing.
- Teflon or polyurethane catheters appear to be associated with fewer infectious complications than

catheters made of polyvinyl chloride or polyethylene.[3]

Care and Maintenance of Infusion Systems

- Maintain a closed system. Access the system through ports rather than open hubs.
- Cleanse catheter injection hubs and connections or sampling ports with 70% alcohol before accessing the system.[3, 11]
- In-line filters are unnecessary because they have not been shown to prevent infections associated with infusion systems.[3, 9]
- Use needleless devices or a protected-needle system.
- Use only sterile caps on stopcocks. Do not reuse caps. Apply an end cap after an infusion is complete.[12]
- Do not use antibiotic lock solutions routinely.
- Use aseptic technique for all manipulations of the system including flushing IV tubing and device.

Care of the Site

- Patients with poor personal hygiene habits should be taught how to improve and maintain their personal hygiene.
- An antiseptic (e.g., 2% chlorhexidine, povidone iodine, or alcohol) should be used to cleanse the insertion site with each dressing change. Chlorhexidine is the most effective.[3, 13]
- Manipulation of a catheter should be performed in a manner that minimizes contamination.
- If there is need for a dressing, use either a sterile gauze or a transparent dressing to cover the catheter site. Avoid touch contamination of the insertion site when the dressing is replaced. Change dressings when the device is removed or replaced, or when the dressing becomes damp, loosened, or soiled.[3]
- Do not use ointment routinely; studies on its use are contradictory.[3]
- Do not submerge the catheter under water. Showering may be permitted if precautions can be taken to reduce the likelihood of introducing microbes into the catheter, such as using an impermeable covering for the catheter site and the connecting device during the shower.[3]

Prevention Procedures

Use of Barrier Precautions and Hand Hygiene

- Use Standard Precautions for all patients (see Chapter 6).
- Cleanse hands with an alcohol-based product or antibacterial soap and water before and after patient care.[3, 14] Patient care activities include palpation, insertion, replacement, manipulation, and dressing any VAD (see Chapter 5).
- Gloves are to be used for all vascular access procedures, including drawing blood. Use needleless or safety devices for IV catheters and phlebotomy.[15–16]
- Gloves must be changed between patients.[15]
- Care must be taken to avoid touching surfaces with gloved hands that will later be touched with ungloved hands.
- Healthcare workers (HCW) must wear gowns and face protection when performing procedures during which spattering of blood might occur.[15]
- Resuscitation devices should be readily accessible.
- Hepatitis B vaccination is recommended for all staff members who may have contact with blood or body fluids.[15]

Fluids

- Check all containers of fluid for visible turbidity, leaks, cracks, particulate matter, and the expiration date prior to use.[11]
- Develop protocols outlining appropriate hang-time for various fluids.[3]

Pharmacy[17–18]

- All sterile medications for use in the ambulatory care facility should be prepared in a suitable environment by appropriately trained personnel and labeled appropriately for the user.[3]
- Quality control and quality assurance procedures for the preparation of sterile products should exist, including periodic assessment of personnel on aseptic technique.

- All sterile products should be prepared with sterile equipment (e.g., syringes and vials) and sterile ingredients and solutions.
- Procedures should address personnel education and training, competency evaluation, product acquisition, storage and handling of products and supplies, storage and delivery of final products, use and maintenance of facilities and equipment, appropriate garb and conduct of personnel working in the controlled area, process validation, preparation technique, labeling, documentation, quality control, and material movement.
- Solutions, drugs, supplies, and equipment must be stored according to the manufacturer or United States Pharmacopeia requirements.
- Clean room garb must be worn inside the controlled area. Attire consists of a low-shedding coverall or low-particulate clean clothing covers such as clean gowns or a coverall with sleeves having elastic cuffs, head cover, facemask, gloves, gowns, masks, and shoe covers. Garb will differ for various risk categories.
- Personnel must scrub their hands and forearms for an appropriate period at the beginning of each aseptic compounding process.
- Personnel preparing sterile products must scrub their hands and arms with an antimicrobial soap.
- Hand, finger, and wrist jewelry must be minimized or eliminated. Nails are to be kept clean and trimmed.

Patient-Care Equipment

- Between patients, infusion pumps and chairs must be cleaned with a cleaner/disinfectant.
- Multiple-use patient care items must be cleaned between uses whenever soiled.

Use of Medications and Multiple-Dose Vials (MDVs)

- Use single-dose vials of parenteral additives or medications whenever possible.
- The access diaphragm of MDVs should be wiped with 70% alcohol prior to puncture.[3]
- Use a new sterile safety device for any access into the medication vial.[3]

Cleaning Environmental Surfaces

- If an item is visibly contaminated with blood, a low-level disinfectant should be used (see Chapter 3).
- Blood spills should be cleaned immediately with a cloth soaked with a low-level disinfectant. After all visible blood is cleaned, a new cloth or towel should be used to apply disinfectant a second time (see Chapter 3).

Waste Management

- Any waste contaminated with blood, hazardous substances, and sharp items must be discarded according to local and state regulations.
- Environmental services staff members should promptly remove trash and medical waste and should maintain an environment that enhances patient care.

Isolation Precautions

The background on this subject is outlined in Chapter 6. Practices specific to infusion centers follow.

Antibiotic-Resistant Microorganisms

1. Wash hands whenever anything in the vicinity of the patient was touched, including environmental surfaces.
2. Use gloves for *any* patient contact.
3. If the patient's skin integrity is intact (i.e., no open, draining wounds) and his or her clothes are clean, a protective gown is not required for staff.
4. Multiple-use patient care equipment that has contact with the patient or that may have been contaminated must be cleaned or disinfected before being used by another patient.
5. Bedside equipment (e.g., stethoscope, sphygmomanometer, and thermometer) must remain in the patient's area while the patient is in the center, and then cleaned and disinfected when the patient leaves. If such devices must be used on other patients during this time, they must first be cleaned and disinfected.

Airborne-Spread Disease

1. There should be an isolation room to separate patients who have or are suspected of having a communicable disease spread through the air.[1]
2. Diseases of concern are chicken pox, measles, rubella, and tuberculosis.
3. Appropriate masks must be available for staff and patients (see Chapter 6).

Education

- Provide ongoing education and training of staff regarding use of intravascular devices and appropriate infection prevention and control measures.[3]
- Appropriate annual infection prevention and control training is required for staff.

- Educate patients regarding the infusion procedure and care of the VAD, emphasizing the importance of good hygiene and keeping the catheter site clean.

SURVEILLANCE

An active surveillance system can assist with early detection of infectious complications[19] (see Chapter 20). Definitions of VAD-related infections should be standardized for the facility. The clinical definitions for catheter-related infections from the CDC guidelines are outlined in Table 10.1. Definitions should include criteria to distinguish between a hospital, home care, or infusion center infection. A record-keeping system (e.g., a logbook or electronic file) should be in place where the following information is recorded:

- Incidence of bloodstream infection

Table 10.1 Examples of Clinical Definitions for Catheter-Related Infections**

Localized catheter colonization	Significant growth of a microorganism (>15 CFU*) from the catheter tip, subcutaneous segment of the catheter, or catheter hub
Exit site infection	Erythema or induration within 2 cm of the catheter exit site, in the absence of concomitant bloodstream infection and without concomitant purulence
Clinical exit site infection or tunnel infection	Tenderness, erythema, or site induration >2 cm from the catheter site along the subcutaneous tract of a skin tunneled catheter, in the absence of concomitant bloodstream infection
Pocket infection	Purulent fluid in the subcutaneous pocket of a totally implanted intravascular device that may or may not be associated with spontaneous rupture and drainage or necrosis of the overlaying skin, in the absence of concomitant bloodstream infection
Infusate-related bloodstream infection	Concordant growth of the same microorganism from the infusate and blood cultures (preferably percutaneously drawn) with no other identifiable source of infection
Catheter-related bloodstream infection	Bacteremia/fungemia in a patient with an intravascular catheter with at least one positive blood culture and with clinical manifestations of infections (i.e., fever, chills, and/or hypotension) and no apparent source for the bloodstream infection except the catheter or any of the following: 1. A positive semiquantitative (>15 CFU/catheter segment) or quantitative (>10^3 CFU/catheter segment catheter) culture whereby the same microorganism (species and antibiogram) is isolated from the catheter segment and peripheral blood 2. Simultaneous quantitative blood cultures with a >5:1 ratio (central venous catheter [CVC] vs. peripheral) 3. Differential time period of CVC culture vs. peripheral blood culture positive of >2 hours.

*CFU: Colony-forming units

**Adapted from Centers for Disease Control and Prevention. Guidelines for the Prevention of Intravascular Catheter-Related Infections, 2002. MMWR. 2002; 51(RR-10):1–32. http://www.cdc.gov/ncidod/hip/IV/Iv.htm.

- Incidence of vascular access site infection

A staff person should be designated to review surveillance data periodically. In addition, a record that includes the location of the infusion station used for each session and the names of staff members who connect and disconnect the patient to the infusion should be maintained for each patient. There should be a protocol outlining the actions required when changes occur in rate of infections.

Other performance indicators[3] to evaluate quality of care include:

- Implementation of educational programs
- Use of maximal sterile barrier precautions
- Use of 2% chlorhexidine for skin antisepsis
- Rates of catheter discontinuation when no longer required

References

1. Mortlock, N. Intravenous Therapy in the Alternative Care Setting. In: Hankins, J., Lonsway, R. A. W., Hedrick, C., and Perdue, M. B., eds. *Infusion Therapy in Clinical Practice*. 2nd Ed. St. Louis: W. B. Saunders Co.; 2001: 535–560.

2. Mortlock, N. J., and Schleis, T. Outpatient parenteral antimicrobial therapy technology. *Infect Dis Clin North Am*. 1998; 12:861–877.

3. Centers for Disease Control and Prevention. Guidelines for the prevention of intravascular catheter-related infections, 2002. *MMWR*. 2002: 51(RR-10):1–32. *http://www.cdc.gov/ncidod/hip/IV/Iv.htm.*

4. Maki, D. G., and Mermel, L. A. Infections Due to Infusion Therapy. In: Bennett, J. V., and Brachman, P. S., eds. *Hospital Infections*. 4th Ed. Philadelphia: Lippincott-Raven, Inc.; 1998: 689–742.

5. Howell, P. B., Walters, P. E., Donowitz, G. R., and Farr, B. M. Risk factors for infection of adult patients with cancer who have tunneled central venous catheters. *Cancer*. 1995; 75:1367–1375.

6. Pegues, D. A., Carson, L. A., Anderson, R. L., Norgard, M. J., Argent, T. A., and Jarvis, W. R., et al. Outbreak of *Pseudomonas cepacia* bacteremia in oncology patients. *Clin Infect Dis*. 1993; 16:407–411.

7. Maki, D. G. Infections caused by intravascular devices: Pathogenesis, strategies for prevention. In: Maki, D. G., ed. *Improving Catheter Site Care*. London: Royal Society of Medicine Services Ltd.; 1991: 3–27.

8. Tokars, J. I., Cookson, S. T., McArthur, M. A., Boyer, C. L., McGeer, A. J., and Jarvis, W. R. Prospective evaluation of risk factors for bloodstream infection in patients receiving home infusion therapy. *Ann Intern Med*. 1999; 131:340–347.

9. Mermel, L. A. Prevention of intravascular catheter-related infections. *Ann Int Med*. 2000; 132:391–402.

10. Maxson, J. H., and Wolk, J. E. Principles of Preparation, Administration, and Disposal of Antineoplastic Agents. In: Itano, J. K., and Taoka, K. N., eds. *Core Curriculum for Oncology Nursing*. 3rd Ed. Philadelphia: W.B. Saunders Co.; 1998: 657–661.

11. Nolet, B. R. Office- and clinic-based ambulatory infusion programs: Opportunities for the infusion nurse. *J Intraven Nurs*. 2000; 23:S32–S41.

12. Moureau, N. Preventing complications with vascular access. *Nursing*. 2001; 31:52–55.

13. Calfee, D. R. Infection control aspects of long-term vascular catheters. *Semin Infect Control*. 2001; 1:224–233.

14. Centers for Disease Control and Prevention. Guideline for hand hygiene in health-care settings: Recommendations of the Healthcare Infection Control Practices Advisory Committee and the HICPAC/SHEA/APIC/IDSA Hand Hygiene Task Force. *MMWR*. 2002; 51 (No. RR-16):1–44.

15. Occupational Exposure to Bloodborne Pathogens: Final Rule. *Fed Reg*. 1991; 56 (Dec. 6):64175–64182.

16. Occupational Exposure to Bloodborne Pathogens; Needlestick and Other Sharps Injuries: Final Rule. *Fed Reg*. 2001; 66:5317–5325.

17. ASHP Guidelines: *Minimum Standard for Pharmaceutical Services in Ambulatory Care*, 1999. American Society of Health-System Pharmacists, Inc., *http://www.ashp.org/bestpractices/guidelines.cfm?cfid =14030335&CFToken=27461495.*

18. *ASHP Guidelines on Quality Assurance for Pharmacy-Prepared Sterile Products*, 2000. American Society of Health-System Pharmacists, Inc., *http://www.ashp.org/bestpractices/guidelines.cfm?cfid= 140303 35&CFToken=27461495.*

19. Smith, T. L., Pullen, G. T., Crouse, V., Rosenberg, J., and Jarvis, W. R. Bloodstream infections in pediatric oncology outpatients: A new healthcare systems challenge. *Infect Control Hosp Epidemiol*. 2002; 23:239–243.

CHAPTER 11

Invasive Cardiology

BACKGROUND

Cardiac catheterization procedures involve the introduction of special catheters into the central arterial and/or central venous circulatory system to diagnose or treat conditions of the heart or vascular system.[1] Cardiac catheterization laboratories have evolved from highly specialized research laboratories into procedure rooms in which diagnostic tests and therapeutic interventional procedures are performed. Improvements in the quality of imaging equipment, potent antiplatelet agents, and coronary stent technology have resulted in a high degree of safety for most interventional procedures. The majority of routine diagnostic procedures performed occur in the outpatient setting. Improvements in X-ray systems and the development of digital processing capabilities have facilitated "noncardiac" vascular investigations and interventions in other areas of the vascular system.[2]

CAUSES OF INFECTION

Infection is rare after invasive cardiovascular procedures.[3] In a retrospective study of 385 laboratories an overall infection rate of 0.35% was noted, with the incidence for cut-downs 10 times higher than that for percutaneous sites (0.62% vs. 0.06%).[4] Laboratories that performed 150 or fewer cutdowns per year had more infections than those performing more procedures. Microorganisms may come from contaminated instruments, solutions, or breaks in technique.[5] It is presumed that when infection occurs, bacteria are introduced at the time of percutaneous transarterial puncture.

Local and systemic infectious complications due to cardiac catheterization procedures include bloodstream infection, endarteritis, pacemaker infections, and puncture site infections.[6–17] Endotoxin reactions after catheterization have also been reported.[18–20] There have also been reports of infections involving coronary stents.[21–22]

RISKS

As noted, invasive cardiology procedures have the potential for infection transmission although the risk is low. Generally, risk factors include:[8]

- Repuncture of the ipsilateral vascular access site within three to seven days of the first procedure
- Vascular sheath dwelling in the vessel for more than 24 hours
- Prolonged duration of the procedure
- Number of catheter passes performed through the arterial sheath
- Vascular complications such as bleeding, hematoma, pseudoaneurysm, or dissection at the access site
- Immunocompromised host (e.g., diabetes, human immunodeficiency virus, renal failure)
- Obesity
- Prosthetic heart valves

The potential for staff exposure to blood or other possibly infectious material exists in virtually any invasive procedure. Splashing or spraying of blood may occur during cardiac catheterization. In addition, sharp instruments are used in these procedures and pose a risk.

PREVENTION

Procedures

General

All procedures must be conducted as though there was a risk of infection, and Standard Precautions (see Chapter 6) must be used routinely with all patients. Staff must be trained in surgical asepsis, aseptic technique, and methods for preventing exposure to blood and body fluids.

Hand Hygiene

For invasive procedures, anyone who will touch the surgical field, sterile instruments, or wound site should perform a surgical scrub.[1]

- An operator should start the day with a hand scrub of at least two minutes. For subsequent cases, a full scrub using a brush may not be necessary.[23] However, thorough handwashing must be performed using an antimicrobial soap or alcohol-based product with persistent activity designed for surgical scrubs.
- Remove debris by thoroughly cleaning underneath fingernails.[24–25]
- Fingernails should not extend past the fingertips and should be kept free of artificial nails.[25]
- Remove all rings and bracelets before scrubbing.[24]

Staff/Patient Preparation

Cardiac catheterization laboratory operators must perform an appropriate hand scrub and wear a scrub suit or uniform,[23] a sterile nonporous long-sleeved gown, surgical cap, mask, and gloves.[1–2]

- Technicians and nurses involved in the procedure room should wear scrub suits, caps, and masks.[23]
- There is controversy regarding the wearing of caps or masks during percutaneous cardiac catheterization procedures.[26–27] If caps are worn, they should completely cover and contain hair.

- Visitors may wear a cover (bunny) suit in place of a scrub suit.[23]
- Nonporous drapes (i.e., those that resist liquid penetration) should be used to cover the area surrounding the wound.[25] Drapes must be large enough to minimize contamination of the sterile field.

Use sterile technique before inserting catheters.

- If it is necessary to remove hair at the wound site, it should be done with a clipper or depilatory on the day of the procedure.[23]
- Cleanse the skin site and then apply an antiseptic agent before device insertion.[2, 23] Principles for maintaining a sterile field should be practiced.
- A vascular sheath should be used to minimize vascular trauma, especially when multiple catheter changes are anticipated.[2]

In cases where greater wound exposure is necessary, such as pacemaker implantation or brachial cut-downs, full surgical sterile technique must be used, including scrub suit, cap, and mask.[1–2, 23]

- Sterile gloves should be pulled over a long-sleeved gown.
- Other staff should wear scrub suits, masks, and caps.
- Visitors should wear a cap and mask and either a scrub suit or a cover suit.[1]

Antibiotic prophylaxis for cardiac catheterization generally is not recommended.[1]

Personal Protective Equipment

Gloves must be worn when there is potential for exposure to blood or body fluids. The significant increase in the rate of perforation when gloves are worn more than two hours suggests that gloves should routinely be changed at or before two hours of wear.[28]

- Change gloves routinely after 90 minutes, as well as any time they are contaminated or perforation is suspected.[29]
- Double-gloving should be practiced if the operator has a break in skin integrity.[30]
- Double-gloving may be helpful in reducing chances of a puncture.
- Remove gloves before touching uncovered equipment control panels or other items.

Masks, gowns, eye/face protection, and protective caps are important for preventing exposure to the patient's blood that might splatter onto the operator during invasive procedures.[2, 23, 31] These barriers also decrease the risk of patient infection when cutdown procedures are performed.[4] Given the potential for splashing during invasive procedures, gowns are also needed. Eye/face protection should be used when removing a vascular catheter at the end of a procedure.[30]

To prevent mucous membrane contact during resuscitation, a mouth-bag or mouth-mask device should be kept in each examination and procedure room or in a crash cart.

When there is a reasonable risk of exposure to blood or bloody fluid during any vascular or interventional procedure, additional protective clothing is recommended, including shoes worn only for performing procedures, shoe covers or gaiters to cover lower legs and feet, and hair covering.[30]

Any barrier that becomes saturated with blood must be removed and replaced as soon as patient safety permits.[1] All personal protective equipment must be removed upon exiting the unit.

Sterile Items

The sterile field should be prepared as close to the procedure time as possible. Large equipment (e.g., overhead lights) in the vicinity of the procedure table that may need to be handled should be covered with a sterile cover. Intravascular devices and sheaths must be handled using meticulous aseptic technique.[1]

Dressings/Site

A standard protocol should be developed using guidelines for vascular catheters.[32] The indwelling sheath or catheter should be removed as early as possible.[23] Dressings can be removed after sheaths are withdrawn, when wound edges are approximated, and when the wound is no longer draining.[1] Patients should be educated to inspect the site and report any signs and symptoms of infection.

Flush Solutions

Small amounts of flush solution can be poured from larger containers. The larger container must be dated and timed when first opened and discarded within 24

hours of opening. An operator's gloved hand should not dip into the flush solution when filling a syringe.[1]

Contaminated fluids must be handled carefully to avoid splashing or spilling. Closed flush systems are preferable. A good system of fluid management involves the use of a manifold via an extra port that contains a one-way valve. The discarded fluid enters a disposal bag that constitutes a closed system with the manifold.[23]

Sharp Items

There must be procedures to safely handle contaminated sharps and minimize percutaneous and skin or mucosal exposure. These procedures can include various practices, including the following:

- Do not recap needles.
- Sharps containers should be conveniently located.
- Evaluate and use, as appropriate, devices to prevent exposures. These include disposable safety scalpels, needleless IV systems, closed flush systems, self-sheathing needles, and needle-holding devices.
- Use a container to hold reusable sharp instruments.[1]
- When needles must be removed from syringes or exchanged, use a clamp, forceps, or other mechanical device.[30]
- Use a no-touch method to pass sharp instruments between individuals by placing instruments on the table and avoiding hand-to-hand transfer.[33]
- There should be a designated area for placement of sharp items (e.g., needles and blades) that may be used throughout a case.[1]

Medications and Multiple-Dose Vials (MDVs)

- Use single-dose vials of parenteral additives or medications whenever possible.[32]
- The access diaphragm of MDVs should be wiped with 70% alcohol prior to puncture.[32]
- Use a new sterile device for any access to the medication vial.
- Disposal containers for syringes should be located as close as practical to the location of syringe use.

Physical Space

Procedure rooms should be designed so there is ease of movement without the potential to compromise sterile items or fields. Traffic in areas where invasive procedures are performed should be kept to a minimum.[23] Scrubbed personnel should remain close to the sterile field and should not leave the room during the procedure.[1]

The doors to procedure rooms should be closed during procedures except for required movement of staff and equipment.[23] There should be handwashing sinks equipped with foot pedals or elbow/wrist blades easily available for staff to use.

The ventilation system should provide at least 15 air exchanges per hour, three of which must be of outside air.[25, 34] Air should be introduced at the ceiling and exhausted near the floor.[25] Maintain positive-pressure ventilation in the procedure room with respect to the corridors and adjacent areas.[30]

The careful disposal of all needles, catheters, sheaths, tubing, and any other instruments, as well as body fluids, is important. Local, state, and federal medical waste rules must be followed. Closed flush-and-waste containment systems should be used. Glass containers (e.g., contrast media bottles) should be handled separately from regular waste to reduce injury to environmental services staff.[30]

The procedure room should be thoroughly cleaned daily. Spot cleaning of any blood or body fluid should occur between each case.

Decontamination of Equipment

Catheters must always be sterile for use and are typically disposable. Devices labeled as single-use by manufacturers may only be reprocessed using the guidance procedures outlined by the Food and Drug Administration (*http://www.fda.gov/cdrh/reuse/index.html*). Several studies have reviewed the risk of infection from use of reuseable cardiac catheters. Generally they note that with standardized cleaning and sterilization methods the reuse of catheters did not increase the risk of infection.[35–37]

If catheters are reusable, they must be properly cleaned and sterilized. The use of single-use catheters has eliminated the problem of pyrogenic reactions. If catheters are reused, they should be rinsed with sterile water to reduce this problem.[5] Sinks used for cleaning must be separate from handwashing sinks.

Potentially contaminated work surfaces (e.g., exam tables) should be cleaned and disinfected at the end of each procedure.[30] A material that can be discarded or disinfected between patients should cover surfaces that may be difficult to disinfect, such as switches and control panels.[38]

Communicable Diseases in Patients

Patients may present to the cardiac catheterization laboratory with both diagnosed and undiagnosed infections. Contamination of equipment and the environment with microorganisms from patients undergoing procedures may occur and result in subsequent spread to other patients and to healthcare workers. *Mycobacterium tuberculosis* may spread via the airborne route from a patient with unrecognized tuberculosis to other patients and healthcare workers. It is important that referring staff inform the area that a patient may have a communicable disease and may require special precautions.

Patients with antibiotic-resistant microorganisms should be managed so that spread of microorganisms is minimized (see Chapter 6). However, additional special practices in the catheterization laboratory are not necessary.

References

1. Vander Hyde, K. Cardiac Catheterization. In: *APIC Text of Infection Control and Epidemiology*. Washington, DC: Association for Professionals in Infection Control and Epidemiology; 2000: 62:1–7.

2. Bashore, T. M., Bates, E. R., Berger, P. B., Clark, D. A., Cusma, J. T., and Dehmer, G. J., et al. Cardiac catheterization laboratory standards: A report of the American College of Cardiology Task Force on Clinical Expert Consensus Documents (ACC/SCA&I Committee to Develop an Expert Consensus Document on Catheterization Laboratory Standards). *J Am Coll Cardiol*. 2001; 37:2170–2214.

3. Sande, M. A., Levinson, M. E., Lukas, D. S., and Kaye, D. Bacteremia associated with cardiac catheterization. *N Engl J Med*. 1969; 281:1104–1106.

4. Leaman, D. M., and Zelis, R. F. What is the appropriate "dress code" for the cardiac catheterization laboratory? *Cathet Cardiovasc Diagn*. 1983; 9:33–38.

5. Weinstein, R. A., and Welbel, S. F. Other Procedure-Related Infections. In: Bennett, J.V., and Brachman, P.S., eds. *Hospital Infections*. 4th Ed. Philadelphia: Lippincott-Raven Publishers; 1998: 741–759.

6. Wiener, R. S., and Ong, L. S. Local infection after percutaneous transluminal coronary angioplasty: Relation to early repuncture of ipsilateral femoral artery. *Cathet Cardiovasc Diagn.* 1989; 16:180–1.

7. Evans, B. H., and Goldstein, E. J. Increased risk of infection after repeat percutaneous transluminal coronary angioplasty. *Am J Infect Control.* 1987; 15:125–126.

8. Sankari, A., Kumar, A. N., Kabins, S., Chandna, H., and Lieb, D. Staphylococcal pericarditis following percutaneous transluminal coronary angioplasty. *Cathet Cardiovasc Interv.* 2000; 50:71–73.

9. Cleveland, K. O., and Gelfand, M. S. Invasive Staphylococcal infections complicating percutaneous transluminal coronary angioplasty: Three cases and review. *Clin Inf Dis.* 1995; 21:93–96.

10. McCready, R. A., Siderys, H., Pittman, J. N., Herod, G. T., Halbrook, H. G., and Fehrenbacher, J. W., et al. Septic complications after cardiac catheterization and percutaneous transluminal coronary angioplasty. *J Vasc Surg.* 1991; 14:170–174.

11. Frazee, B. W., and Flaherty, J. P. Septic endarteritis of the femoral artery following angioplasty. *Rev Infect Dis.* 1991; 13:620–623.

12. Malanoski, G. J., Samore, M. H., Pefanis, A., and Karchmer, A. W. *Staphylococcus aureus* catheter-associated bacteremia. Minimal effective therapy and unusual infectious complications associated with arterial sheath catheters. *Arch Intern Med.* 1995; 155:1161–1166.

13. Shea, K. W., Schwartz, R. K., Gambino, A. T., Marzo, K. P., and Cunha, B. A. Bacteremia associated with percutaneous transluminal coronary angioplasty. *Cathet Cardiovasc Diagn.* 1995; 36:5–9.

14. Rubin, S. J., Lyons, R. W., and Murcia, A. J. Endocarditis associated with cardiac catheterization due to a gram-positive coccus designated *Micrococcus mucilaginosus incertae sedis. J Clin Microbiol.* 1978; 7:546–549.

15. Strampfer, M. J., Ullman, R. F., Sacks-Berg, A., and Cunha, B. A. Group B streptococcal bacteremia after cardiac catheterization. *Crit Care Med.* 1987; 15:625–626.

16. Dimarco, J. P., Garan, H., and Ruskin, J. N. Complications in patients undergoing cardiac electrophysiologic procedures. *Ann Int Med.* 1982; 97:490–493.

17. Chamis, A. L., Peterson, G. E., Cabell, C. H., Corey, G. R., Sorrentino, R. A., and Greenfield, R. A., et al. *Staphylococcus aureus* bacteremia in patients with permanent pacemakers or implantable cardioverter-defibrillators. *Circulation.* 2001; 104:1029–1033.

18. Reyes, M. P., Ganguly, S., Fowler, M., Brown, W. J., Gatmaitan, B. G., Friedman, C., and Lerner, A. M. Pyrogenic reactions after inadvertent infusion of endotoxin during cardiac catheterizations. *Ann Int Med.* 1980; 93:32–35.

19. Lee, R. V., Drabinsky, M., Wolfson, S., Cohen, L. S., and Atkins, E. Pyrogen reactions from cardiac catheterization. *Chest.* 1973; 63:757–761.

20. Endotoxic Reactions Associated with the Reuse of Cardiac Catheters—Massachusetts. *MMWR.* 1979; 28:25–27.

21. Leroy, O., Martin, E., Prat, A., Decoulx, E., Georges, H., and Guilley, J., et al. Fatal infection of coronary stent implantation. *Cathet Cardiovasc Diagn.* 1996; 39:168–170.

22. Bouchart, F., Dubar, A., Bessou, J. P., Redonnet, M., Berland, J., and Mouton-Schleifer, D., et al. *Pseudomonas aeruginosa* coronary stent infection. *Ann Thoracic Surg.* 1997; 64:1810–1813.

23. Heupler, F. A., Heisler, M., Keys, T. F., Serkey, J., and Society for Cardiac Angiography and Interventions Laboratory Performance Standards Committee. Infection prevention guidelines for cardiac catheterization laboratories. *Cathet Cardiovasc Diagn.* 1992; 25:260–263.

24. Centers for Disease Control and Prevention. Guideline for hand hygiene in health-care settings: Recommendations of the Healthcare Infection Control Practices Advisory Committee and the HICPAC/SHEA/APIC/IDSA Hand Hygiene Task Force. *MMWR.* 2002; 51 (No. RR-16):1–44.

25. Mangram, A. J., Horan, T. C., Pearson, M. L., Silver, L. C., and Jarvis, W. R. Guideline for prevention of surgical site infection, 1999. *Am J Infect Control.* 1999; 27:97–134.

26. Laslett, L. J., and Sabin, A. Wearing of caps and masks not necessary during cardiac catheterization. *Cathet Cardiovasc Diagn.* 1989; 17:158–160.

27. Perry, P. Dress code—the right cath garb sparks IC success. *Materials Management.* 1997; 6:46.

28. Hansen, M. E., McIntire, D. D., and Miller, G. L., 3rd. Occult glove perforations: Frequency during interventional radiologic procedures. *AJR. Am J Roentgenol.* 1992; 159:131–135.

29. Hansen, M. E. Bloodborne pathogens and procedure safety in interventional radiology. *Semin Ultrasound CT MR.* 1998; 19:209–214.

30. Hansen, M. E., Bakal, C. W., Dixon, G. D., Eschelman, D. J., Horton, K. M., and Katz, M., et al. Guidelines regarding HIV and other bloodborne pathogens in vascular/interventional radiology. *J Vasc Interv Radiol.* 1997; 8:667–676. Society of Cardiovascular and Interventional Radiology. *http://www.sirweb.org/clinical/T51.htm.*

31. Dehmer, G. J., Arani, D., Noto, T., Scanlon, P., Hildner, F., Clark, D., and Sheldon, W. Lessons learned from the review of cardiac catheterization laboratories: A report from the Laboratory Survey Committee of the Society for Cardiac Angiography and Interventions. *Cathet Cardiovasc Interv.* 1999; 46:24–31.

32. Centers for Disease Control and Prevention. Guidelines for the prevention of intravascular catheter-related infections, 2002. *MMWR.* 2002: 51(RR-10):1–32.

33. Klein, J. S., and Sandu, J. Interventional Procedures in the AIDS Patient. *Radiology Clinics NA.* 1997; 35:1223–1243.

34. AIA. *Guidelines for Design and Construction of Hospital and Health Care Facilities.* Washington, DC: The American Institute of Architects and the Facilities Guidelines Institute; 2001.

35. Ravin, C. E., and Koehler, P. R. Reuse of disposable catheters and guide wires. *Radiology.* 1977; 122:577–579.

36. Jacobson, J. A., Schwartz, C. E., Marshall, H. W., Conti, M., and Burke, J. P. Fever, chills, and hypotension following cardiac catheterization with single- and multiple-use disposable catheters. *Cathet Cardiovasc Diagn.* 1983; 9:39–46.

37. Frank, U., Herz, L., and Daschner, F. D. Infection risk of cardiac catheterization and arterial angiography with single and multiple use disposable catheters. *Clin Cardiol.* 1988; 11:785–787.

38. Ribner, B. S. Nosocomial Infections Associated with Procedures Performed in Radiology. In: Mayhall, C. G., ed. *Hospital Epidemiology and Infection Control.* Baltimore: Williams & Wilkins; 1996: 783–789.

CHAPTER 12

Dentistry

BACKGROUND

Dental and oral surgical procedures are the most frequently performed minor surgical procedures in the United States.[1] Dental healthcare workers and patients may be exposed to a wide variety of microbes because of contact with blood and oral/respiratory secretions and contaminated equipment and surfaces.[2] Patients may shed herpes simplex virus, carry hepatitis B virus (HBV), or have tuberculosis. In addition, scientific articles and increased publicity about the potential for transmitting infectious agents in dentistry have focused attention on dental instruments as possible agents for disease transmission.[3,4]

CAUSES OF INFECTION

A variety of microorganisms are found in the oral cavity. Infections following surgery to the gums or teeth or involving mucosal incisions made in the mouth are caused by a combination of these microbes. Infections may be localized (e.g., dental abscess), result from direct extension of a localized infection (e.g., osteomyelitis of the mandible or maxilla), or distant infections that develop secondary to an oral infection (e.g., liver abscesses).[1] Health care-associated infections have been identified after extraction of teeth, dental implants, osteotomy, and temporomandibular joint surgery.[5–9] Oral infection may also lead to septicemia.[10]

Infections in the dental environment may be spread by at least three methods:[11]

1. Direct contact with blood or body fluids;
2. Indirect contact with contaminated instruments or equipment; or
3. Droplet contact from body fluid splatter or aerosol.

Although the possibility of transmission of blood-borne infections from dental workers to patients is considered to be small,[12–15] precise risks have not been evaluated in the dental setting. Reports published from 1970 through 1987 note nine clusters in which patients were infected with HBV associated with treatment by infected dental workers.[16–25] In addition, transmission of human immunodeficiency virus (HIV) to six patients of a dentist with acquired immunodeficiency syndrome has been reported.[26–27] Transmission of HBV from dentists to patients has not been reported since 1987, possibly reflecting such factors as incomplete reporting, increased adherence to Standard Precautions, and increased use of hepatitis B vaccine. Epidemiological and laboratory data indicate that both HBV and HIV infections were probably transmitted from dental healthcare workers to patients rather than from one patient to another.[26, 28]

Pathways for potential contamination and infection in the dental arena include:[2, 29]

- Patient to dental team
- Dental team to patient
- Patient to patient through equipment
- Dental facility to community

DEVICES

A number of sources of contaminated aerosols exist in dental offices. Procedures and equipment include ultrasonic scaling and use of high-speed hand pieces.[30]

External and internal surfaces of high-speed hand pieces, low-speed hand-piece components, and prophylaxis angles may become contaminated with patient material during use. This retained patient material then may be expelled intraorally during subsequent uses.[31–33] Contamination of internal parts of a hand piece may originate from saliva or the air/water supply.[34]

Dental unit water lines (the plastic tubing that connects the high-speed hand piece, air/water syringe, and sonic and ultrasonic scaler to the water supply) have been shown to harbor a wide variety of microorganisms. These microbes colonize and replicate on the interior surfaces of the waterline tubing, resulting in adherent microbial accumulations termed "biofilms."[35] Units may be supplied with municipal water or from separate reservoirs with either distilled or sterile water. Elevated bacterial counts have been found in water from these systems.[36] The presence of potential human pathogens in the water is a concern. There is one report of infections in immunocompromised patients with exposure to dental-unit water.[37]

RISKS

There are multiple sources of microorganisms that can lead to contamination or infection. These include:[2]

- Exposure to blood, saliva, or other secretions during dental treatment procedures
- Indirect contact via contaminated instruments, hand pieces, equipment, or supplies
- Aerosolization of microbes in droplet splatter from patient's blood and/or saliva while using air/water sprays, or high-speed or ultrasonic equipment

Serologic surveys evaluating staff risks have indicated that 10 to 30% of healthcare or dental workers show evidence of past or present HBV infection, while infection in U.S. adults is only 1 to 2%.[38]

PREVENTION

A comprehensive infection prevention and control program should focus on the various methods of spread of microorganisms and prevention techniques.

Procedures

Use of Barrier Precautions and Hand Hygiene

- Use Standard Precautions for all patients (see Chapter 6).
- Hand hygiene
  - Hands must be washed routinely before and after treatment of each patient and after removal of gloves.[38–39]
  - For routine dental procedures, such as examinations and nonsurgical techniques, handwashing with plain soap is adequate. When hands are not visibly soiled, an alcohol-based hand rub may be used. For surgical procedures, an antimicrobial surgical hand scrub should be used[38–39] (see Chapter 5).
  - Dental health care workers who have exudative lesions or weeping dermatitis, particularly on the hands, should refrain from all direct patient care and from handling dental equipment until the condition resolves.[38]
- Gloves
  - Gloves are required when there is potential for contacting blood, blood-contaminated saliva, or mucous membranes.[40]
  - Clean gloves are appropriate for examinations and other nonsurgical procedures; sterile gloves should be used for surgical procedures.
  - Gloves must be changed between patients.
  - Gloves can become punctured during oral surgery procedures. Double-gloving during bone removal and soft tissue repair might be reasonable.[41]
  - Care must be taken to avoid touching clean surfaces with soiled, gloved hands that will later be touched with ungloved hands. Use a non-touch technique (e.g., transfer forceps) if necessary. Alternatively, another glove may be worn.[29]
  - Precut supplies (e.g., floss, cellulose acetate strips, gingival retraction cord, and articulating

paper) can reduce the need to remove gloves to obtain these items.

- Face shields or masks and protective eyewear should be worn when aerosols are likely to be generated. When a mask is used, it should be changed between patients or during patient treatment if it becomes moist. Face shields or protective eyewear should be washed with soap and water and disinfected between patients when visibly soiled.
- Protective clothing, such as reusable or disposable gowns, laboratory coats, or uniforms, should be worn when clothing is likely to be soiled with blood or other body fluids. Reusable protective clothing should be washed using a normal laundry cycle. Protective clothing should be changed at least daily or as soon as it becomes visibly soiled.
- Protective garments and devices (including gloves, masks, and eye and face protection) should be removed before personnel exit areas of the dental office used for laboratory or patient-care activities.
- Appropriate use of rubber dams, high-velocity air evacuation, and proper patient positioning can minimize the formation of aerosols during patient treatment.[2, 38] In addition, splash shields should be used in the dental laboratory.[38]
- Disposable airway equipment or resuscitation devices should be available for use.

Sharps

- Use protective devices (e.g., safety dental syringes/injectors) to minimize exposure to blood.[42]
- Sharp items (e.g., needles, scalpel blades, and wires) contaminated with blood or saliva should be considered as potentially infectious and handled with care to prevent injuries.[38]
- For procedures involving multiple injections with a single needle, the unsheathed needle should be placed where it will not become contaminated or contribute to unintentional needle sticks between injections. If it is necessary to recap a needle between injections, a one-handed "scoop" technique or a mechanical device designed to hold the needle sheath is recommended.[38]

- Disposable needles, scalpels, or other sharp items must be placed intact into puncture-resistant containers before disposal.

Patient-Care Equipment

(Also see Chapter 3 regarding this topic.)

- There should be a designated sink for instrument cleaning, separate from a handwashing sink.[29]
- Instruments[43]
  - Instruments should be placed into a presoak solution immediately after use to prevent drying of organic material.[1]
  - Surgical and other instruments used to penetrate soft tissue or bone should be sterilized or discarded after each use. These devices include forceps, scalpels, bone chisels, scalers, and surgical burs.[38, 44] Use only Food and Drug Administration-cleared medical devices for sterilization.
  - Items such as mirrors, air/water syringes, and amalgam condensers that do not penetrate soft tissues or bone but contact oral tissues should be high-level disinfected, at a minimum, after each use.[38, 44]
  - Instruments or medical devices such as external components of X-ray heads that come into contact only with intact skin may be cleaned between patients with intermediate- or low-level disinfection, depending on the nature of the surface and the degree and nature of the contamination.[38]
  - Specific information on instrument processing in dentistry is available on the Organization for Safety and Asepsis Procedures (OSAP) Web site at *http://www.osap.org/issues/pages/position/pp-ip.htm.*
- Routine between-patient use of sterilization is recommended for all high-speed dental hand pieces, low-speed hand-piece components used intraorally, and reusable prophylaxis angles. These devices have a number of moving parts and cracks and crevices that make them difficult to clean. Surface disinfection by wiping or soaking in liquid chemical germicides is not an acceptable method for reprocessing these items.[38]

- Hand pieces
  - High-speed hand pieces should be run to discharge water and air for a minimum of 20 to 30 seconds after use on each patient. This procedure is intended to aid in physically flushing out patient material that may have entered the turbine and air or water lines.[34] Use of an enclosed container or high-velocity evacuation should be considered to minimize the spread of aerosols generated during discharge procedures.
  - Thoroughly clean the internal and external surfaces of the hand piece. Sterilize according to manufacturer's directions.
  - Hand pieces that cannot be heat sterilized should be retrofitted to attain heat tolerance or not used.[44]
  - There is evidence that overnight or weekend microbial accumulation in water lines can be reduced substantially by removing the hand piece and allowing water lines to run and to discharge water for several minutes at the beginning of each clinic day.[45-46]
- Because retraction valves in dental unit water lines may cause aspiration of patient material back into the hand piece and water lines, anti-retraction valves (one-way flow check valves) may be installed to prevent fluid aspiration and to reduce the risk of transfer of potentially infectious material. Routine maintenance of anti-retraction valves is necessary to ensure effectiveness. This risk may not be an issue if up-to-date equipment is used.[47]
- Use water that meets standards set by the Environmental Protection Agency for drinking water (fewer than 500 colony-forming units/ml of heterotrophic water bacteria) for routine dental treatment.
- Sterile saline or sterile water should be used as a coolant/irrigator when surgical procedures involving the cutting of bone are performed. Discard any remaining solution.
- Other reusable intraoral instruments attached to, but removable from, the dental unit air or water lines—such as ultrasonic scaler tips and component parts and air/water syringe tips—should be cleaned and sterilized after treatment of each patient in the same manner as hand pieces.[38]
- Some dental instruments have components that are heat-sensitive or are permanently attached to dental unit water lines. Some items may not enter the patient's oral cavity; however, they are likely to become contaminated with oral fluids during treatment procedures (e.g., handles or dental unit attachments of saliva ejectors, high-speed air evacuators, and air/water syringes). These components should be covered with impervious barriers that are changed after each use or, if the surface permits, carefully cleaned and then treated with an intermediate-level disinfectant (see Chapter 3).
- Single-use disposable instruments (e.g., prophylaxis angles, prophylaxis cups and brushes, tips for high-speed air evacuators, saliva ejectors,[48] and air/water syringes) should be used for one patient only and then discarded.
- Radiography
  - Wear gloves when placing films in a patient's mouth.
  - Use disposable covers or disinfect positioning devices after use.[11, 49] Avoid contaminating the sleeves and external and internal components of the processor.[50]
  - Transport films in a paper cup or towel.
  - Open film packets with gloves. After all packets are opened, remove gloves so that darkroom equipment is not contaminated.[11]
- Laboratories
  - Dental laboratories should institute appropriate infection prevention and control programs. Such programs should be coordinated with the dental office.[45] Dental laboratories can be maintained as isolated areas and require all prostheses, impressions, and other laboratory work to be disinfected before entering the laboratory; or, the laboratory can have a receiving area to isolate, evaluate, and decontaminate all materials entering the laboratory.[51]
  - Laboratory materials and other items that have been used in the mouth (e.g., impressions, bite registrations, fixed and removable prostheses, and orthodontic appliances) should be cleaned and disinfected before being manipulated in the laboratory.[45, 52] These items also should be cleaned and disinfected after being manipulated in the dental laboratory and before placement in the patient's mouth. Because chemicals may damage some materials, review the manufacturer's instructions prior to disinfection.

- Items such as impressions, jaw relation records, casts, prosthetic restorations, and devices that have been in the patient's mouth should be properly disinfected prior to shipment to a dental laboratory.[45]
- A list of disinfectants can be found in Chapter 3.

Use of Medications and Multiple-Dose Vials (MDVs)

- When MDVs are used, individual patient doses should be prepared in a clean area.
- The diaphragm of MDVs should be wiped with alcohol prior to puncture.[53]
- Use a new sterile device for access to the medication vial.[53]
- If trays are used to distribute medications, they must be cleaned between patients.

Cleaning Environmental Surfaces

- If an item is visibly contaminated with blood, a low-level disinfectant should be used (see Chapter 3).
- Blood spills should be cleaned immediately with a cloth soaked in low-level disinfectant. After all visible blood is cleaned, a new cloth or towel should be used to apply disinfectant a second time.
- Countertops, chair switches, light handles, and dental unit surfaces that may have become contaminated with body fluids should be cleaned with disposable toweling using a cleaning product after each patient treatment. Surfaces then should be disinfected with a low-level disinfectant.[38] A product such as a quaternary ammonium compound may combine both cleaning and disinfecting agents.
- Impervious-backed paper, drapes, aluminum foil, or plastic covers should be used to protect items and surfaces (e.g., light handles, switches, or X-ray unit heads) that may become contaminated by blood or saliva during use and that are difficult or impossible to clean and disinfect. Between patients the coverings should be removed using gloves, discarded, and replaced (after ungloving and washing of hands) with clean material. The surfaces should be disinfected at the end of the day.[44]
- The most frequently contaminated surfaces in dental surgery include the aspirator tube, edge of the spittoon, ultrasonic scaler hand piece, and surgery work surface.[54] These areas need to be cleaned with a disinfectant after each patient.

Physical Space

There must be handwashing sinks conveniently available for staff. They can be placed in or adjacent to work areas. All areas must have surfaces that are easy to clean.

Dental unit water systems should be of suitable water quality.[35] It is important to control biofilm formation and resulting contamination;[36] the goal is less than 200 colony-forming units per milliliter.[2] Water lines to all instruments should be flushed thoroughly (for 20–30 seconds) after the treatment of each patient; flushing at the beginning of each clinic day for several minutes is also recommended.[11, 38] There are various products available to help improve the microbial quality of dental unit water.[55–56]

Waste Management

- Environmental services staff members in the dental facility should promptly remove trash and medical waste and maintain an environment that enhances patient care.
- Follow local requirements for handling regulated waste (e.g., items soaked with blood or body fluids).
- Blood, suctioned fluids, or other liquid waste may be poured carefully into a drain connected to a sanitary sewer system.

Evaluation and Management of Communicable Diseases

General—Communicable Diseases

Patients infected with bloodborne pathogens can be safely treated in the dental office using Standard Precautions.[57] Dental healthcare workers are at risk for exposure to and possible transmission of vaccine-preventable diseases. Vaccination against influenza, measles, mumps, rubella, chicken pox, and tetanus may be appropriate.[58]

Tuberculosis

A medical history for all new patients should be completed to evaluate for signs or symptoms of pulmonary tuberculosis.[1] All dental healthcare workers should have a tuberculin test at least annually. Determine the frequency based on a risk assessment.[59] Educate staff regarding the recognition of signs and symptoms and transmission risk of tuberculosis. Defer elective treatment until the patient is noninfectious.

Employee-Focused Prevention Techniques— Vaccination and Education

- Hepatitis B vaccination is recommended for all dental healthcare workers.[40]
- Appropriate annual infection prevention and control training is required for staff. This information should include procedures to minimize risks and proper sterilization/disinfection practices. Only two-thirds of respondents in one survey reported that they always used a combination of gloves, masks, and eye protection appropriately when treating patients.[60] Thus, education and compliance of staff are crucial components of infection prevention.
- Develop a policy outlining required and recommended immunizations, work restrictions and exclusions, and management of employees with known contact dermatitis.

SURVEILLANCE

An active surveillance system can assist with early detection of infectious complications.

Note: Draft Recommended Infection Control Practices for Dentistry were published for public comment by the Centers for Disease Control and Prevention on February 12, 2003.

References

1. Hamory, B. H. Nosocomial Infections in Dental, Oral, and Maxillofacial Surgery. In: Mayhall, C. G., ed. *Hospital Epidemiology and Infection Control*. Baltimore: Williams & Wilkins; 1996: 585–592.

2. Molinari, J. A. Dental. In: *APIC Text of Infection Control and Epidemiology*. Washington, DC: Association for Professionals in Infection Control and Epidemiology; 2000: 42:1–18.

3. Lewis, D. L., Arens, M., Appleton, S. S., Nakashima, K., Ryu, J., and Boe, R. K., et al. Cross-contamination potential with dental equipment. *Lancet.* 1992; 340:1252–1254.

4. Lewis, D. L., and Boe, R. K. Cross-infection risks associated with current procedures for using high-speed dental handpieces. *J Clin Microbiol.* 1992; 30: 401–406.

5. Osbourne, T. P., Frederickson, G., Small, I. A., and Torgerson, T. S. A prospective study of complications related to mandibular third molar surgery. *J Oral Maxillofac Surg.* 1985; 43:767–769.

6. Larsen, P. E. Role of antimicrobials for dentoalveolar surgery. *J Oral Maxillofac Surg.* 1993; 51(Suppl 3):155.

7. Larsen, P. E. Antibiotic prophylaxis for placement of dental implants. *J Oral Maxillofac Surg.* 1993; 51(Suppl 3):194.

8. Dingaman, R. O., Dingaman, D. L., and Lawrence, D. A. Surgical correction of lesions in the temporomandibular joint. *Plastic Reconstruct Surg.* 1978; 55:335.

9. Tarro, A. W. Arthroscopic treatment of anterior disc displacement: A preliminary report. *J Oral Maxillofac Surg.* 1989; 47:353.

10. Bergmann, O. J. Oral infections and septicemia in immunocompromised patients with hematologic malignacies. *J Clin Microbiol.* 1988; 26:2105–2109.

11. Terezhalmy, G. T., and Gitto, C. A. Today's minimal requirements for a practical dental office infection control and exposure control program. *Dental Clin North Am.* 1998; 42:629–642.

12. CDC. Recommendations for preventing transmission of human immunodeficiency virus and hepatitis B virus during exposure-prone invasive procedures. *MMWR.* 1991; 40(No. RR-8):1–9.

13. CDC. Update: Investigations of patients who have been treated by HIV-infected health-care workers. *MMWR.* 1992; 41:344–346.

14. Chamberland, M. E., and Bell, D. M. HIV transmission from health care worker to patient: What is the risk? *Ann Intern Med.* 1992; 116:871–873.

15. Siew, C., Chang, B., Gruninger, S. E., Verrusio, A. C., and Neidle, E. A. Self-reported percutaneous injuries in dentists: Implications for HBV, HIV transmission risk. *J Am Dent Assoc.* 1992; 123:37–44.

16. Ahtone, J., and Goodman, R. A. Hepatitis B and dental personnel: Transmission to patients and prevention issues. *J Am Dent Assoc.* 1983; 106:219–222.

17. Hadler, S. C., Sorley, D. L., Acree, K. H., Webster, H. M., Schable, C. A., Francis, D. P., and Maynard, J. E. An outbreak of hepatitis B in a dental practice. *Ann Intern Med.* 1981; 5:133–138.

18. CDC. Hepatitis B among dental patients—Indiana. *MMWR.* 1985; 34:73–75.

19. Levin, M. L., Maddrey, W. C., Wands, J. R., and Mendeloff, A. L. Hepatitis B transmission by dentists. *JAMA.* 1974; 228:1139–40.

20. Rimland, D., Parkin, W. E, Miller, G. B., and Schrack, W. D. Hepatitis B outbreak traced to an oral surgeon. *N Engl J Med.* 1977; 296:953–958.

21. Goodwin, D., Fannin, S. L., and McCracken, B. B. An oral surgeon-related hepatitis B outbreak. *Calif Morbid.* 1976; 14.

22. Reingold, A. L., Kane, M. A., Murphy, E. L., Checko, P., Francis, D. P., and Maynard, J. E. Transmission of hepatitis B by an oral surgeon. *J Infect Dis.* 1982; 145:262–268.

23. Goodman, R. A., Ahtone, J. L., and Finton, R. J. Hepatitis B transmission from dental personnel to patients: Unfinished business. *Ann Intern Med.* 1982; 96:119.

24. Shaw, F. E., Barrett, C. L., Hamm, R., Peare, R. B., Coleman, P. J., and Hadler, S. C., et al. Lethal outbreak of hepatitis B in a dental practice. *JAMA.* 1986; 255:3261–3264.

25. CDC. Outbreak of hepatitis B associated with an oral surgeon, New Hampshire. *MMWR.* 1987; 36:132–3.

26. Ciesielski, C., Marianos, D., Ou, C. Y., Dumbaugh, R., Witte, J., and Berkelman, R., et al. Transmission of human immunodeficiency virus in a dental practice. *Ann Intern Med.* 1992; 116:798–805.

27. CDC. Investigations of persons treated by HIV-infected health-care workers—United States. *MMWR.* 1993; 42:329–31, 337.

28. Gooch, B., Marianos, D., Ciesielski, C., Dumbaugh, R., Lasch, A., and Jaffe, H., et al. Lack of evidence for patient-to-patient transmission of HIV in a dental practice. *J Am Dent Assoc.* 1993; 124:38–44.

29. Palenik, C. J., Burke, F. J. T., and Miller, C. H. Strategies for dental clinic infection control. *Dental Update.* 2000; 27:7–15.

30. Leggat, P. A., and Kedjarune, U. Bacterial aerosols in the dental clinic: A review. *Intern Dental J.* 2001; 51:39–44.

31. Lewis, D. L., and Boe, R. K. Cross infection risks associated with current procedures for using high-speed dental handpieces. *J Clin Microbiol.* 1992; 30:401–406.

32. Crawford, J. J., and Broderius, R. K. Control of cross infection risks in the dental operatory: Prevention of water retraction by bur cooling spray systems. *J Am Dent Assoc.* 1988; 116:685–687.

33. Lewis, D. L., Arens, M., Appleton, S. S., Nakashima, K., Ryu, J., and Boe, R. K., et al. Cross-contamination potential with dental equipment. *Lancet.* 1992; 340:1252–1254.

34. Larsen, T., Andersen, H. K., and Fiehn, N. E. Evaluation of a new device for sterilizing dental high-speed handpieces. *Oral Surg Oral Med Oral Pathol Oral Radiol Endodont.* 1997; 84:513–516.

35. ADA Statement on Dental Unit Waterlines. Chicago: American Dental Association. 1995. *http://www.ada.org/prof/prac/issues/statements/lines.html.*

36. Donlan, R. M., and Costerton, J. W. Biofilms: Survival mechanisms of clinically relevant microorganisms. *Clin Micro Rev.* 2003; 15:167–193.

37. Martin, M. V. The significance of the bacterial contamination of dental unit water systems. *Br Dent J.* 1987; 163:152–153.

38. Centers for Disease Control and Prevention. Recommended infection-control practices for dentistry, 1993. *MMWR.* 1993; 42 (RR-8): 1–12.

39. Centers for Disease Control and Prevention. Guideline for hand hygiene in health-care settings: Recommendations of the Healthcare Infection Control Practices Advisory Committee and the HICPAC/SHEA/APIC/IDSA Hand Hygiene Task Force. *MMWR.* 2002; 51 (No. RR-16):1–44.

40. Department of Labor, Occupational Safety and Health Administration. 29 CFR Part 1910.1030, Occupational exposure to bloodborne pathogens: Final rule. *Fed Reg.* 1991; 56:64004–64182.

41. Burke, F. J. T., Baggett, F. J., and Lomax, A. M. Assessment of the risk of glove puncture during oral surgery procedures. *Oral Surg Oral Med Oral Pathol Oral Radiol Endodont.* 1996; 82:18–21.

42. Occupational Exposure to Bloodborne Pathogens; Needlestick and Other Sharps Injuries: Final Rule. *Fed Reg.* 2001; 66:5317–5325.

43. Palenik, C. J. Dental instrument sterilization: A six-step process, CDE. *J Contemp Dent Pract.* (Electronic Resource) 2001; 2:84.

44. Rutala, W. A. APIC Guideline for selection and use of disinfectants. *Am J Infect Control.* 1996; 24:313–342.

45. ADA. Infection Control Recommendations for the Dental Office and the Dental Laboratory. Chicago: American Dental Association. *http://www.ada.org/prof/prac/issues/topics/icontrol/ic-recs/index.html.*

46. Scheid, R. C., Kim, C. K., Bright, J. S., Whitely, M. S., and Rosen, S. Reduction of microbes in handpieces by flushing before use. *J Am Dent Assoc.* 1982; 105:658–660.

47. ADA Statement on Backflow Prevention and the Dental Office. Chicago: American Dental Association, 1996. *http://www.ada.org/prof/prac/issues/statements/backflow.html.*

48. ADA Statement on Saliva Ejectors. Chicago: American Dental Association, 2000. *http://www.ada.org/prof/prac/issues/statements/saliva.html.*

49. Hubar, J. S., and Gardiner, D. M. Infection control procedures used in conjunction with computed dental radiography. *Int J Computerized Dentistry.* 2000; 3:259–267.

50. OSAP Research Foundation. Infection Control in Dentistry Guidelines, September 1997, Annapolis, MD: Office Safety & Asepsis Procedures. *http://www.osap.org/resources/IC/icguide.pdf.*

51. OSAP Position Paper: Laboratory Asepsis: November 1998. Annapolis, MD: Organization for Safety & Asepsis Procedures. *http://www.osap.org/issues/pages/position/LAB.htm.*

52. Council on Dental Materials, Instruments, and Equipment; Dental Practice; and Dental Therapeutics. American Dental Association. Infection control recommendations for the dental office and the dental laboratory. *J Am Dent Assoc.* 1988; 1126:241–248.

53. Centers for Disease Control and Prevention. Guidelines for the prevention of intravascular catheter-related infections. *MMWR.* 2002; 51(No. RR-10):1–32.

54. Edmunds, L. M., and Rawlinson, A. The effect of cleaning on blood contamination in the dental surgery following periodontal procedures. *Aust Dental J.* 1998; 43:349–353.

55. Lee, T. K., Waked, E. J., Wolinsky, L. E., Mito, R. S., and Danielson, R. E. Controlling biofilm and microbial contamination in dental unit waterlines. *J Calif Dent Assoc.* 2001; 29:679–684.

56. Pederson, E. D., Stone, M. E., Ragain, J. C., Jr., and Simecek, J. W. Waterline biofilm and the dental treatment facility: A review. *Gen Dentistry.* 2002; 50:190–195.

57. ADA Policy Statement on Bloodborne Pathogens, Infection Control and the Practice of Dentistry. Chicago: American Dental Association, 1999. *http://www.ada.org/prof/prac/issues/statements/blood.html.*

58. Centers for Disease Control and Prevention. Immunization of health-care workers: Recommendations of the Advisory Committee on Immunization Practices (ACIP) and the Hospital Infection Control Practices Advisory Committee (HICPAC). *MMWR.* 1997; 46 (No. RR-18):1–42.

59. Centers for Disease Control and Prevention: Guidelines for preventing the transmission of *Mycobacterium tuberculosis* in health-care facilities,1994. *MMWR.* 1994; 43(RR-13):i–v, 1–132.

60. McCarthy, G. M., and MacDonald, J. K. A comparison of infection control practices of different groups of oral specialists and general dental practitioners. *Oral Surg Oral Med Oral Pathol Oral Radiol Endodont.* 1998; 85:47–54.

CHAPTER 13

Dialysis

BACKGROUND

Peritoneal dialysis (PD) and hemodialysis (HD) are treatment modalities for individuals with chronic renal failure or end stage renal disease. The procedures mimic kidney function by removing metabolic waste products and fluid. A balanced electrolyte solution (dialysate) is introduced on one side of a semipermeable membrane and blood flows on the other side. Waste solutes are removed from the blood into the dialysate by diffusing down a concentration gradient, by movement of solutes and fluid through convective transport and/or by movement from introduced pressures. Peritoneal dialysis uses the peritoneum as the semipermeable membrane and the peritoneal capillary bed as bloodstream access; hemodialysis uses an artificial membrane or dialyzer kidney and vascular access to the bloodstream.[1-2]

Different types of equipment are used to perform HD; however, all have similar basic components, including a purified water system, dialysate concentrate, a dialyzer, a circulation apparatus, and access to the patient's blood.[3] The PD system for exchanging dialysate may include an automated cycling machine and/or intermittent gravity-feed, with connection to a surgically implanted catheter in the patient's peritoneal cavity. Peritoneal renal treatment modalities are used by approximately 15% of dialysis patients in the United States.[4]

Approximately 70% of chronic dialysis procedures occur in freestanding centers in the United States. Hemodialysis centers are potentially hazardous settings for both patients and staff. Chronic HD patients are at high risk for infection because the process of hemodialysis requires vascular access for prolonged periods, blood is circulated through dialyzers that may be reprocessed for reuse, and there is potential exposure to nonsterile dialysate.[3, 5]

Bacterial infections, especially those involving vascular access, are the most frequent infectious complication of HD.[6] In 1999, the Centers for Disease Control and Prevention (CDC) initiated a surveillance system for bloodstream and vascular access infections in outpatient centers.[7] In the 1990s, the prevalence of antibiotic-resistant bacteria, such as methicillin-resistant *Staphylococcus aureus* (MRSA) and vancomycin-resistant enterococci (VRE), increased in dialysis units.[8] Pyrogenic reactions and gram-negative sepsis are the most common complications associated with contaminated dialysis fluid.[8-9] Because of the potential exposure to blood in the environment of these units, there is also a risk of bloodborne pathogen transmission for both patients and staff.[10-11]

In 1972, the CDC began conducting surveillance for dialysis-associated hepatitis. Other hemodialysis-associated diseases were included over the years, including pyrogenic reactions and vascular access infections.[8] The National Kidney Foundation (*www.kidney.org*) has published clinical practice guidelines on various topics (e.g., vascular access) and has an associated Kidney Disease Outcomes Quality Initiative (KDOQI) (*http://www.kidney.org/professionals/doqi/index.cfm*). In the KDOQI guideline section on infection rates, the goal is <10% risk of infection for life use of fistulae and grafts. The current data indicate a rate of 1 to 4% for fistulae and 11 to 20% for grafts. The goal for tunneled catheters is <10% at three months and <50% at one year.[12]

97

Recommendations for the control of hepatitis B in hemodialysis centers were first published in 1977.[13] A recent update focuses on preventing infections in chronic dialysis patients.[5] Measures include the use of Standard Precautions and additional practices specific to the dialysis setting. Specific information is outlined in the prevention section of this chapter.

CAUSES OF INFECTION

Infectious complications for patients include infection of the access site or of the bloodstream.[6, 8, 11] Dialysis staff is at risk for exposure to blood, especially through needle-stick injuries.[14] Communicable diseases of concern include bloodborne pathogens, such as hepatitis B, C, D, or G and human immunodeficiency virus (HIV), tuberculosis, and influenza.[15–20]

The mechanisms of infection for hemodialysis include:[21]

- Contamination or inadequate disinfection of dialyzers during processing[22–27]
- Leaks in the dialyzer membrane[28–30]
- Contamination of priming saline or dialysate[21, 31–35]
- Inadequate aseptic technique, access site preparation, and environmental contamination[36–47]
- Causative microbe found in treated water or dialysate[48–54]

Peritoneal dialysis infections are associated with maintenance and use of the access site and contamination of dialysis fluid. During the exchange process there is a high potential for infection.[1] Peritonitis is the most common complication, with rates of infections that vary between 0 and 2%.[55] Patients on PD may also develop an exit-site infection with or without sinus tract involvement. The total healing time for a freshly implanted catheter is approximately six weeks; infection risk is greater during this period.[56] Patients acquire most of these infections from their endogenous microorganisms.[57]

DEVICES

A typical hemodialysis system consists of a water supply, a system for mixing water and concentrated dialysis fluid, and a machine to pump dialysis fluid through the dialyzer. Purified water is created using a combination of reverse osmosis and/or deionization systems, filters, and tanks. The main components of dialysis are also the risk factors for infection and other complications. They include:

- Access to the bloodstream
- Dialyzer (the semipermeable membrane)
- Dialysate (purified water with chemicals added)

Hemodialysis access types include:

- Vascular access (temporary if < 3 weeks is anticipated or cuffed for ≥3 weeks)
- Native arteriovenous fistula
- Synthetic arteriovenous graft

Typically, the type of peritoneal dialysis used today is chronic ambulatory peritoneal dialysis (CAPD), continuous-cyclical peritoneal dialysis (CCPD), or chronic intermittent peritoneal dialysis (CIPD). CAPD can be self-administered by the patient. All PD patients will have a surgically implanted catheter through which dialysis is performed.

RISKS

In a dialysis center there is opportunity for spread of microbes through contaminated devices, equipment and supplies, environmental surfaces, or hands of personnel. Various issues related to access for dialysis affect the potential for infection. These include duration of catheterization, the type of fistula or graft, the type of dressing, the number of needle-access events, movement of the site, and personal hygiene of the patient.[4, 58] Infection rates have been shown to be highest among temporary catheters and lowest among permanent native arteriovenous fistulae or synthetic grafts.[59–62] Rates for bacteremia per 1000 days range from 0.07 to 0.09 for arteriovenous fistulae, 0.15 to 0.23 for grafts, 1.3 to 2.4 for tunneled catheters, and 2.2 to 4.5 for nontunneled catheters.[61, 63–64]

An increase in the reuse of dialyzers was aided by the development of automated reprocessing machines so that by 1996, 81% of chronic hemodialysis centers reprocessed dialyzers.[65–66] Dialyzer reuse improves biocompatibility, decreases "first use syndrome," and is cost-effective. However, there will be a decline in function and performance of the dialyzer over time and an increased risk of infection or pyrogenic reaction.

Microorganisms, especially Gram-negative bacteria, commonly are found in water used for hemodialysis. Therefore, water used for the production of dialysis fluid must be treated to remove microbial contaminants.[11]

Bloodborne pathogens, including hepatitis B, hepatitis C, and HIV, have been transmitted in hemodialysis centers. The risk for hepatitis B has decreased dramatically over the past 20 years, primarily due to the adoption of Standard Precautions and use of hepatitis B vaccine.[67] However, the risk for hepatitis C has increased during this period. The prevalence of hepatitis C virus in one study of dialysis patients[8] was 9.3%, whereas only 1.8% infection was noted in the U.S. population.[68] The risk of bloodborne virus spread can be high if proper infection prevention and control measures are not practiced.

PREVENTION

Environmental prevention techniques focus on the design and maintenance of dialysis systems, treated water, and dialysate and dialyzer reprocessing. Patient-focused prevention techniques include care of the access site (including access technique), aseptic procedures (e.g., dressing changes, initiation and discontinuation, blood drawing), and evaluation and management of communicable diseases. Employee-focused prevention techniques include vaccination, handwashing, appropriate use of personal protective equipment, competencies, and education.

Care and Maintenance of Dialysis Systems

- The total dialysis system, including water treatment system, distribution system, and dialysis machine, needs to be included in the disinfection process. Manufacturer's recommendations must be followed.
- Water storage tanks, if used, should be drained, cleaned (including scrubbing the sides of the tank to remove bacterial biofilm), and disinfected frequently.[11]
- For single-pass machines, perform rinsing and disinfection procedures daily. The disinfectant must reach all parts of the system's fluid pathways.[4]
- For batch recirculating machines, drain, rinse, and disinfect machines after each use.[5]
- Chlorine-based disinfectants (e.g., sodium hypochlorite solutions) are convenient and effective when used before the start of hemodialysis. Chlorine products cannot be left in a machine because of corrosion issues. Formaldehyde, peracetic acid, or glutaradehyde may be used if disinfection occurs at the end of the day.[4] These products are not as corrosive; however, there are environmental or toxicity concerns related to their use. Testing to assure chemical removal by flushing post-disinfection should be performed and documented. Some dialysis systems use water heated to 80°C (176°F) for disinfection. If hot water disinfection is used, weekly treatment with sodium hypochlorite to remove build-up may be necessary per the dialysis machine manufacturer's instructions.[11]
- External venous and arterial pressure transducer filters/protectors should be used for each patient treatment to prevent blood contamination of the dialysis machine's pressure monitors. The filters/protectors are to be changed between each patient treatment and not reused.[5, 11]
- If the external transducer protector becomes wet, it should be replaced immediately. If fluid is visible on the side of the transducer protector that faces the machine, open the machine after the treatment is completed and check for contamination. If contamination has occurred, the machine must be taken out of service and disinfected using either 1:100 dilution of bleach or a comparable disinfectant before reuse.[5]
- Internal transducer filters do not need to be changed routinely between patients.

Treated Water and Dialysate

- Routine bacteriologic assays of water, dialysis fluids, and reuse water should be performed at least monthly according to the recommendations of the Association for the Advancement of Medical Instrumentation (AAMI)[69] (see Table 13.1).

Table 13.1 AAMI Microbiologic and Endotoxin Standards

Source	Acceptable Level
Dialysate	<2,000 CFU/ml
Water used to prepare dialysate	<200 CFU/ml
Water used to rinse and reprocess dialyzer	<200 CFU/ml or 1ng/ml (5 EU/ml)*
Water used to prepare dialyzer disinfectant	<200 CFU/ml or 1ng/ml (5 EU/ml)*

*Endotoxin units/milliliter

AAMI: Association for the Advancement of Medical Instrumentation

CFU: Colony-forming units

- Water samples should be collected at the point where water enters the dialysate concentrate-proportioning unit.[11]
- Dialysis fluid samples should be taken from the entry or exit point of the dialyzer during or at termination of dialysis.
- If acceptable levels are exceeded, disinfection of the water system must occur and repeat samples taken prior to use.
- Containers used to mix bicarbonate concentrate should be cleaned and disinfected routinely.[70]
- Concentrate should be nonpyrogenic.
- There should be written procedures outlining all the testing procedures and methods, a description of activities performed if contamination levels are exceeded, and how documentation and records are maintained.[11]

Dialyzer Reprocessing

In 1987, the U.S. Public Health Service adopted AAMI's guidelines for reusing dialyzers[69] and recommended them to the Centers for Medicare & Medicaid Services (formerly known as the Health Care Financing Administration). These guidelines are conditions of participation in Medicare/Medicaid (Chapter 42 of the Code of Federal Regulations, Part 405.2150).[4] There may also be state regulations associated with dialyzer reprocessing.

General guidelines are as follows:

- There should be written protocols detailing processing procedures.[71]
- For dialyzers and blood tubing that will be reprocessed, the dialyzer ports should be capped and all tubing should be clamped for transport to the reprocessing area. Caps may be either new or disinfected.[69]
- All used dialyzers and tubing should be placed in leak-resistant containers for transport from the dialysis station to the reprocessing or disposal area.[5]
- It is important to clean, rinse, and do a performance check and leak test of dialyzers between uses.[4]
- There must be a system to label and track dialyzers to ensure that each is dedicated for single-patient use.
- High-level disinfection must be used following AAMI recommendations. Disinfectants may include formaldehyde, glutaraldehyde, or paracetic acid/hydrogen peroxide. If 4% formaldehyde is used, the contact time is at least 24 hours.[69]
- Disinfectant must be rinsed from the dialyzer to below toxic levels. Perform testing to confirm.[69]
- The reprocessing procedure must include a protocol to discard dialyzers when the maximum number of reprocessing cycles is reached or for leak test failure, whichever comes first.
- The reprocessing room should be set up so that work flow progresses from dirty to clean.
- There must be a dedicated storage area for reprocessed dialyzers that protects them from contamination (e.g., dust, splashes).

Insertion of Hemodialysis Catheters[72]

- Use a cuffed central venous catheter if the period of temporary access is anticipated to be longer than three weeks.
- Use aseptic technique, including use of a cap, mask, sterile gown and gloves, and a large sterile sheet during insertion.

Care of the Access Site[72]

- Patients with poor personal hygiene habits should be taught how to improve and maintain their personal hygiene.
- Clean technique should be used for all needle cannulation procedures. Hands must be washed prior to cannulation.
- An antimicrobial product (e.g., 2% chlorhexidine or povidone iodine) should be used to clean the access site.[12]
- Replace catheter-site dressing when the dressing becomes damp, loosened, or soiled. Routinely change the dressing every two days for gauze and at least every seven days for transparent dressings.
- Apply povidone-iodine ointment to the catheter exit site at the end of each dialysis session. For patients with an allergy to iodine, alternate agents, such as polyantimicrobial gel, can be substituted. These agents must have activity against *S. aureus*, the most common microbe involved in infections in these patients. Catheter material, such as polyurethane, may be damaged by alcohol or oils; check the manufacturer's recommendations regarding compatible agents.
- Minimize manipulation of the catheter to prevent contamination.
- Do not use intravascular catheters for applications other than hemodialysis except during dialysis itself or under emergency conditions.

Aseptic Procedures

Use of Barrier Precautions and Hand Hygiene

- Use Standard Precautions for all patients (see Chapter 6).
- Hands must be washed routinely before and after patient care, especially if visibly soiled. If hands are not visibly soiled, use of an alcohol-based hand rub is recommended.[5, 73]
- Gloves are required whenever caring for a patient or when touching the dialysis equipment and accessories, such as when handling machine control panels. Gloves must be used when drawing blood.[74]
- Gloves must be changed between patients and stations.

- Care must be taken to avoid touching surfaces with gloved hands that will later be touched with ungloved hands.
- Healthcare workers (HCW) must wear gowns and face protection when performing procedures during which spurting or spattering of blood might occur, such as initiation and termination of dialysis and cleaning of dialyzers.[5, 74]
- To prevent mucous membrane contact during resuscitation, a mouth-bag or mouth-mask device should be kept in each examination and procedure room or in a crash cart.

Initiation and Discontinuation[12]

- During initiation and disconnection procedures and dressing changes, staff should wear eye/face protection.[70] Staff should wear clean gloves during all connect and disconnect procedures.
- The catheter hub caps or bloodline connectors should be soaked for three to five minutes in iodophor[1] and then allowed to dry prior to separation. To prevent contamination, the lumen and tip should never remain open to the air. A cap or syringe should be placed on or within the catheter lumen, while maintaining a clean field under the catheter connectors.
- Extracorporeal circuits should not be prepared more than two hours before initiation of therapy.[70]

Patient-Care Equipment

- Items taken into the dialysis area should be disposable, dedicated for use on only a single patient, or cleaned and disinfected before being taken to a common clean area or used on another patient.[5]
- Nondisposable items that cannot be cleaned and disinfected (e.g., adhesive tape, cloth-covered blood pressure cuffs) should be dedicated for use only on a single patient.
- If a common cart is used for supplies, it should not be taken into patient treatment areas.[5]

---

1. *Author's Note:* Iodophors such as povidone iodine are antiseptics, designed to be used on skin. However, all official recommendations outlining dialysis procedures describe its use as a disinfectant in the manner described.

Use of Medications and Multiple-Dose Vials (MDVs) and Supplies[5, 11]

- When MDVs are used, individual patient doses should be prepared in a clean area away from dialysis areas.
- The access diaphragm of MDVs should be wiped with alcohol prior to puncture.[72]
- MDVs should not be carried from station to station.
- Unused medications or supplies (e.g., syringes, alcohol swabs) taken to a patient's dialysis area should not be returned to a common area or used on another patient.
- Medication carts should not be used to deliver medications to patients.
- If trays are used to distribute medications, they must be cleaned between patients.
- Medications and supplies should not be carried in healthcare workers' pockets.

Sharp Items

There must be a procedure to safely handle contaminated sharp items and minimize percutaneous and skin or mucous membrane exposure.[75] These procedures include various practices such as the following:

- Do not recap needles.
- Sharps containers should be conveniently located.
- Evaluate and use, as appropriate, devices to prevent exposures. These include safety needles/syringes, guarded needles,[76] and safety medication fill needles.

Cleaning Environmental Surfaces[5]

- After each patient treatment, environmental surfaces (e.g., the dialysis bed or chair, countertops, and external surfaces of the dialysis machine including panels and containers associated with the prime waste) should be cleaned and disinfected. Special attention should be given to cleaning control panels on the dialysis machines and other surfaces that are frequently touched and potentially contaminated with patient blood.

- A low-level disinfectant may be used for cleaning. Check local and state regulations for any special requirements. See Chapter 3 for additional information.
- Medical equipment (e.g., hemostats, clamps, blood pressure cuffs, and stethoscopes) should be disinfected with a low-level disinfectant between uses. The item should be cleaned first. Blood pressure cuffs and stethoscopes may be wiped with a disinfectant-soaked cloth.
- If an item is visibly contaminated with blood, bleach at 1:100 dilution (500 ppm) or an intermediate-level disinfectant should be used.
- Blood spills should immediately be cleaned with a cloth soaked in a 1:100 dilution of household bleach or an intermediate-level disinfectant. After all visible blood is cleaned, a new cloth or towel should be used to apply disinfectant a second time.
- Allow disinfectant to remain wet on all surfaces for the time recommended by the manufacturer. Allow bleach to dry and then rinse with water.
- Discard all priming fluid.[11]

Peritoneal Dialysis

- Perform aseptic manipulation of the sterile disposable lines that deliver dialysis fluid into the peritoneal cavity for peritoneal dialysis and aseptic connection of the tubing to the patient's catheter.
- Wear gloves whenever there is any potential contact with dialysis effluent, during exit-site care, and when drawing blood or taking dialysate samples. Wear gloves, gown, and face shield when disposing of the effluent.[70]
- Cleanse the catheter exit site during the post-insertion period with an antiseptic agent. A general cleansing agent may be used for chronic care.[77] Cleanse beginning at the catheter site and moving outward in a circular motion.
- Gentle care when cleansing, handling the catheter, and changing the dressing is recommended for sites less than six weeks post-insertion.[56]
- Stabilize and secure the catheter to reduce friction.

- Dressings help to keep the exit site clean and immobilize the catheter. Non-occlusive gauze dressings are recommended.[78]
- Peritoneal effluent should be considered potentially infectious for bloodborne pathogens.
- Cleanse the catheter prior to connecting it to dialysate and connections (e.g., catheter adapter/transfer set).
- Use a twin-bag system and/or a Y-connector system to minimize contamination during connections.[78]

Waste and Specimen Management[5]

- Environmental services staff members in the dialysis facility should keep the area clean and promptly remove potentially infectious waste to maintain an environment that enhances patient care.
- All disposable items should be placed in bags thick enough to prevent leakage or in leak-resistant containers.
- Waste generated from a hemodialysis facility should be considered potentially infectious and handled according to local and state regulations governing medical waste disposal. It must be placed in appropriately constructed and labeled receptacles (e.g., sharps disposal boxes and outer shipping containers).
- No special precautions for laboratory specimens are required beyond a leak-resistant container.

- Label transport containers with a standard biohazard symbol.

Evaluation and Management of Communicable Diseases

- Tests for hepatitis B surface antigen (HBsAg), total hepatitis B core antibody (anti-HBc), and hepatitis B surface antibody (anti-HBs) should be obtained on all patients before admission to the hemodialysis center (see Table 13.2).
- If a patient's hepatitis B virus (HBV) serologic status is not known at the time of admission, testing should be completed within seven days. Until the status is known, the patient should be managed as though he or she is a hepatitis carrier.[79]
- For transferred patients, HBV test results should be obtained before the patient is transferred.
- Testing for hepatitis C virus (HCV) infection should be obtained on all patients before admission to the hemodialysis center.
- Routine HCV testing should include use of both an enzyme immunoassay (EIA) and supplemental or confirmatory testing with an additional, more specific assay (e.g., recombinant immunoblot assay).
- Baseline alanine aminotransferase (ALT) level should be obtained at the time of baseline HCV-antibody testing.
- Polymerase chain reaction (PCR) testing for HCV ribonucleic acid (RNA) is not recommended as

Table 13.2 Schedule for Routine Testing for Hepatitis B Virus (HBV) and Hepatitis C Virus (HCV) in Dialysis Units[5]

Patient Status	On Admission	Monthly	Semiannual	Yearly
All patients	HBsAg; anti-HBc, anti-HBs; anti-HCV, ALT			
HBV-susceptible		HBsAg		
Anti-HBs positive *and* anti-HBc negative				anti-HBs
Anti-HBs *and* anti-HBc positive		No HBV testing is needed		
Anti-HCV negative		ALT	anti-HCV	

ALT: Alanine aminotransferase

HBsAg: Hepatitis B surface antigen

Anti-HBc: Antibody to hepatitis B core antigen

Anti-HBs: Antibody to hepatitis B surface antigen

Anti-HCV: Antibody to hepatitis C

the primary test for routine screening because few HCV infections will be identified in HCV antibody–negative patients. However, if ALT levels are persistently abnormal in patients who are HCV antibody–negative in the absence of another etiology, testing for HCV RNA should be considered.

- Routine HIV testing for the purposes of infection prevention and control is not recommended.[5]
- Patients with chronic renal failure have an increased risk of developing tuberculosis (TB). Therefore, prior to admission there should be a facility/community risk assessment for TB and consideration for two-step baseline skin testing of patients using the Mantoux TB test.[80]
- Patients should be educated regarding participation in their care including treatment compliance (e.g., site care, diet, medications, hygiene) and reporting of signs/symptoms of infection or disease.

Use of Hepatitis B Vaccine

- All susceptible chronic hemodialysis patients should receive hepatitis B vaccine.
- Vaccination also is recommended for all patients receiving peritoneal or home dialysis, because such patients may require in-house dialysis at some point.
- If an adult predialysis patient begins the vaccine series with a standard dose but does not finish the series before moving to hemodialysis, the series should be completed using a higher dose.[5]
- If the vaccination series is interrupted after the first dose, the second dose should be administered as soon as possible.
- If the third dose is delayed, it may be administered when convenient.
- Refer to the manufacturer's recommendation for dosing.

Postvaccination Testing for HBV

- All vaccinated individuals should be tested for anti-HBs one to two months after completing the vaccination series.
- Adequate response is defined as 10 mIU/ml or more.
- Patients who do not respond to the primary series should receive a second three-dose series and then be retested for anti-HBs.

- Patients who do not respond to the second series should be considered susceptible to hepatitis B and not be given further doses of vaccine.
- Patients who respond to the vaccine should be tested annually for anti-HBs; if antibody levels decline to less than 10 mIU/ml, a booster dose of vaccine should be given. Retesting after the booster dose is not necessary (although annual testing should be continued).

Other Patient Immunizations

Patients should be evaluated for and encouraged to participate in vaccination against pneumococcus, influenza, and other pertinent communicable diseases.

Isolation Precautions

HBV Infection[5]

Patients who are HBsAg-positive are considered infectious for HBV. The following isolation precautions are recommended:

- A separate room should be provided for treatment.
- Machines, equipment, instruments, supplies, and medications should be dedicated.
- Staff members caring for HBsAg-positive patients should not care for susceptible patients at the same time, including during the period when dialysis is terminated on one patient and initiated on another.
- If the facility cannot provide separate rooms, HBsAg-positive patients should be separated from HBV-susceptible patients in an area removed from the mainstream of activity and should undergo dialysis on dedicated machines.[81] Alternatively, HBV-immune patients may undergo dialysis in the same area as HBsAg-positive patients, or immune patients may serve as a geographic buffer between HBsAg-positive and HBV-susceptible patients.
- Dialyzers should not be reused on HBsAg-positive patients to eliminate risk of transmission of HBV during reprocessing.
- Consideration should be given to separating HBsAg-negative and delta-positive patients from HBsAg-positive and delta-negative patients.[20]

HCV Infection[5]

- Patients who are anti-HCV–positive (or HCV RNA–positive) do not have to be isolated from other patients or dialyzed separately on dedicated machines.
- Anti-HCV–positive patients may participate in dialyzer reuse programs.
- If more than one patient seroconverts to anti-HCV during a six-month period, more frequent testing of anti-HCV–negative patients is warranted (i.e., every one to three months instead of every six months). If ongoing HCV infection is documented, an investigation should be conducted to identify potential sources of transmission.

HIV Infection[5]

- HIV-infected patients do not have to be isolated from other patients or dialyzed separately on dedicated machines.
- HIV-infected patients may participate in dialyzer reuse programs.

Antibiotic-Resistant Microorganisms

- In 1997, the prevalence of vancomycin-resistant enterococci (VRE) in dialysis patients ranged from 1 to 8% in one study.[82]
- Vancomycin-intermediate *S. aureus* was identified in a patient on long-term ambulatory peritoneal dialysis. The first clinical isolate of *S. aureus* that is fully resistant to vancomycin was identified in a dialysis patient in 2002. Widespread use of antimicrobials, such as vancomycin, is a major contributing factor for the emergence of vancomycin-resistant microorganisms, including VRE.[83–85]
- The potential for environmental contamination is greater in hospitalized dialysis patients than in dialysis outpatients. Exposure to the hospital environment is known to contribute to the increase of VRE among chronic dialysis patients.[83–85]
- General dialysis center precautions should be used. In addition, enhanced attention to environmental cleaning and patient separation is prudent for patients with poor hygiene or infectious material (e.g., fecal incontinence or wound drainage)

that cannot be contained. Specific practices for patients with noncontainable infectious material include:

1. Wash hands whenever anything in the vicinity of the patient was touched (including environmental surfaces).
2. Use gloves for any patient contact.
3. If the patient's skin integrity is intact (no open, draining wounds) and clothes are clean, a gown is not required. However, if contact with moist body substances is anticipated, then a fluid-resistant gown must be worn to protect clothing and all areas of exposed skin (following Standard Precautions).
4. Use of a designated dialysis machine is not necessary.
5. Bedside equipment (stethoscope, sphygmomanometer, thermometer) must remain in the patient's area while the patient is in dialysis. If such devices must be used on other patients, they must first be cleaned and disinfected.

Employee-Focused Prevention Techniques—Vaccination and Education

- Routine testing of staff members for HBV, HCV, or HIV is not recommended.[5]
- Hepatitis B vaccination is recommended for all staff members. Staff should be aware of their immune status. Staff members who do not respond to the primary series should receive a second three-dose series and then be retested for anti-HBs. No additional doses are warranted if there is still no response.[5] See Chapter 19 for details.
- Safety sharp devices should be evaluated with the assistance of staff and put into use to reduce risk of percutaneous exposure to blood or body fluids.[75]
- Annual influenza vaccination should be encouraged.
- Staff should be evaluated by occupational health for recommendations regarding immunizations against pneumococcus, varicella, tetanus, diphtheria, measles, mumps, and rubella.
- Appropriate annual infection prevention and control and safety training is required for staff.[5, 74]
- Policies and procedures should be in place and followed for communicable disease post-exposure evaluation and treatment (see Chapter 19).

Surveillance

An active surveillance system can assist with early detection of infectious complications. A record-keeping system (logbook or electronic file) should be in place with the following information recorded:[5, 11]

- Vaccination status and response to vaccination for patients
- Serologic testing results for viral hepatitis for patients
- Incidence of bacteremia or vascular access site infection
- Frequency of pyrogenic reactions
- Water culture results
- Adverse events (e.g., blood leaks and spills, dialysis machine malfunctions)

Consistent definitions of surveillance indicators are critical to ensure comparability of data (see Chapter 20). A staff person should be designated to review surveillance data periodically. In addition, a record that includes the location of the dialysis station and machine number used for each dialysis session as well as the names of staff members who connect and disconnect the patient to and from the machine should be maintained for each patient. This information may be important during outbreak or exposure investigations. There should be a procedure outlining the actions required when changes occur in test results or rate of infections.

Other indicators to evaluate quality of care might focus on procedures, such as compliance with reprocessing procedures or use of personal protective equipment.[3]

References

1. Dialysis. *Pocket Guide to Infection Prevention and Safe Practice.* Schaffer, S. D., Garzon, L. S., Heroux, D. L., and Korniewicz, D. M., eds. St. Louis: Mosby-Year Book, Inc.; 1996: 351–362.

2. Habach, G., and Port, F. K. Dialyzers, dialysate, and delivery devices. In: Massry, S. G., and Glassock, R. J., eds., *Massry & Galssocks's Textbook of Nephrology.* Vol 2, 3rd Ed. Baltimore: Williams & Wilkins; 1995: 1525–1531.

3. Arnow, P. M., and Garcia-Houchins, S. Dialysis Units. In: Abrutyn, E., Goldmann, D. A., and Scheckler, W. E., eds. *Saunders Infection Control Reference Service.* 2nd Ed. Philadelphia: W.B. Saunders Co., 2001: 161–165.

4. Favero, M. S., Alter, M. J., and Bland, L. A. Nosocomial Infections Associated with Hemodialysis. In: Mayhall, C. G., ed. *Hospital Epidemiology and Infection Control.* Baltimore: Williams & Wilkins; 1996: 693–714.

5. Recommendations for preventing transmission of infections among chronic hemodialysis patients. *MMWR.* 2001; 50(RR05):1–43. *http://www.cdc.gov/mmwr/PDF/rr/rr5005.pdf.*

6. National Institutes of Health. *1999 Annual Data Report. U.S. Renal Data System.* Bethesda, MD: U.S. Department of Health and Human Services, National Institutes of Health, National Institute of Diabetes and Digestive and Kidney Diseases, April 1999.

7. Tokars, J. I. Description of a new surveillance system for bloodstream and vascular access infections in outpatient hemodialysis centers. *Semin Dial.* 2000; 13:97–100.

8. Tokars, J. I., Miller, E. R., Alter, M. J., and Arduino, M. J. National surveillance of dialysis-associated diseases in the United States, 1997. *Semin Dial.* 2000; 13:75–85.

9. Favero, M. S., Petersen, N. J., Carson, L. A., Bond, W. W., and Hindman, S. H. Gram-negative water bacteria in hemodialysis systems. *Health Lab Sci.* 1975; 12:321–334.

10. Petrosillo, N., Puro, V., Jagger, J., and Ippolito, G. The risks of occupational exposure and infection by human immunodeficiency virus, hepatitis B virus, and hepatitis C virus in the dialysis setting. *Am J Infect Control.* 1995; 23:278–285.

11. Tokars, J. I., Arduino, M. J., and Alter, M. J. Infection control in hemodialysis Units. *Infect Dis Clin North Am.* 2001; 15:797–812.

12. Work Group of the NKF-KDOQI. Clinical practice guidelines for vascular access. *Am J Kidney Dis.* 2002; 37[Suppl 1]:S137–S181.

13. CDC. *Hepatitis: Control measures for hepatitis B in dialysis centers.* Atlanta, GA: U.S. Department of Health, Education, and Welfare, Public Health Services, CDC, 1977. HEW publication no. (CDC) 78-8358 (Viral Hepatitis Investigations and Control Series).

14. Perry, J., Parker, G., and Jagger, J. Reducing sharps injuries in dialysis settings. *Nursing.* 2001; 31:78.

15. Forseter, G., Wormser, G. P., Adler, S., Lebovics, E., Calmann, M., and O'Brien, T. A. Hepatitis C in the health care setting. II. Seroprevalence among hemodialysis staff and patients in suburban New York City. *Am J Infect Control.* 1993; 21:5–8.

16. Masuko, K., Mitsui, T., Iwano, K., Yamazaki, C., Okuda, K., and Meguro, T., et al. Infection with hepatitis GB virus C in patients on maintenance hemodialysis. *N Engl J Med.* 1996; 334:1485–1490.

17. de Lamballerie, X., Charrel, R. N., and Bussol, B. Hepatitis GB virus C in patients on hemodialysis. *N Engl J Med.* 1996; 334:1549.

18. Sivapalasingam, S., Malak, S. F., Sullivan, J. F., Lorch, J., and Sepkowitz, K. A. High prevalence of hepatitis C infection among patients receiving hemodialysis at an urban dialysis center. *Infect Control Hosp Epidemiol.* 2002; 23:319–324.

19. Fabrizi, F., Lunghi, G., and Ponticelli, C. Epidemiology of human immunodeficiency virus (HIV) infection in dialysis: Recent insights. *Int J Art Organs.* 2001; 24:425–433.

20. Fabrizi, F., Lunghi, G., and Martin, P. Epidemiology of hepatitis delta virus (HDV) infection in the dialysis population. *Int J Art Organs.* 2002; 25:8–17.

21. Arnow, P. M., Garcia-Houchins, S., Neagle, M. B., Bova, J. L., Dillon, J. J., and Chou, T. An outbreak of bloodstream infections arising from hemodialysis equipment. *J Infect Dis.* 1998; 178:783–791.

22. Gordon, S. M., Tipple, M., Bland, L. A., and Jarvis, W. R. Pyrogenic reactions associated with the reuse of disposable hollow-fiber hemodialyzers. *JAMA.* 1988; 260:2077–81.

23. Rudnick, J. R., Arduino, M. J., Bland, L. A., Cusick, L., McAllister, S. K., Aguero, S. M., and Jarvis, W. R. An outbreak of pyrogenic reactions in chronic hemodialysis patients associated with hemodialyzer reuse. *Artificial Organs.* 1995; 19:289–294.

24. Bolan, G., Reingold, A. L., Carson, L. A., Silcox, V. A., Woodley, C. L., and Hayes, P. S., et al. Infections with *Mycobacterium chelonei* in patients receiving dialysis and using processed hemodialyzers. *J Infect Dis.* 1985; 152:1013–1019.

25. Beck-Sague, C. M., Jarvis, W. R., Bland, L. A., Arduino, M. J., Aguero, S. M., and Verosic, G. Outbreak of gram-negative bacteremia and pyrogenic reactions in a hemodialysis center. *Am J Nephrol.* 1990; 10:397–403.

26. Flaherty, J. P., Garcia-Houchins, S., Chudy, R., and Arnow, P. M. An outbreak of gram-negative bacteremia traced to contaminated O-rings and reprocessed dialyzers. *Ann Intern Med.* 1993; 119:1072–1078.

27. Lowry, P. W., Beck-Sague, C. M., Bland, L. A., Aguero, S. M., Arduino, M. J., and Minuth, A. N. *Mycobacterium chelonae* infection among patients receiving high-flux dialysis in a hemodialysis clinic in California. *J Infect Dis.* 1990; 161:85–90.

28. Snydman, D. R., Bryan, J. A., London, W. T., Werner, B., Bregman, D., and Blumberg, B. S., et al. Transmission of hepatitis B associated with hemodialysis: Role of malfunction (blood leaks) in dialysis machines. *J Infect Dis.* 1976; 134:562–570.

29. CDC. Epidemiologic notes and reports. Bacteremias associated with reuse of disposable hollow-fiber hemodialyzers. *MMWR.* 1986; 35:417–418.

30. Murphy, J., Parker, T., Carson, L., Bland, L., and Solomon, S. Outbreaks of bacteremia in hemodialysis patients associated with alteration of dialyzer membranes following chemical disinfection [abstract]. *ASAIO Transactions.* 1987; 16:51.

31. Humar, A., Oxley, C., Sample, M. L., and Garber, G. Elimination of an outbreak of gram-negative bacteremia in a hemodialysis unit. *Am J Infect Control.* 1996; 24:359–363.

32. Jochimsen, E. M., Frenette, C., Delorme, M., Arduino, M., Aguero, S., and Carson, L., et al. A cluster of bloodstream infections and pyrogenic reactions among hemodialysis patients traced to dialysis machine waste-handling option units. *Am J Nephrol.* 1998; 18:485–489.

33. Olver, W. J., Webster, C., Clements, H., Weston, V., and Boswell, T. Two cases of *Enterococcus faecalis* bacteremia associated with a hemodialysis machine. *J Infect Dis.* 1999; 179:1312.

34. CDC. Outbreaks of gram-negative bacterial bloodstream infections traced to probable contamination of hemodialysis machines—Canada, 1995; United States, 1997; and Israel, 1997. *MMWR.* 1998; 47:55–59.

35. Goetz, A., Yu, V. L., Hanchett, J. E., and Rihs, J. D. *Pseudomonas stutzeri* bacteremia associated with hemodialysis. *Arch Intern Med.* 1983; 143:1909–1912.

36. Longfield, R. N., Wortham, W. G., Fletcher, L. L., and Nauscheutz, W. F. Clustered bacteremias in a hemodialysis unit: Cross-contamination of blood tubing from ultrafiltrate waste. *Infect Control Hosp Epidemiol.* 1992; 13:160–164.

37. Danzig, L. E., Tormey, M. P., Sinha, S. D., Robertson, B. J., Lambert, S., and Itano, A., et al. Common source transmission of hepatitis B virus infection in a hemodialysis unit. *Infect Control Hosp Epidemiol.* 1995; 16(S):P19, Abstract 24.

38. CDC. Outbreaks of hepatitis B virus infection among hemodialysis patients—California, Nebraska, and Texas, 1994. *MMWR.* 1996; 45:285–289.

39. Niu, M. T., Alter, M. J., Kristensen, C., and Margolis, H. S. Outbreak of hemodialysis-associated non-A, non-B hepatitis and correlation with antibody to hepatitis C virus. *Am J Kidney Dis.* 1992; 19:345–352.

40. Welbel, S. F., Schoendorf, K., Bland, L. A., Arduino, M. J., Groves, C., and Schable, B., et al. An outbreak of gram-negative bloodstream infections in chronic hemodialysis patients. *Am J Nephrol.* 1995; 15:1–4.

41. Wang, S. A., Levine, R. B., Carson, L. A., Arduino, M. J., Killar, T., and Grillo, F. G., et al. An outbreak of gram-negative bacteremia in hemodialysis patients traced to hemodialysis machine waste drain ports. *Infect Control Hosp Epidemiol.* 1999; 20:746–751.

42. Keroack, M. A., and Kotilainen, H. R. A cluster of pyrogenic reactions and yeast colonization of hemodialysis machines. *Infect Control Hosp Epidemiol.* 1996; 17(S):474. Abstract LB-5.

43. Hutin, Y. J., Goldstein, S. T., Varma, J. K., O'Dair, J. B., Mast, E. E., Shapiro, C. N., and Alter, M. J. An outbreak of hospital-acquired hepatitis B virus infection among patients receiving chronic hemodialysis. *Infect Control Hosp Epidemiol.* 1999; 20:731–735.

44. Snydman, D. R., Bryan, J. A., Macon, E. J., and Gregg, M. B. Hemodialysis-associated hepatitis: Report of an epidemic with further evidence on mechanisms of transmission. *Am J Epidemiol.* 1976; 104:563–570.

45. Niu, M. T., Penberthy, L. T., Alter, M. J., Armstrong, C. W., Miller, G. B., and Hadler, S. C. Hemodialysis-associated hepatitis B: Report of an outbreak. *Dialysis Transpl.* 1989; 18:542–555.

46. Delarocque-Astagneau, E., Baffoy, N., Thiers, V., Simon, N., de Valk, H., and Laperche, S., et al. Outbreak of hepatitis C virus infection in a hemodialysis unit: Potential transmission by the hemodialysis machine? *Infect Control Hosp Epidemiol.* 2002; 23:328–334.

47. Price, C. S., Hacek, D., Noskin, G. A., and Peterson, L. R. An outbreak of bloodstream infections in an outpatient hemodialysis center. *Infect Control Hosp Epidemiol.* 2002; 23:725–729.

48. Hindman, S. H., Favero, M. S., Carson, L. A., Petersen, N. J., Schonberger, L. B., and Solano, J. T. Pyrogenic reactions during haemodialysis caused by extramural endotoxin. *Lancet.* 1975; 2:732–734.

49. Egwari, L. O., and Mendie, U. E. Incidence of pyrexia in patients undergoing haemodialysis. *West African J Med.* 1996; 15:101–106.

50. Jackson, B. M., Beck-Sague, C. M., Bland, L. A., Arduino, M. J., Meyer, L., and Jarvis, W. R. Outbreak of pyrogenic reactions and gram-negative bacteremia in a hemodialysis center. *Am J Nephrol.* 1994; 14:85–89.

51. CDC. Nontuberculous mycobacterial infections in hemodialysis patients—Louisiana, 1982. *MMWR.* 1983; 32:244–245.

52. CDC. An outbreak of bacteremia and pyrogenic reactions in a dialysis unit—Pennsylvania. *MMWR.* 1978; 27:307–309.

53. Uman, S. J., Johnson, C. E., Beirne, G. J., and Kunin, C. M. *Pseudomonas aeruginosa* bacteremia in a dialysis unit. *Am J Med.* 1977; 62:667–671.

54. Petersen, N. J., Boyer, K. M., Carson, L. A., and Favero, M. S. Pyrogenic reactions from inadequate disinfection of a dialysis fluid distribution system. *Dialysis Transplant.* 1978; 7:52–60.

55. Spencer, M., and Bird, G. Device-related, nonintravascular infections. *Crit Care Clin North Am.* 1995; 7:685–693.

56. Twardowski, Z. J., and Prowant, B. F. Exit-site healing post catheter implantation. Peritoneal catheter exit-site morphology and pathology. *Perit Dialy International.* 1996; 16 Suppl 3:S51–S68.

57. Vas, S., and Oreopoulos, D. G. Infections in patients undergoing peritoneal dialysis. *Infect Dis Clin North Am.* 2001; 15:743–774.

58. Epidemiology of hemodialysis vascular access infections from longitudinal infection surveillance data: Predicting the impact of NKF-DOQI clinical practice guidelines for vascular access. *Am J Kid Dis* (online). 2002; 39:549–555.

59. Stevenson, K. B., Adcox, M. J., Mallea, M. C., Narasimhan, N., and Wagnild, J. P. Standardized surveillance of hemodialysis vascular access infections: 18-month experience at an outpatient, multifacility hemodialysis center. *Infect Control Hosp Epidemiol.* 2000; 21:200–203.

60. Marr, K. A., Sexton, D. J., Conlon, P. J., Corey, G. R., Schwab, S. J., and Kirkland, K. B. Catheter-related bacteremia and outcome of attempted catheter salvage in patients undergoing hemodialysis. *Ann Intern Med.* 1997; 127:275–280.

61. Stevenson, K. B., Hannah, E. L., Lowder, C. A., Adcox, M. J., Davidson, R. L., and Mallea, M. C., et al. Epidemiology of hemodialysis vascular access catheter infections from longitudinal infection surveillance data: Predicting the impact of NKF-DOQI Clinical Practice Guidelines for Vascular Access. *Am J Kid Dis.* 2002; 39:549–555.

62. Dopirak, M., Hill, C., Oleksiw, M., Dumigan, D., Arvai, J., and English, E., et al. Surveillance of hemodialysis-associated primary bloodstream infections: The experience of ten hospital-based centers. *Infect Control Hosp Epidemiol.* 2002; 23:721–724.

63. Taylor, G., Gravel, D., Johnston, L., Embil, J., Holton, D., and Paton, S., et al. Prospective surveillance for primary bloodstream infections occurring in Canadian hemodialysis units. *Infect Control Hosp Epidemiol.* 2002; 23:716–720.

64. Tokars, J. I., Miller, E. R., and Stein, G. A new national surveillance system for hemodialysis-associated infections: Initial results. *Am J Infect Control.* 2002; 30:288–295.

65. Tokars, J. I., Miller, E. R., Alter, M. J., and Arduino, M. J. *National surveillance of dialysis-associated diseases in the United States, 1999.* Atlanta, GA: Centers for Disease Control and Prevention: 1999; 1–60, *http://www.cdc.gov/ncidod/hip/Dialysis/dialysis99.pdf.*

66. Module V. I. Dialyzer Reprocessing. Dahlin, J., and Beckett-Tharp, D., eds. *Core Curriculum for the Dialysis Technician.* Madison, WI: Medical Media Associates, Inc.; 1998.

67. Arduino, M. J., Tokars, J. I., Lyerla, R., and Alter, M. J. Prevention of healthcare-associated transmission of bloodborne viruses in hemodialysis facilities. *Semin Infect Control.* 2001; 1:49–60.

68. Alter, M. J., Kruszon-Moran, D., Nainan, O., McQuillan, G. M., Gao, F., and Moyer, L. A., et al. The Prevalence of hepatitis C virus infection in the United States, 1988 through 1994. *N Engl J Med.* 1999; 341:556–562.

69. *AAMI Standards and Recommended Practices for Dialysis.* Arlington, VA: Association for the Advancement of Medical Instrumentation, 2001.

70. Module V. Hemodialysis Procedures and Hemodialysis Complications. Arslanian, J., Swartzendruber, D., and Peacock, E., eds. *Core Curriculum for the Dialysis Technician.* Madison, WI: Medical Media Associates, Inc.; 1998.

71. Lancaster, L. E., ed. *Core Curriculum for Nephrology Nursing*, 3rd Ed. Pitman, NJ: American Nephrology Nurses Association; 1995: 221–224.

72. Centers for Disease Control and Prevention. Guidelines for the prevention of intravascular catheter-related infections, 2002. *MMWR.* 2002; 51(RR-10):1–32.

73. Centers for Disease Control and Prevention. Guideline for hand hygiene in health-care settings: Recommendations of the Healthcare Infection Control Practices Advisory Committee and the HICPAC/SHEA/APIC/IDSA Hand Hygiene Task Force. *MMWR.* 2002; 51 (No. RR-16):1–44.

74. Occupational exposure to bloodborne pathogens: Final rule. *Fed Reg.* 1991; 56 (Dec. 6):64175–64182, *http://www.osha-slc.gov/pls/oshaweb/owadisp.show_document?p_table=STANDARDS&p_id=10051&p_text_version=FALSE.*

75. Occupational Exposure to Bloodborne Pathogens; Needlestick and Other Sharps Injuries; Final Rule. *Fed Reg.* 2001; 66:5317–5325.

76. McCleary, J., Caldero, K., and Adams, T. Guarded fistula needle reduces needlestick injuries in hemodialysis. *Nephrol News Issues.* 2002; 16:66–72.

77. Lewis, S. L., Prowant, B. F., Douglas, C., and Cooper, C. L. Nursing practice related to peritoneal catheter exit site care and infections. *ANNA J.* 1996; 23:609–615.

78. Oliver, M. J., and Schwab, S. J. Infections Related to Hemodialysis and Peritoneal Dialysis. In: Waldvogel, F. A., and Bisno, A. L., eds. *Infections Associated with Indwelling Medical Devices.* 3rd Ed. Washington, DC: ASM Press; 2000: 345–372.

79. Standards for patients with renal failure. *Nurs Standard.* 1998; 12:32–33.

80. Screening for tuberculosis and tuberculosis infection in high-risk populations. *MMWR.* 1995; 44 (RR-11):19–32.

81. Favero, M. S. Preventing transmission of hepatitis B infection in health care facilities. *Am J Infect Control.* 1989; 17:168–171.

82. *Staphylococcus aureus* with reduced susceptibility to vancomycin—United States, 1997. *MMWR.* 1997; 46:765–766.

83. Tokars, J. I., Gehr, T., Jarvis, W. R., Anderson, J., Armistead, N., and Miller, E. R., et al. Vancomycin-resistant enterococci colonization in patients at seven hemodialysis centers. *Kidney Int.* 2001; 60:1511–1516.

84. Roghmann, M. C., Fink, J. C., Polish, L., Maker, T., Brewrink, J., and Morris, J. G., et al. Colonization with vancomycin-resistant enterococci in chronic hemodialysis patients. *Am J Kidney Dis.* 1998; 32:254–257.

85. *Staphylococcus aureus* resistant to vancomycin—United States, 2002. *MMWR.* 2002; 51:565–567.

CHAPTER 14

Ophthalmology/Optometry

BACKGROUND

Eye care in the outpatient setting covers a broad range of patient care activities, from routine optometry exams to complicated, multi-procedure eye surgery. Ophthalmic surgery is among the most common, with 1.3 to 1.5 million cataract extractions performed in the United States annually and approximately 1.5 million laser in situ keratomileusis (LASIK) procedures performed worldwide annually.[1–3] Although reported rates of infection post-cataract surgery[4–5] and eye examination-related adenovirus conjunctivitis[6] are decreasing, numerous outbreaks of infections associated with ophthalmologic surgery, examination, and equipment have been described.

CAUSES AND RISKS

Epidemic keratoconjunctivitis (EKC), an acute adenovirus conjunctivitis, is one of the most commonly reported causes of outbreaks in ophthalmology and optometry.[7–15] Adenovirus is a hardy virus that can remain viable for up to 35 days on nonporous surfaces.[16–17] It has been recovered from the hands of patients with culture-proven EKC.[18–19] EKC has a prolonged period of communicability, from late in the incubation period of three to 30 days[7] to 14 or more days after onset of symptoms.[15, 20] Spread of EKC has been linked to use of contaminated diagnostic lenses,[12] pneumotonometry,[7, 8, 13, 19] delay in applying control measures,[9, 13–14] lack of handwashing or contact with infected healthcare workers,[19] and a combination of these factors.

Multi-dose eye drop solutions[21] and containers can become contaminated during use (e.g., inside container rims and caps, tips, and droppers)[22–24] and have been linked to bacterial infections such as *Serratia marcescens*[25] and Pseudomonas aeruginosa.[26] One study found that the frequency of contamination of medications increased with increasing duration of use and recommended replacing eyedrops on a regular basis.[23] Another study found the incidence of microbial contamination of in-use therapeutic, preservative containing eyedrops was increased at 14 days versus seven days, but concluded that the increase (6 to 9% of bottles) and the range of contamination (1 to 162 colony-forming units/ml of drops) was insignificant.[21] Another study found that adenovirus inoculated into fluorescein survived up to 21 days.[27] However, other studies of both in-use[28–29] and artificially contaminated solutions[29–30] show a lack of sustained microbial growth.

Ophthalmologic surgery is complicated by infection in less than 0.5% of cases.[1, 4, 5, 31–35] However, infection often leads to sight loss with endophthalmitis among the most devastating complications following eye surgery. Patient factors that increase risk of infection include diabetes, immune suppression, and inflammation or infection of the eye, eyelid, or around the eye.[4] Intra-operative factors that contribute to infection risk include surgery duration of more than 60 minutes[4] and type of lenses implanted for cataract surgery.[36] Clusters of endophthalmitis have been related to contaminated donor corneas,[37] contaminated special ophthalmology surgical equipment,[1, 38–41] contaminated ocular irrigating solution,[42] improperly sterilized surgical supplies,[43–45] inadequate operating room air filtration,[46] and hospital construction.[47] Several reports described infections after simultaneous bilateral LASIK procedures in which the same set of instruments was used on both eyes.[48] A wide variety of microorganisms, including Pseudomonas,[39–40] Serratia,[38] Enterobacter,[43] Acremonium,[46] nontuberculous Mycobacterium,[48] Candida,[42] and Aspergillus[47] have been identified in these outbreaks. Background or endemic cases are most often associated with skin flora, such as coagulase-negative Staphylococcus.[2, 32–33, 36] In addition, isolates from some cases have been resistant to perioperative prophylactic antibiotics.[49]

During the first years of the acquired immunodeficiency syndrome (AIDS) epidemic, when human immunodeficiency virus (HIV) was found in tears,[50] potential spread of HIV via ophthalmologic examination presented special concerns. However, levels of HIV found in tears, conjunctiva, cornea, and contact lenses of infected patients are so low that transmission is highly unlikely to occur.[51] HIV present on environmental surfaces is not difficult to inactivate, unlike EKC, and routine reprocessing of devices that contact the eye, use of Standard Precautions (see Chapter 6), and handwashing are effective measures to prevent spread.[52–53]

More recently, concern about transmission of hepatitis C via tear fluid has arisen, based on finding hepatitis C virus in tear fluid.[54] Theoretically, failure to effectively decontaminate reusable devices that contact the eye could spread hepatitis C. After inoculation of Goldmann tonometer tips with hepatitis C virus, soaking in 3% hydrogen peroxide or 70% isopropyl alcohol followed by cold-water rinsing were most effective at virus removal; dry gauze, alcohol wipes, and povidone iodine wipes were ineffective.[54]

INFECTION PREVENTION AND CONTROL MEASURES

Implementation of routine, formal infection prevention and control measures are effective in reducing spread of infection. In one university-affiliated eye center, nosocomial cases of EKC were significantly reduced from 54.1 to 5.7 per 100,000 visits by instituting standard methods of handwashing, instrument disinfection, medication distribution, furlough of infected employees, and patient screening and isolation.[6]

Hand Hygiene and Gloving

Hands should be washed before and after eye examination and after removing gloves; see Chapter 5 for details on procedure and products. For all cases of conjunctivitis or suspected eye infection, gloves should be worn when touching the eye, drainage, items soiled with drainage, and when administering eye medications. Staff with open wounds or lesions on their hands should also wear gloves for any patient care activities. Patients should be taught to wash hands before and after administering eye drops and before inserting contact lenses.

Instrument Disinfection

High-level disinfection should be a standard procedure for all devices that contact the eye; see Chapter 3 for details on procedures and products. Because patients with unrecognized or incubating infections are likely to be examined, the same disinfection practices should apply to *all* patients, regardless of a known diagnosis. The "gold standard" for tonometer tips is removal, cleaning with instrument detergent, soaking for a specified time in disinfectant, thorough rinsing with fresh water, drying, and storage to prevent contamination. Recommended disinfectant and soak times are summarized in Table 14.1.

It is common to merely wipe the tonometer tip with 70% isopropyl alcohol, either using small, individually packaged wipes or an alcohol-soaked gauze. However, there is little evidence that this practice is consistently effective in inactivating adenovirus; the studies showing efficacy were very small in number and were conducted in a controlled laboratory setting.[55] Reports describing damage to tonometer tips by extended soaking in alcohol have also been published;[56] however, with a timed soak and thorough drying, damage is minimized. In addition, special soaking containers are available from optical suppliers.

Table 14.1 Tonometer Tip Disinfection

Disinfectant	Soak Time	Procedure	Reference
Bleach, 1:100 dilution (500 parts per million chlorine)	5–10 minutes	Prepare fresh solution daily. Or, double the concentration (1:50), store for 30 days[57] in an opaque plastic container to preserve efficacy, label with expiration date, and pour into clean soaking dish each day of use. Rinse tips thoroughly with water after soaking.	Nagington, 1983[58] Koo, 1989[7] Jernigan, 1993[19] Rutala, 1996[55]
Alcohol, 70% isopropyl or ethyl	5–10 minutes	Pour fresh daily into a clean soaking dish from the original bottle. Allow tips to dry thoroughly before use.	Craven, 1987[59] AOA, 1993[60] Rutala, 1996[57]
Hydrogen peroxide, 3%	5–10 minutes	Pour fresh daily into a clean soaking dish from the original bottle. Rinse tips thoroughly with water after soaking.	Craven, 1987[59] Threlkeld, 1993[61] AOA, 1993[60] Rutala, 1996[55]

Although bleach is often recommended as a dilution of 1:10,[59–61] at least one report has described eye injury at this concentration in which crystal deposits had formed on the tonometer tip.[62] Therefore, bleach at 1:100 dilution is recommended as effective and less likely to cause injury or damage.[57]

Some pressure-measuring device tips (e.g., tonopens) can be covered with a disposable cover during use. A new cover is used for each patient and the "pen" surface can be wiped with a surface disinfectant/cleaner or alcohol as for other handheld devices.

Other lenses (e.g., gonio, yag, or Zeiss lenses) and applanation or Schiotz tonometers must also be soaked after patient contact; it is essential to follow the manufacturer's directions for each type and brand of lens to avoid damage. After disinfection, lenses should be stored dry in a clean container to prevent damage or contamination. Fitting contact lenses that are labeled for single use must not be reused. High-level disinfection is the standard of care for reusable trial contact lenses; standard heat treatment is most effective.[63]

Ancillary equipment (e.g., lid retractors) should also be soaked in high-level disinfectant at a minimum; alcohol wipes provide inadequate disinfection.[64] This includes lid retractors and other instruments that may be taken from the clinic for use in neonatalogy or other in-patient units. Because in-patient units are rarely staffed or equipped to perform disinfection, enough clean devices should be supplied to the ophthalmology team for each patient who will be examined, along with a container to transport them back to the clinic.

Modalities such as certain laser equipment and devices that measure pressure via a "puff" of air are not designed to touch the eye surface and need only decontamination if inadvertently touched to the eye. Before disinfecting these devices, the manufacturer must be consulted to determine safe disinfectants and reprocessing procedures.

Environmental Surfaces

Surfaces in examination rooms, such as countertops, examination chairs, and eye examining equipment, should be cleaned with a low-level disinfectant or disinfectant cleaner; see Chapter 3 for details and recommended products. The slit lamp surfaces that contact forehead and chin can be cleaned after each patient with the same disinfectant used for the rest of the room. Pads of paper tissues are sometimes used on the chin rest, with the top tissue removed to expose a fresh tissue for each patient. Because the tissues are thin paper, drainage potentially can seep through one layer. Therefore, based on common sense, it is best either to use no tissue and wipe the surface after each patient or, if patient comfort is a concern, to place several sheets from the pad onto the chin rest and discard them after each patient.

Certain chemicals may damage devices, such as laser equipment; therefore, it is essential to read the manufacturer's instructions outlining safe disinfectants and procedures.

Medications

If the clinic is associated with a hospital facility, pharmacy policies for expiration dating of multipatient use medications should be adopted. There may also be state regulations to follow. In any case, if the tip of the container or dropper touches the eye or becomes contaminated, the container must be discarded. The medications must also be disposed of according to the manufacturer's expiration date. Although written guidelines are scarce, in some settings an arbitrary expiration date, such as 30 days, may be practical.[65] After opening, label the container to expire according to this date. Medications containing no preservatives and/or labeled as unit dose must be discarded after a single use.

Employee Health

Any staff member with conjunctivitis should be prohibited from working directly with patients for the duration of symptoms.[20, 66]

Epidemic Keratoconjunctivitis (EKC) Prevention and Outbreak Control

Following the standard procedures described should eliminate the risk of EKC spread. However, because EKC is very contagious and environmentally hardy, the following more stringent measures may be needed to halt an outbreak:

1. Develop a specific protocol before an outbreak occurs that is reviewed and approved by administrative, clinical, and infection control staff.
2. Define health care-associated cases and how they are to be recognized. For example, a case definition may be any patient with onset of conjunctivitis symptoms within three to 30 days after a visit where an eye infection was not diagnosed at the visit. If staff members develop conjunctivitis, they will also need to be included in a case definition.
3. Define when the protocol will be instituted. For example, if even one patient returns with symptoms compatible with EKC, the patient should be evaluated clinically and cultured. If results are compatible with EKC, the protocol will be implemented.

4. Reinforce the necessity of prohibiting personnel with conjunctivitis from patient contact and the patient care environment for the duration of symptoms.
5. During an outbreak, add glove usage for all patient contacts.
6. Triage patients with suspected EKC to an assigned waiting area and examination rooms to decrease opportunity for contact between infected and uninfected persons.
7. During an outbreak, monitor cleaning procedures to assure that environmental surfaces in examination rooms are decontaminated with an approved disinfectant cleaner after each patient. Eliminate use of paper pads on chin rests of the slit lamps. *Note:* There has been no evidence that allowing a room to sit empty or "air out" between patients is effective in preventing spread of infection.
8. Monitor disinfection procedures to ensure that tonometers and other lenses or devices contacting the eye are reprocessed adequately. Tonometer tips should be removed and soaked in disinfectant as a standard procedure, regardless of patient diagnosis.
9. Use unit-dose eye medications.[67]
10. If the outbreak continues, reevaluate the protocol to ensure that it is being followed and to determine whether any changes are needed.

Ophthalmologic Surgery

To the degree possible, patient risk factors, such as diabetes, conjunctivitis, or other eye-related infection or inflammation, should be treated preoperatively. Patient teaching, including information on applying eye drops, avoidance of touching the tip of the dropper to any surface including skin or eye, and information on applying eye covers or pads, should be done preoperatively and postoperatively.

Other preventive measures include impeccable aseptic technique. For any eye surgery performed in the operating room, such as cataract surgery, the surgical team should wear masks. A study reported in 2002[68] found significantly fewer microorganisms cultured on the sterile field during eye surgery when the surgeon used a face mask. Standard surgical hand antisepsis, as described in Chapter 5, should be performed and sterile gloves worn for all eye surgery. Because risk of infection post-cataract surgery is greater for procedures longer than 60 minutes,[4] it is important to limit the time of routine surgery.

Thorough skin antispesis of the surgical site with 5 to 10% povidone-iodine is the standard eye presurgical preparation and has been shown to be safe and effective.[2, 4, 48, 69] Other antiseptics must be used with caution, only after thorough review of ophthalmologic surgical literature and product information for safety and efficacy. There has been at least one report of chlorhexidine causing corneal damage.[70] All solutions and medications used during surgery need to be sterile. Plastic drapes to isolate eyelashes and lid margins from the surgical field should be used.[48]

Perioperative antibiotics are commonly applied prophylactically directly to the eye before, during, and after surgery. Standard doses, timing, formulations, and types vary widely. Changing philosophies about prophylactic antibiotics reflect growing concerns about antibiotic resistance; studies are equivocal on the optimum antibiotic regimen that will prevent infection.[2, 4] Regardless of the specific regimen favored by a particular surgeon or institution, any antibiotic needs to be applied in an aseptic manner and the dose, time, and type must be recorded on the surgical notes.

All instruments and equipment must be sterilized. Reusable equipment needs to be cleaned with instrument detergent and sterilized after each case; cleaning and sterilization must be consistent with the principles discussed in Chapter 3. Any hand controls manipulated by the surgeon should be fitted with sterile covers, including light handles or laser hand controls. Surgical sets or trays should be sterilized for each patient. Additionally, if simultaneous bilateral procedures are planned, microkeratome blades and surgical sets should be packaged and sterilized separately for each eye.[35, 48] Before using or reprocessing any new equipment, manufacturer's instructions must be reviewed thoroughly. Of special concern is any equipment with tubing, pumps, reservoirs, and/or irrigating fluid that could become contaminated with water microorganisms, because of several outbreaks due to these devices.[1, 38–41] To avoid contamination and/or build up of biofilm, purchase devices with tubing and fluid reservoirs that are designed to be discarded after each patient. Use fresh, sterile solution for each patient. Types and lot numbers of implants should be recorded to determine any link between infection or other negative outcomes and specific implants. The type of incision and suture, if used, should also be described in the surgical notes to determine whether any new technique is contributing to endophthalmitis.

An active surveillance plan to prevent and detect cases of postoperative endophthalmitis should be developed.[71] Cultures should be taken from any suspected case. All isolates should be analyzed for antibiotic susceptibility to establish whether isolates are resistant to any of the perioperative antibiotic drops or ointments. Isolates of non-skin bacteria, such as Pseudomonas, Mycobacteria, or other microorganisms that commonly live in water should alert staff to suspect contamination of any perioperative fluids or devices that are potentially exposed to tap water. There should be close communication between the ophthalmologists and the infection control staff to follow up on any suspected cases. Even a cluster of only a few infections should alert staff to a potential outbreak. See Chapter 21 on outbreak investigation.

Professional Resources

American Optometric Association (AOA), *http://www.aoa.org.*
American Academy of Ophthalmology (AAO),. *http://www.aao.org.*

References

1. Hoffmann, K. K., Weber, D. J., Gergen, J. F., Rutala, W. A., and Tate, G. *Pseudomonas aeruginosa*-related postoperative endophthalmitis linked to a contaminated phacoemulsifier. *Arch Ophthalmol.* 2002; 120:90–93.

2. Ciulla, T. A., Starr, M. B., and Masket, S. Bacterial endophthalmitis prophylaxis for cataract surgery. *Ophthalmol.* 2002; 109:13–26.

3. Melki, S. A., and Azar, D. T. LASIK complications: Etiology, management, and prevention. *Surv Ophthalmol.* 2001; 46:95–116.

4. Mamalis, N., Nagpal, M., Nagpal, K., and Nagpal, P. N. Endophthalmitis following cataract surgery. *Ophthalmol Clin North Am.* 2001; 14:661–674.

5. Montan, P. G., Wejde, G., Koranyi, G., and Tylander, M. Efficacy in preventing endophthalmitis after cataract surgery. *J Cataract Refract Surg.* 2002; 28:977–981.

6. Gottsch, J. D., Froggatt, J. W., 3rd, Smith, D. M., Dwyer, D. M., and Borenstein, P. Prevention and control of EKC in a teaching eye institute. *Ophthalmic Epidemiol.* 1999; 6:29–39.

7. Koo, D., Bouvier, B., Wesley, M., Courtright, P., and Reingold, A. EKC in a university medical center ophthalmology clinic; need for re-evaluation of the design and disinfection of instruments. *Infect Control Hosp Epidemiol.* 1989; 10:547–552.

8. Keenlyside, R. A., Hierholzer, J. C., and D'Angelo, L. J. Keratoconjunctivitis associated with adenovirus type 37; an extended outbreak in an ophthalmologist's office. *J Infect Dis.* 1983; 147:191–198.

9. Richmond, S., Burman, R., Crosdale, E., Cropper, L., Longson, D., Enoch, B. E., and Dodd, C. L. A large outbreak of keratoconjunctivitis due to adenovirus type 8. *J Hygiene.* 1984; 93:285–291.

10. Gottsch, J. D. Surveillance and control of epidemic keratoconjunctivitis. *Transactions Am Ophthalmol Soc.* 1996; 94:539–587.

11. Curtis, S., Wilkinson, G. W., and Westmoreland, D. An outbreak of epidemic keratoconjunctivitis caused by adenovirus type 37. *J Med Microbiol.* 1998; 47:91–94.

12. Montessori, V., Scharf, S., Holland, S., Werker, D. H., Roberts, F. J., and Bryce, E. Epidemic keratoconjunctivitis outbreak at a tertiary referral eye care clinic. *Am J Infect Control.* 1998; 26:399–405.

13. Colon, L. E. Keratoconjunctivitis due to adenovirus type 8: Report on a large outbreak. *Ann Ophthalmol.* 1991; 23:63–65.

14. Klapper, P. E., and Cleator, G. M. Adenovirus cross-infection: A continuing problem. *J Hosp Infect.* 1995; 30 Suppl:262–267.

15. Warren, D., Nelson, K. E., Farrar, J. A., and Hurwitz, E., et al. A large outbreak of epidemic keratoconjunctivitis: Problems in controlling nosocomial spread. *J Infect Dis.* 1989; 160:938–943.

16. Nauheim, R. C., Romanowski, E. G., Cruz, T. A., Kowalski, R. P., Turgeon, P. W., Stopak, S.S., and Gordon, Y.J. Prolonged recoverability of desiccated adenovirus type 19 from various surfaces. *Ophthalmol.* 1990; 97:1450–1453.

17. Gordon, Y. J., Gordon, R. Y., Romanowski, E. G., and Cruz, T. A. Prolonged recovery of desiccated adenoviral serotypes 5, 8, and 19 from plastic and metal surfaces in vitro. *Ophthalmol.* 1993; 100:1835–1840.

18. Azar, M. J., Dhaliwal, D. K., Bower, K. S., Kowalski, R. P., and Gordon, Y. J. Possible consequences of shaking hands with your patients with EKC. *Am J Ophthalmol.* 1996; 121:711–712.

19. Jernigan, J. A., Lowry, B. S., Hayden, F. G., Kyger, S. A., and Conway, B. P. Adenovirus type 8 epidemic keratoconjunctivitis in an eye clinic: Risk factors and control. *J Infect Dis.* 1993; 167:1307–1313.

20. Chin, J., ed. *Control of Communicable Diseases Manual.* Washington, DC: American Public Health Association; 2000: 122.

21. Livingstone, D. J., Hanlon, G. W., and Dyke, S. Evaluation of an extended period of use for preserved eye drops in hospital practice. *Brit J Ophthalmol.* 1998; 82:473–475.

22. Hovding, G., and Sjursen, H. Bacterial contamination of drops and dropper tips of in-use multidose eye drop bottles. *Acta Oph.* 1982; 60:213–222.

23. Geyer, O., Gottone, E. J., Podos, S. M., Schumer, R. A., and Asbell, P. A. Microbial contamination of medications used to treat glaucoma. *Brit J Ophthalmol.* 1995; 79:376–379.

24. Schein, O. D., Hibberd, P. L., Starck, T., Baker, A. S., and Kenyon, K. R. Microbial contamination of in-use ocular medications. *Arch Ophthalmol.* 1992; 110:82–85.

25. Templeton, W. C., III, Eiferman, R. A., Snyder, J. W., Melo, J. C., and Raff, M. J. *Serratia* keratitis transmitted by contaminated eyedroppers. *Am J Ophthalmol.* 1982; 93:723–726.

26. Alfonso, E., Kenyon, K. R., Ormerod, D., Stevens, R., Wagoner, M. D., and Albert, D. M. *Pseudomonas* corneoscleritis. *Am J Ophthalmol.* 1987; 103:90–98.

27. Kowalski, R. P., Romanowski, E. G., Waikhom, B., and Gordon, Y. J. The survival of adenovirus in multidose bottles of topical fluorescein. *Am J Ophthalmol.* 1998; 126:835–836.

28. Wessels, I. F., Bekendam, P., Calvin, W. S., and Zimmerman, G. J. Open drops in ophthalmology offices: Expiration and contamination. *Ophthalmic Surg Lasers.* 1999; 30:540–546.

29. Palmberg, R., Gutierrez, Y. S., Miller, D., Feuer, W. J., and Anderson, D. R. Potential bacterial contamination of eyedrops used for tonometry. *Am J Ophthalmol.* 1994; 117:578–582.

30. Coad, C. T., Osato, M. S., and Wilhelmus, K. R. Bacterial contamination of eyedrop dispensers. *Am J Ophthalmol.* 1984; 98:548–551.

31. Dattan, H. M., Flynn, H. W., Jr., Pflugfelder, S. C., Robertson, C., and Forster, R. K. Nosocomial endophthalmitis survey. Current incidence of infection after intraocular surgery. *Ophthalmol.* 1991; 98:227–238.

32. Somani, S., Grinbaum, A., and Slomovic, A. R. Postoperative endophthalmitis: Incidence, predisposing surgery, clinical course and outcome. *Can J Ophthalmol.* 1997; 32:303–310.

33. Heaven, C. J., Mann, P. J., and Boase, D. L. Endophthalmitis following extracapsular cataract surgery: A review of 32 cases. *Brit J Ophthalmol.* 1992; 76:419–423.

34. Aaberg, T. M., Jr., Flynn, H. W., Jr., Schiffman, J., and Newton, J. Nosocomial acute-onset postoperative endophthalmitis survey. A 10-year review of incidence and outcomes. *Ophthalmol.* 1998; 105:1004–1010.

35. Sugar, A., Rapuano, C. J., Culbertson, W. W., Huang, D., Varley, G. A., and Agapitos, P. J., et al. Laser in situ keratomileusis for myopia and astigmatism: Safety and efficacy. *Ophthalmol.* 2002; 109:175–187.

36. Montan, P., Lundstrom, M., Stenevi, U., and Thorburn, W. Endophthalmitis following cataract surgery in Sweden. The 1998 national prospective survey. *Acta Ophthalmol Scand.* 2002; 80:258–261.

37. Cameron, J. A., Badr, I. A., Miguel Risco, J., Abboud, E., and Gonnah, el-S. Endophthalmitis cluster from contaminated donor corneas following penetrating keratoplasty. *Can J Ophthalmol.* 1998; 33:8–13.

38. Kappstein, I., Schneider, C. M., Grundmann, H., Scholz, R., and Janknecht, P. Long-lasting contamination of a vitrectomy apparatus with *Serratia marcescens. Infect Control Hosp Epidemiol.* 1999; 20:192–195.

39. Zaluski, S., Clayman, H. M., Karsenti, G., and Bourzeix, S., et al. *Pseudomonas aeruginosa* endophthalmitis caused by contamination of the internal fluid pathways of a phacoemulsifier. *J Cataract Refract Surg.* 1999; 25:540–545.

40. Cruciani, M., Malena, M., Amalfitano, G., Monti, P., and Bonomi, L. Molecular epidemiology in a cluster of cases of postoperative *Pseudomonas aeruginosa* endophthalmitis. *Clin Infect Dis.* 1998; 26:330–333.

41. Mino de Kastar, H., Grasbon, T., and Kampik, A. Automated surgical equipment requires routine disinfection of vacuum control manifold to prevent postoperative endophthalmitis. *Ophthalmol.* 2000; 107:685–690.

42. O'Day, D. M., Head, W. S., and Robinson, R. D. An outbreak of *Candida prarpsilosis* endophthalmitis: Analysis of strains by enzyme pro-

file and antifungal susceptibility. *Brit J Ophthalmol.* 1987; 71:126–129.

43. Mirza, G. E., Karakucuk, S., Doganay, M., and Caglayangil, A. Postoperative endophthalmitis caused by an Enterobacter species. *J Hosp Infect.* 1994; 26:167–172.

44. Kreisler, K. R., Martin, S. S., Young, C. W., Anderson, C. W., and Mamalis, N. Postoperative inflammation following cataract extraction caused by bacterial contamination of the cleaning bath detergent. *J Cataract Refract Surg.* 1992; 18:106–110.

45. Janknecht, P., Schneider, C. M., and Ness, T. Clinical investigation of outbreak of *Empedobacter brevis* endophthalmitis after cataract extraction. *Graefes Arch Clin Experiment Ophthalmol.* 2002; 240:291–295.

46. Fridkin, S. K., Kremer, F. B., Bland, L. A., Padhye, A., McNeil, M. M., and Jarvis, W. R. *Acremonium kiliense* endophthalmitis that occurred after cataract extraction in an ambulatory surgical center and was traced to an environmental reservoir. *Clin Infect Dis.* 1996; 22:222–227.

47. Tabbara, K. F., and al Jabarti, A. L. Hospital construction-associated outbreak of ocular aspergillosis after cataract surgery. *Ophthalmol.* 1998; 105:522–526.

48. Garg, P., Bansal, A. K., Sharma, S., and Vemuganti, G. K. Bilateral infectious keratitis after laser in situ keratomileusis: A case report and review of the literature. *Ophthalmol.* 2001; 108:121–125.

49. Cosar, C. B., Cohen, E. J., Rapuano, C. J., and Laibson, P. R. Clear corneal wound infection after phacoemulsification. *Arch Ophthalmol.* 2001; 119:1755–1759.

50. Fujikawa, L. S., Salahuddin, S. Z., Ablashi, D., Palestine, A. G., Masur, H., Nussenblatt, R. B., and Gallo, R. C. HTLV-III [HIV] in the tears of AIDS patients. *Ophthalmol.* 1986; 93:1479–1481.

51. Nataloni, R. CDC and AAO offer guidance on safe surgery. *J Ophthalmic Nurs Tech.* 1996; 15:257–258.

52. AAO. *Clinical Alert 2/4: Updated Recommendations for Ophthalmic Practice in Relation to the Human Immunodeficiency Virus.* San Francisco, CA: American Academy of Ophthalmology; 1993.

53. Govig, B., Jackson, W. B., and Gilmore, N. Preventing transmission of HIV in ophthalmologic practice. *Can J Ophthalmol.* 1988; 23:5–7,23.

54. Segal, W. A., Pirnazar, J. R., Arens, M., and Pepose, J. S. Disinfection of Goldmann tonometers after contamination with hepatitis C virus. *Am J Ophthalmol.* 2001; 131:184–187.

55. Rutala, W. A. APIC guidelines for selection and use of disinfectants. *Am J Infect Control.* 1996; 24:313–342.

56. Maldonado, M. J. Corneal epithelial alterations resulting from use of chlorine-disinfected contact tonometer after myopic photorefractive keratectomy. *Ophthalmol.* 1998; 105:1546–1549.

57. Rutala, W. A., Cole, E. C., Thomann, C. A., and Weber, D. J. Stability and bactericidal activity of chlorine solutions. *Infect Control Hosp Epidemiol.* 1998; 19:323–327.

58. Nagington, J., Sutehall, G. M., and Whipp, P. Tonometer disinfection and viruses. *Brit J Ophthalmol.* 1983; 67:674–676.

59. Craven, E. R., Butler, S. L., McCulley, J. P., and Luby, J. P. Applanation tonometer tip sterilization for adenovirus type 8. *Ophthalmol.* 1987; 94:1538–1540.

60. American Optometric Association Primary Care and Ocular Disease Committee. Infection control: Guidelines for the optometric practice. *J Am Optom Assoc.* 1993; 64:853–857.

61. Threlkeld, A. B., Froggatt, J. W., III, Schein, O. D., and Forman, M. S. Efficacy of a disinfectant wipe method for the removal of adenovirus 8 from tonometer tips. *Ophthalmol.* 1993; 100:1841–1845.

62. Chronister, C. L., and Russo, P. Effects of disinfecting solutions on tonometer tips. *Optometry Vision Sci.* 1990; 67:818–821.

63. Simmons, P. A., Edrington, T. B., Lao, K. F., and LeConcepcion, L. The efficacy of disinfection systems for in-office storage of hydrogel contact lenses. *Int Contact Lens Clin.* 1996; 23:94–97.

64. Woodman, T. J., Coats, D. K., Paysse, E. A., Demmler, G. J., and Rossmann, S. N. Disinfection of eyelid speculums for retinopathy of prematurity examination. *Arch Ophthalmol.* 1998; 116:1195–1198.

65. Kellogg Eye Center, University of Michigan Hospitals and Health Centers, verbal communication, 2003.

66. Bolyard, E. A., Tablan, O. C., Williams, W. W., Pearson, M. L., Shapiro, C. N., and Deitchman, S. D., et al. Guidelines for infection control in health care personnel, 1998. *Am J Infect Control.* 1998; 26:289–354.

67. Editorial Note. Epidemic keratoconjunctivitis in an ophthalmology clinic. *MMWR.* 1990; 39:598–601.

68. Alwitry, A., Jackson, E., Chen, H., and Holden, R. The use of surgical facemasks during cataract surgery: Is it necessary? *Brit J Ophthalmol.* 2002; 86:975–977.

69. Speaker, M. G., and Menikoff, J. A. Prophylaxis of endophthalmitis with topical povidone-iodine. *Ophthalmol.* 1991; 98:1769–1775.

70. Anders, N., and Wollensak, J. Inadvertent use of chlorhexidine instead of balanced salt solution for intraocular irrigation. *J Cataract Refract Surg.* 1997; 23:959–962.

71. Baird, D. R., Henry, M., Liddell, K. G., Mitchell, C. M., and Sneddon, J. G. Post-operative endophthalmitis: The application of hazard analysis critical control points (HACCP) to an infection control problem. *J Hosp Infect.* 2001; 49:14–22.

CHAPTER 15

Physical Medicine and Rehabilitation

BACKGROUND

Physical medicine and rehabilitation (PM&R) emphasizes the prevention, diagnosis, and treatment of disorders—particularly those of the musculoskeletal, cardiovascular, and pulmonary systems—that may produce temporary or permanent impairment. PM&R includes the following practices:

- Physical therapy
- Occupational therapy
- Therapeutic recreation
- Speech-language pathology
- Art and music therapy
- Vocational evaluation and counseling
- Orthotics
- Prosthetics
- Rehabilitation engineering
- Special diagnostic techniques, such as electromyography, nerve conduction studies

Some of these PM&R practices may be accredited by the Commission on Accreditation of Rehabilitation Facilities (CARF), *http://www.carf.org.*

CAUSES OF INFECTION

PM&R activities are seldom implicated in cross-infections; the major exception is hydrotherapy. Hydrotherapy has been associated with outbreaks of infection, especially with *Pseudomonas* species.[1-6] Potential routes of infection include accidental ingestion of water, sprays, and aerosols, and direct contact with wounds and skin. (7–8) Patients may also be at risk of developing aspiration pneumonia as a result of dysphagia evaluations by communicative disorder specialists.[9]

Another area of concern is related to *Burkholderia cepacia,* a significant microorganism causing disease in cystic fibrosis patients. It is spread most commonly as a result of intimate or prolonged contact between cystic fibrosis patients. It can also be spread via the hands of healthcare workers if proper handwashing does not occur or by patients touching contaminated environmental surfaces and inoculating themselves. There is some evidence that *B. cepacia* is disseminated into the environment when patients are receiving physiotherapy.[10]

Electromyography (EMG) is a medical diagnostic procedure that involves insertion of needle electrodes into muscle mass with exploration of the muscle as it contracts and relaxes. Needles or surface electrodes are also used in electrodiagnostic testing. An outbreak of infections due to *Mycobacterium fortuitum* associated with EMG was associated with reprocessing of needle electrodes.[11]

RISKS

The risk of infection in PM&R may be a result of therapists having direct physical contact with patients or the various treatments and/or equipment used in physical medicine. Areas of concern include aquatics and hydrotherapy, electrodiagnostic testing, thermal pharyngeal stimulation, wound care, and intermittent urinary catheterization. Treatments and equipment used in these procedures pose a risk.

Hydrotherapy involves the use of hydrotherapy pools, immersion tanks (e.g., full-body tanks or Hubbard tanks), therapeutic extremity tanks, or therapeutic whirlpools. These tanks use pumps to agitate water and provide heating, massage, and gentle debridement. The major concern for infections has been the use of immersion or Hubbard tanks because they are used for severely ill patients with open wounds. The tank may become contaminated with microorganisms carried in the wound. In addition, the water may become contaminated with a patient's organic material, and the water temperature may then promote bacterial growth. Accessory equipment (e.g. parallel bars, plinths, Hoyer lifts, and wheelchairs) may be used in hydrotherapy. Aquatic pools are designed for use by many individuals at the same time and also may become contaminated with organic matter.

PREVENTION

Procedures

General

All procedures must be conducted assuming that there was a risk of infection, and Standard Precautions (see Chapter 6) must be used routinely.

Hand Hygiene[12]

- Hands should be washed before and after each patient contact and after removing gloves.
- Wash hands with an antiseptic agent before palpating, inserting, changing, or dressing any intravascular device or providing wound care.[13]
- Handwashing should occur before and after any procedure.[14–15]
- Alcohol-based hand rub products may be used when hands are not visibly soiled.

Personal Protective Equipment

Gloves must be used for all activities where there is potential for exposure to blood or body fluids. This includes examining abraded or non-intact skin, having contact with mucous membranes, working with contaminated instruments, suctioning, and when the healthcare worker has non-intact skin. Gloves should be changed whenever they are contaminated.

Masks, eye/face protection, and gowns must be worn if there is a likelihood of exposure to droplets of blood or body fluids or to contaminated water. To prevent mucous membrane contact during resuscitation, a mouthbag or mouth-mask device should be kept in each examination and procedure room or in a crash cart.

Sharp Items

There must be procedures established to safely handle contaminated sharp items and to minimize percutaneous and skin or mucosal exposure. These procedures can include various practices such as the following:

- Do not recap needles.
- Sharps containers should be conveniently located.
- Evaluate and use devices, as appropriate, to prevent exposures; these include disposable or safety needles.
- Use a container to hold nondisposable sharp items.
- Remove scalpel blades with a hemostat or clamp or use safety scalpels.
- Discard pins used for sensory testing after each use.

Medications and Multiple-Dose Vials (MDVs)

- Use single-dose vials of parenteral additives or medications whenever possible.
- The access diaphragm of MDVs should be wiped with 70% alcohol prior to puncture.[13]
- Use a new sterile device for any access to a medication vial.[13]

Physical Space

There must be sufficient space for equipment and treatment areas. All work surfaces (e.g., mats and tabletops) must be covered with a surface that can be easily cleaned.[16] Handwashing sinks should be located in areas so that staff can wash their hands conveniently between patients, such as within or at each treatment space. One handwashing station may serve several treatment stations or cubicles.[17]

Careful disposal of all needles and instruments, as well as body fluids, is important. Therefore, waste-handling areas should be designed with staff safety in mind, including convenient disposal containers.

Decontamination of Equipment

Cleaning supplies should be readily available to staff. Potentially contaminated work surfaces (e.g., exam tables and mats) should be cleaned and disinfected at the end of each procedure, unless covered with linen. Other items should be cleaned after use, including evaluation tools, splints, and splinting pans. Any equipment soiled with blood or body fluids must be promptly cleaned and then disinfected. See Chapter 3 for information about disinfection.

It is preferable to use disposable needles; however, if it is necessary to reuse needles, protocols must be established outlining safe handling and sterilization methods. Any instrument used in a sterile manner (e.g., for minor debridement) must be reprocessed and sterilized according to routine procedures. Make sure items used and reprocessed are not labeled for single-patient use. See Chapter 3 for information about sterilization.

Pharyngeal/laryngeal visualization, pharyngeal thermal stimulation, and EMG equipment should be single-patient–use equipment. Any reusable equipment must be appropriately cleaned and disinfected between patient use. Items used for oral examinations or manipulations must be thoroughly rinsed of disinfectant residue to protect patients.

Food preparation areas must be managed safely.[9] Food used for dysphagia evaluations must be stored and handled appropriately. Dishes and utensils should be washed and dried between use. Refrigerators/freezers must be monitored regularly to ensure appropriate temperatures. Temperatures are considered out of range if a refrigerator is greater than 41°F/5°C or a freezer is greater than 0°F/−17.8°C. There are state requirements for food safety; check with the state government for specific information.

Paraffin units should be cleaned routinely with hot water. When using molding materials and adaptive and supporting devices, place a barrier between the patient's non-intact skin and the molding medium. Drain, clean, and disinfect molding pans on a regular basis.[9] Keep a hydrocollator at 160°F (71°C) to minimize bacterial growth. Change the water on a routine basis, and clean the hydrocollator with a nonabrasive cleaner. Use a towel between the device and the patient's skin.

Launder covers between each patient if a towel is not used, on a routine schedule, and whenever soiled.

Aquatic Pools

Proper management is needed to maintain the correct balance of water conditioning and disinfection of pools. Generally, requirements are similar to public swimming pools.[7] The pool requires maintenance of a proper level of chlorine, bromine, or other appropriate disinfectant. The equivalent of 1.5 to 2 parts per million (ppm) of free chlorine at a pH of 7.5 to 7.8 is crucial.[9] Water should be filtered continuously.[16] There may be local or state regulations to follow for pool maintenance. Consider a change in schedule for patients with fecal incontinence, open wounds, healing stomas, or skin lesions.[9]

If the pool becomes contaminated, use the following guidelines:[9]

1. Terminate treatment in the pool.
2. Remove all foreign matter.
3. Shock-disinfect the pool (raise chlorine levels to 10 ppm or more for a limited time), and then measure chlorine levels hourly.
4. Let patients return to the pool when level returns to normal.

Hydrotherapy Tanks: Immersion (Hubbard) Tanks and Whirlpools

Personal protective equipment, such as elbow-length or longer gloves, fluid-impervious gowns, and face protection, should be used for staff providing wound care and performing cleaning procedures.[14]

Drain and clean the tank between each patient use. Clean by scrubbing all inside tank surfaces, including agitator, turbine, and thermometer shafts, with a detergent. Rinse with clean water. After cleaning with detergent and rinsing the tank, apply disinfectant to all surfaces. Use a scrub brush and a bucket of disinfectant.

If the tank is used on a patient with intact skin, the following disinfectants may be used afterward:[14]

- Ethyl or isopropyl alcohol (70 to 90%)
- Sodium hypochlorite (100 ppm available chlorine)
- Phenolic germicide
- Quaternary ammonium germicide

If the tank is used on a patient with non-intact skin, the following disinfectants may be used afterward:[14]

- Ethyl or isopropyl alcohol (70 to 90%)
- Phenolic germicide

The disinfection exposure time must follow the manufacturer's directions. Ensure that agitator jets are cleaned and disinfected; the agitator can be placed into a bucket with disinfectant solution[7, 14] and then rinsed in a bucket of hot water. Finally, rinse the tank. Dry the inside surfaces with a clean towel.

Wipe all tank stretchers, hoist cables, and seats with disinfectant after each use.[14] Tub liners and plastic covers for stretchers and seats are available for use with individual patients. However, these liners do not eliminate the need for proper cleaning. Use of disposable plastic liners with channels for agitation with compressed air may avoid the difficulties in cleaning agitators.[16] Some facilities add disinfectants to the tub water while in use, the most common choice being a hypochlorite. If used, a residual chlorine level of 15 ppm should be maintained.

Communicable Diseases in Patients

Patients may present to PM&R areas with both diagnosed and undiagnosed infections. They can contaminate the environment, items used in procedures, or the air. It is important that referring staff inform the PM&R area that a patient may have a communicable disease and may require special precautions. In addition, patients should be assessed for signs and symptoms of communicable diseases, such as a rash, open skin lesions, or productive cough. Treatment may need to be delayed if a patient is suspected of having a communicable disease.

Contraindications for pool therapy include:[14]

- Exposed subepidermal tissue or blisters
- Wounds and skin lesions
- Skin eruptions
- Unmanaged bladder or bowel, except for indwelling catheters and external catheters in conjunction with a controlled bladder program (patients using external catheters should not be allowed in the pool if they have bladder infections)
- Infectious or communicable disease

Patients with cystic fibrosis who are *B. cepacia*-positive should be separated from other cystic fibrosis patients.[10]

Tuberculosis

Due to the potential of caring for patients who might have unrecognized tuberculosis, PM&R staff should have, at least, an annual tuberculin skin test.

Antibiotic-Resistant Microorganisms

Patients may attend therapy if the site of microbial colonization can be contained, such as if a dressing adequately covers a wound.[14] Equipment used by patients must be disinfected after use.

References

1. Ringham, S. A whirlpool of bacteria . . . *Nurs Times*. 1989; 85:77–80.
2. Jacobson, J. A. Pool-associated *Pseudomonas aeruginosa* dermatitis and other bathing-associated infections. *Infect Control*. 1985; 6:398–401.
3. Schlech, W. F., 3rd, Simonsen, N., Sumarah, R., and Martin, R. S. Nosocomial outbreak of *Pseudomonas aeruginosa* folliculitis associated with a physiotherapy pool. *Can Med Assoc J*. 1986; 134:909–913.
4. McGuckin, M. B., Thorpe, R. J., and Abrutyn, E. Hydrotherapy: An outbreak of *Pseudomonas aeruginosa* wound infections related to Hubbard tank treatments. *Arch Phys Med Rehabil*. 1981; 62:283–285.
5. Mayhall, C. G., Lamb, V. A., Gayle, W. E., Jr., and Haynes, B. W., Jr. *Enterobacter cloacae* septicemia in a burn center: Epidemiology and control of an outbreak. *J Infect Dis*. 1979; 139:166–171.
6. Tredget, E. E., Shankowsky, H. A., Joffe, A. M., Inkson, T. I., Volpel, K., and Paranchych, W., et al. Epidemiology of infections with *Pseudomonas aeruginosa* in burn patients: The role of hydrotherapy. *Clin Infect Dis*. 1992; 15:941–949.
7. *CDC Draft Guideline for Environmental Infection Control in Healthcare Facilities*. Atlanta, GA: Centers for Disease Control and Prevention; 2001.
8. Rimland, D. Nosocomial infections with methicillin and tobramycin resistant *Staphylococcus aureus*—implication of physiotherapy in hospital-wide dissemination. *Am J Med Sci*. 1985; 290:91–97.
9. Temple, R. S. Physical and Occupational Therapy and Rehabilitation Medicine. In: *APIC Text of Infection Control and Epidemiology*. Washington, DC: Association for Professionals in Infection Control and Epidemiology; 2000; 69:1–8.

10. Ensor, E., Humphreys, H., Peckham, D., Webster, C., and Knox, A. J. Is *Burkholderia* (Pseudomonas) *cepacia* disseminated from cystic fibrosis patients during physiotherapy? *J Hosp Infect.* 1996; 32:9–15.

11. Nolan, C. M., Hashisaki, P. A., and Dundas, D. F. An outbreak of soft-tissue infections due to *Mycobacterium fortuitum* associated with electromyography. *J Infect Dis.* 1991; 163:1150–1153.

12. Centers for Disease Control and Prevention. Guideline for hand hygiene in health-care settings: Recommendations of the Healthcare Infection Control Practices Advisory Committee and the HICPAC/SHEA/APIC/IDSA Hand Hygiene Task Force. *MMWR.* 2002; 51 (No. RR-16):1–44.

13. Centers for Disease Control and Prevention. Guidelines for the prevention of intravascular catheter-related infections, 2002. *MMWR.* 2002: 51(RR-10):1–32, *http://www.cdc.gov/ncidod/hip/IV/Iv.htm.*

14. APTA. *Hydrotherapy/Therapeutic Pool Infection Control Guidelines.* Alexandria, VA: American Physical Therapy Association; 1995: 1–31.

15. Marcil, W. M. Handwashing practices among occupational therapy personnel. *Am J Occup Therapy.* 1993; 47:523–528.

16. Linnemann, C. C., Jr. Nosocomial Infections Associated with Physical Therapy, Including Hydrotherapy. In: Mayhall, C. G., ed., Hospital Epidemiology and Infection Control. Baltimore: Williams & Wilkins; 1996: 725–730.

17. American Institute of Architects. *The Guidelines for Design and Construction of Hospital and Health Care Facilities.* Washington, DC: American Institute of Architects Press; 2001.

CHAPTER 16

Radiology

BACKGROUND

Radiologists in ambulatory care settings perform a wide variety of diagnostic and therapeutic procedures. These procedures include:[1-2]

- Computed tomography
- Fluoroscopy (e.g., barium enema, cystogram, intravenous pyelogram)
- Diagnostic radiography (e.g., chest, mammography)
- Magnetic resonance imaging
- Nuclear medicine
- Ultrasound (e.g., transvaginal, vascular, abdominal)
- Interventional/invasive (e.g., angiography)

CAUSES OF INFECTION

Infectious complications due to radiologic procedures (e.g., bloodstream infection, exit site infections, and tunnel infections) vary with the procedure. A study of subcutaneous ports inserted in radiology found 6% of patients developed catheter-related infections. The infection rate was 2.1/1000 catheter days. Fifty-eight percent were bloodstream infections, 23% were cutaneous site infections, and 12% were port pocket infections.[3] Tunneled hemodialysis catheters had an infection rate of 3.8/1000 catheter days when placed by radiologists.[4] Groshong catheters placed in radiology suites by ultrasound had an infection rate of 12% in one study.[5] Meningitis after myelography has also been reported.[6-7]

Nosocomial transmission of tuberculosis has been reported in various radiology settings—both patients and staff are at risk.[8-9] A major factor in these exposures was delay in using appropriate precautions with patients infected with *Mycobacterium tuberculosis*.

RISKS

Diagnostic and imaging procedures include techniques that have the potential for spread of infection. Instillation of any fluid into the vascular system carries a potential risk of infection; there have been outbreaks reported of contaminated contrast medium.[10] Nonvascular interventional radiology procedures (e.g., fluid drainage and obstruction removal) have been associated with a high rate of infectious complications; however, many of these patients have preexisting infections.[11-13]

Equipment used in radiology also poses a risk because it can become contaminated.[11] Ultrasound components (e.g., probes or gel) might also be reservoirs of infection.[14-18] Patient-to-patient cross-colonization with *Staphylococcus aureus* via ultrasound probes has been reported.[19]

Invasive radiology procedures also pose a risk for staff. The potential for injury or exposure to blood or body fluids for staff during invasive procedures is generally low.[20-21] However, splashing or spraying of blood occurs in 6.7 to 8.7% of angiographic procedures. Occult glove perforations involve 10% of gloves used in interventional radiology.[22] The risk increases for procedures lasting longer than 30 minutes and for procedures requiring more than two catheter exchanges, as well as for thrombolysis and angioplasty cases.[23-24]

In a survey of interventional radiologists in 1991, 87% reported at least one procedure-related injury, with 58% of injuries due to use of a sharp instrument, 20% due to needle recapping, and 7% due to improper disposal of a sharp instrument. The median number of injuries per year of practice was 0.3.[21]

A survey to determine the frequency of injuries and blood contacts during invasive radiological procedures and to examine procedure-related factors that may increase risk of injury or exposure found that accidental exposure to patients' blood and body fluids occurred in 3% of procedures. The risk of exposure correlated with the duration of the procedure. Most of the exposures in this study were cutaneous and could have been prevented by the use of personal protective equipment such as gloves.[20] Fortunately, the risk of actual transmission of a bloodborne pathogen, whether from patient to healthcare worker or vice versa, is low.[25]

PREVENTION

Procedures

General

All procedures must be conducted as though there was a risk of infection, and Standard Precautions (see Chapter 6) must be used routinely with all patients. Staff must be trained in surgical asepsis, aseptic technique, and methods for preventing exposure to blood and body fluids.

Hand Hygiene

For invasive procedures, anyone who will touch the surgical field, sterile instruments, or wound site should perform a surgical scrub.[26]

- An operator should start the day with a hand scrub of at least two minutes. Subsequent cases may not require a full scrub using a brush.[27–28]
- The first scrub of the day should include a thorough cleaning underneath fingernails.[29]
- Remove all rings and bracelets before scrubbing.
- Subsequent hand preparation should include the use of an antiseptic product.
- Fingernails should not extend past the fingertips and should be kept free of artificial nails.[29]

- Alcohol-based products with persistent activity that are approved for surgical scrubs are available. They should be used according to the manufacturer's directions.

Wash hands with an antiseptic agent before palpating, inserting, changing, or dressing any intravascular device and after removing gloves. In addition, wash hands whenever indicated per unit protocol. When not visibly soiled, an alcohol-based hand rub product may be used.

Staff/Patient Preparation

For invasive procedures the operator should wear a scrub suit, cap, and mask. Sterile gloves should be pulled over a long-sleeved gown. Other staff should wear scrub suits, masks, and caps.[26] Nonporous drapes (that resist liquid penetration) should be used to cover the area surrounding the wound.[29] Drapes must be large enough to prevent contamination of the sterile field. Visitors should wear a cap and mask and either a scrub suit or cover suit.[26]

Use sterile technique before inserting catheters, including sterile scrub suits, gloves, and drapes. Cleanse the skin site with antiseptic before device insertion. Principles for maintaining a sterile field should be practiced, as follows:

- The patient's hair should only be removed if it interferes with the procedure; it should not be a routine practice. If it is necessary to remove hair at the wound site, it should be done with a clipper or depilatory on the day of the procedure.[29]
- Cleanse the skin site and then apply an antiseptic agent before device insertion. A 2% chlorhexidine-based preparation, tincture of iodine, an iodophor, or 70% alcohol may be used.[30]

Nonvascular interventional radiology procedures, such as diagnostic and interventional catheterization, fluid drainage, and obstruction removal, must be performed in an environment like that used for surgical procedures. All personnel involved in the procedure should wear caps, masks, gowns, and gloves.[11] Procedures that do not require complete sterile attire, except for the use of sterile gloves, include shuntograms, thoracentesis, paracentesis, percutaneous biopsies, and arthrograms. Face masks should be used during myelography procedures. Clean technique (i.e., examination gloves) can be used for performing arm and leg venograms.[31]

Personal Protective Equipment

Gloves must be used for all cases where there is potential for exposure to blood or body fluids. The significant increase in the rate of perforation when gloves are worn more than two hours suggests that gloves should routinely be changed at or before two hours of wear.[32]

- Change gloves routinely after 90 minutes as well as any time they are contaminated or perforation is suspected.[25]
- Remove gloves before touching film cassettes or films, equipment control panels, or other similar items.[25]
- Double-gloving should be practiced if the operator has a break in skin integrity.[33]
- Double-gloving may be helpful in reducing chances of a puncture.
- Gloves must be used during blood drawing or intravenous catheter insertion procedures.

Masks, eye/face protection, and protective caps should be worn to keep the patient's blood from splattering onto the operator during invasive procedures.[23–24] These barriers also decrease the risk of patient infection when cut-down procedures are performed.[34] Given the potential for splashing during invasive procedures, gowns are also needed. Eye/face protection should be used when removing a vascular catheter at the end of a procedure.[33]

To prevent mucous membrane contact during resuscitation, a mouth-bag or mouth-mask device should be kept in each examination and procedure room or in a crash cart.

When there is a reasonable risk of exposure to blood or bloody fluid during any vascular or interventional procedure, the following additional protective clothing is recommended in addition to the items listed previously: shoes only worn when performing procedures; a fluid-impermeable gown; shoe covers or gaiters, to cover lower legs and feet; and hair covering.[33]

Any personal protective equipment that becomes saturated with blood must be removed and replaced as soon as patient safety permits. All barriers must be removed upon exiting the unit.

Patient Care Practices

The sterile field should be prepared as close to the procedure time as possible. Set up instrument trays just prior to a case. Large equipment (e.g., overhead lights) in the vicinity of the procedure table that may need to be handled should be covered with a sterile cover. Intravascular devices and sheaths must be handled using meticulous aseptic technique.[26]

A standard protocol should be developed using guidelines for vascular catheters.[30] The indwelling sheath or catheter should be removed as early as possible. Dressings can be removed after sheaths are withdrawn, when wound edges are approximated, and when the wound is no longer draining.[26] Patients should be educated to inspect the site and report any signs and symptoms of infection.

Small amounts of flush solution may be poured from larger containers. The larger container must be dated and timed when first opened and discarded within 24 hours of opening. An operator's gloved hand should not dip into the flush solution when filling a syringe.[26] Contaminated fluids must be handled carefully to avoid splashing or spilling. Closed flush systems are preferable.

Sharp Items

There must be procedures to safely handle contaminated sharp items and to minimize percutaneous and skin or mucosal exposure.[35] These procedures may include:

- Do not recap needles.
- Sharps containers should be conveniently located.
- Evaluate and use, as appropriate, devices to prevent exposures. These include disposable scalpels, needleless intravenous systems, closed flush systems for angiography, self-sheathing needles, and needle-holding devices.
- Use a container to hold reusable sharp instruments.
- Use a foam pad to hold needles that might be reused during a procedure.
- Reassembly of a multi-part needle must be performed carefully or by using an instrument.[25]
- When needles must be removed from syringes or exchanged, use a clamp, forceps, or other mechanical device.[33]

- Carefully remove needles by the hub before the wire is wiped of blood.[36]
- Use a no-touch method to pass sharp instruments between individuals by placing instruments on the table and avoiding hand-to-hand transfer.[22]
- There should be a designated area for placement of sharp items (e.g., needles, blades) that may be used throughout a case.[26]

Medications and Multiple-Dose Vials (MDVs)

- Use single-dose vials of parenteral additives or medications whenever possible.
- The access diaphragm of MDVs should be wiped with 70% alcohol prior to puncture.[30]
- Use a new sterile device for any access to the medication vial.[30]
- Disposal containers for syringes should be located as close as practical to the location of syringe use.

Physical Space

Procedure rooms should be designed so there is ease of movement without the potential to compromise sterile items or fields. Traffic in areas where invasive procedures are performed should be kept to a minimum. Handwashing sinks should be equipped with foot pedals or elbow or wrist blades that are easily available for staff use. Scrubbed personnel should remain close to the sterile field and should not leave the room during the procedure.[26]

The ventilation system for invasive procedure rooms should provide at least 15 air exchanges per hour, three of which must be fresh air.[29,37] Air should be introduced at the ceiling and exhausted near the floor.[29] Positive-pressure ventilation should be maintained in the room with respect to the corridors and adjacent areas.[33] Ventilation in other radiology areas is not as stringent. These rooms should have at least six air exchanges per hour.[37] The doors to the procedure area should be kept closed during a case, except for required movement of staff and equipment.

Radiation-contaminated articles, such as syringes, needles, intravenous tubing, gloves, linen, and clothing, must be placed in separate containers for disposal into appropriate radioactive trash containers and/or radioactive decay in the hot lab. Radioactive syringes must be recapped (using a one-handed technique) and placed inside carriers to be returned to the nuclear pharmacy. Then these are placed into impervious containers and stored for decay. Appropriate containers must be used for radioactive biohazard waste such as injectables, tubing, and needles. Radioactive waste management must comply with appropriate requirements, for example, the Nuclear Regulatory Commission (http://www.nrc.gov/).

Decontamination of Equipment

Catheters must always be sterile and typically are disposable. Devices labeled as single-use by manufacturers may only be reprocessed using the guidance procedures outlined by the Food and Drug Administration (http://www.fda.gov/cdrh/reuse/index.html). If catheters are reusable, they must be cleaned and sterilized properly. Sinks used for cleaning must be separate from handwashing sinks.

Use a disposable cover (e.g., a condom) for vaginal or endocavitary ultrasound probes.[38] Clean probes with enzymatic cleaner and water to remove gel after each use. Endocavitary and vaginal probes should then be high-level disinfected with a product recommended by the probe manufacturer.[39–40] Transducers used on the skin's surface should be cleaned with soap and water or low-level disinfectant sprays or wipes after every examination. Only use disinfectant products recommended by the manufacturer. Use sterile packets of gel. Examiners should wash hands and change gloves after every exam. If there is evidence of an open wound or contamination with moist body fluids, probe cleaning and disinfection should follow endocavitary recommendations.[41]

Closed flush and waste containment systems should be used for angiography. Glass containers (e.g., contrast media bottles) should be handled separately from regular waste to reduce injury to environmental services staff.[33]

Potentially contaminated work surfaces, such as exam tables, should be cleaned and disinfected at the end of each procedure.[32] Surfaces that may be difficult to disinfect, such as switches, computer keyboards, and control panels, should be covered by a material that can be discarded or disinfected between patients.[11]

There are specific requirements related to mammography equipment that has come in contact with blood or other potentially infectious materials. These requirements are outlined in the Food and Drug Administration's Mammography Quality Standards Act of 1992 (*http://www.fda.gov/cdrh/mammography/robohelp/finalregs.htm*). These requirements focus primarily on documentation of infection prevention and control procedures and maintenance of logs indicating when procedures were performed.

Harsh chemicals and disinfectants may damage some equipment; therefore, it is important to follow the manufacturer's directions. Procedures for cleaning and disinfecting specialized equipment, such as computed tomography (CT) units, mammography equipment, magnetic resonance imaging (MRI) machines, and hyperbaric chambers, should be developed, ensuring that corrosive or otherwise damaging agents are avoided. See Chapter 3 for information on various products.

COMMUNICABLE DISEASES IN PATIENTS

Patients may present to the radiology area with both diagnosed and undiagnosed infections. Contamination of radiology equipment and the environment with microorganisms from patients undergoing procedures may occur and result in subsequent spread to other patients and to healthcare workers. *Mycobacterium tuberculosis* may spread via the airborne route from a patient with unrecognized tuberculosis to other patients and healthcare workers. It is important that referring staff inform the radiology area that a patient may have a communicable disease and may require special precautions.

Patients with suspected or confirmed tuberculosis or other airborne-spread infectious disease must wear a surgical or isolation mask when in the radiology area. Schedule the procedure late in the day when traffic in the area is decreased or delay the procedure, if possible. If available, the patient should be treated in a negative-pressure isolation room.

Patients with antibiotic-resistant microorganisms should be managed so that spread of microorganisms is minimized, including appropriate hand hygiene (see Chapter 6). However, special practices in radiology are not necessary.

References

1. Otten, J. E., and Lynch, P. Imaging Services and Radiation Oncology. In: *APIC Text of Infection Control and Epidemiology*. Washington, DC: Association for Professionals in Infection Control and Epidemiology; 2000: 66:1–3.

2. Bansal, S., and Sunshine, J. H. Hospital and office practices of radiology groups. *Radiology*. 1992; 183:729–736.

3. Kuizon, D., Gordon, S., and Dolmatch, B. L. Single-lumen subcutaneous ports inserted by interventional radiologists in patients undergoing chemotherapy: Incidence of infection and outcome of attempted catheter salvage. *Arch Int Med*. 2001; 161:406–410.

4. Obialo, C. I., Conner, A. C., and Lebon, L. F. Tunneled hemodialysis catheter survival: Comparison of radiologic and surgical implantation. *ASAIO Journal*. 2000; 46:771–774.

5. Hull, J. E., Hunter, C. S., and Luiken, G. A. The Groshong catheter: Initial experience and early results of imaging-guided placement. *Radiology*. 1992; 185:803–807.

6. de Jong, J., and Barrs, A. C. Lumbar myelography followed by meningitis. *Infect Control Hosp Epidemiol*. 1992; 13:74–75.

7. Watanakunakorn, C., and Stahl, C. *Streptococcus salivarius* meningitis following myelography. *Infect Control Hosp Epidemiol*. 1992; 13:454.

8. Jarvis, W. R. Nosocomial transmission of multidrug-resistant *Mycobacterium tuberculosis*. *Am J Infect Control*. 1995; 23:146–151.

9. McGowan, J. E. Nosocomial tuberculosis: New progress in control and prevention. *Clin Infect Dis*. 1995; 21:489–505.

10. Sharbaugh, R. J. Suspected outbreak of endotoxemia associated with computerized axial tomography. *Am J Infect Control*. 1980; 8:26–28.

11. Ribner, B. S. Nosocomial Infections Associated with Procedures Performed in Radiology. In: Mayhall, C. G., ed., *Hospital Epidemiology and Infection Control*. Baltimore: Williams & Wilkins; 1996: 783–789.

12. Mueller, P. R., and vonSonnenberg, E. Interventional radiology in the chest and abdomen. *N Engl J Med*. 1990; 322:1364–1374.

13. Joseph, P. K., Bizer, L. S., Sprayregen, S. S., and Gliedman, M. L. Percutaneous transhepatic biliary drainage. Results and complications in 81 patients. *JAMA*. 1986; 255:2763–2767.

14. Ohara, T., Itoh, Y., and Itoh, K. Ultrasound instruments as possible vectors of staphylococcal infection. *J Hosp Infect*. 1998; 40:73–77.

15. Keizur, J. J., Lavin, B., and Leidich, R. B. Iatrogenic urinary tract infections with *Pseudomonas cepacia* after transrectal ultrasound guided needle biopsy of the prostate. *J Urol*. 1993; 149:523–526.

16. Weems, J. J., Usry, G., and Schwab, U. Infections due to rapidly-growing associated with ultrasound directed prostate biopsy. *Infect Control Hosp Epidemiol*. 1996; 17:P50 (abstract).

17. Pyke, M., Hirji, Z., Havill, D., Rawlinson, G., Burt, J., and Conly, J., et al. Ultrasound (U/S) gel—A potential source of microbiologic contamination. *Can J Infect Control*. 2001; 16:9 (abstract).

18. Gaillot, O., Maruéjouls, C., Abachin, E., Lecuru, F., Arlet, G., and Simonet, M., et al. Nosocomial outbreak of *Klebsiella pneumoniae* producing SHV-5 extended spectrum β-lactamase, originating from a contaminated ultrasonography coupling gel. *J Clin Micro*. 1998; 36:1357–1360.

19. O 'Doherty, A. J., Murphy, P. G., and Curran, R. A. Risk of *Staphylococcus aureus* transmission during ultrasound investigation. *J Ultrasound Med.* 1989; 8:619–620.

20. Hansen, M. E., Miller, G. L., 3rd, Redman, H. C., and McIntire, D. D. Needle-stick injuries and blood contacts during invasive radiologic procedures: Frequency and risk factors. *AJR. Am J Roentgenol.* 1993; 160:1119–1122.

21. Hansen, M. E., Miller, G. L., 3rd, Redman, H. C., and McIntire, D. D. HIV and interventional radiology: A national survey of physician attitudes and behaviors. *J Vasc Interv Radiol.* 1993; 4:229–236.

22. Klein, J. S., and Sandu, J. Interventional procedures in the AIDS patient. *Radiology Clin N Am.* 1997; 35:1223–1243.

23. Davidson, I. R., Crisp, A. J., Hinwood, D. C., Whitaker, S. C., and Gregson, R. H. Eye splashes during invasive vascular procedures. *Brit J Radiol.* 1995; 68:39–41.

24. McWilliams, R. G., and Blanshard, K. S. The risk of blood splash contamination during angiography. *Clin Radiol.* 1994; 49:59–60.

25. Hansen, M. E. Bloodborne pathogens and procedure safety in interventional radiology. *Seminars Ultrasound CT MR.* 1998; 19:209–214.

26. Vander Hyde, K. Cardiac Catheterization. In: *APIC Text of Infection Control and Epidemiology.* Washington, DC: Association for Professionals in Infection Control and Epidemiology; 2000: 62:1–7.

27. Centers for Disease Control and Prevention. Guideline for hand hygiene in health-care settings: Recommendations of the Healthcare Infection Control Practices Advisory Committee and the HICPAC/SHEA/APIC/IDSA Hand Hygiene Task Force. *MMWR.* 2002; 51 (No. RR-16):1–44.

28. Heupler, F. A., Heisler, M., Keys, T. F., Serkey, J., and Society for Cardiac Angiography and Interventions Laboratory Performance Standards Committee. Infection prevention guidelines for cardiac catheterization laboratories. *Cathet Cardiovasc Diagn.* 1992; 25:260–263.

29. Mangram, A. J., Horan, T. C., Pearson, M. L., Silver, L. C., and Jarvis, W. R. Guideline for prevention of surgical site infection, 1999. *Am J Infect Control.* 1999; 27:97–134.

30. Centers for Disease Control and Prevention. Guidelines for the prevention of intravascular catheter-related infections, 2002. *MMWR.* 2002: 51(RR-10):1–32, http://www.cdc.gov/ncidod/hip/IV/Iv.htm.

31. Arias, K., and Molavi, A. Radiology, Nuclear Medicine Units, and Medical Imaging. In: Abrutyn, E., Goldmann, D. A., and Scheckler, W. E., eds., *Saunders Infection Control Reference Service.* 2nd Ed. Philadelphia: W. B. Saunders Co.; 2001: 213–217.

32. Hansen, M. E., McIntire, D. D., and Miller, G. L., 3rd. Occult glove perforations: Frequency during interventional radiologic procedures. *AJR. Am J Roentgenol.* 1992; 159:131–135.

33. Hansen, M. E., Bakal, C. W., Dixon, G. D., Eschelman, D. J., Horton, K. M., and Katz, M., et al. Guidelines regarding HIV and other bloodborne pathogens in vascular/interventional radiology. *J Vasc Interv Radiol.* 1997; 8:667–676. Society of Cardiovascular and Interventional Radiology, http://www.scvir.org/clinical/T51.htm.

34. Leaman, D. M., and Zelis, R. F. What is the appropriate 'dress code' for the cardiac catheterization laboratory? *Cathet Cardiovasc Diagn.* 1983; 9:33–38.

35. Occupational Exposure to Bloodborne Pathogens: Needlestick and Other Sharps Injuries: Final Rule. *Fed Register.* 2001; 66:5317–5325, http://www.osha-slc.gov/pls/oshaweb/owadisp.show_document?p_table=FEDERAL_REGISTER&p_id=16265.

36. Wall, S. D., Olcott, E. W., and Gerberding, J. L. AIDS risk and risk reduction in the radiology department. *Am J Radiology.* 1991; 157:911–917.

37. AIA. *Guidelines for Design and Construction of Hospitals and Health Care Facilities.* Washington, DC: The American Institute of Architects and the Facilities Guidelines Institute; 2001.

38. English, J. F., Malone, J. L., Waters, C. L., Brock, N. F., and Vasquez, E. S. Selection and use of disinfectants for transvaginal ultrasound probes. *Am J Infect Control.* 1999; 27:191 (abstract).

39. Goldstein, S. R. Reprocessing of the vaginal probe between patients. *Ultrasound Obs Gyn.* 1996; 7:92–93.

40. Rutala, W. A. APIC guideline for selection and use of disinfectants. *Am J Infect Control.* 1996; 24:313–342.

41. AIUM. *Recommendations for Cleaning Transabdominal Transducers.* Laurel, MD: American Institute of Ultrasound in Medicine: Official Statements and Reports, 1997, http://www.aium.org/consumer/statement_selected.asp?statement=23.

CHAPTER 17

Urgent/Emergency Care Centers

BACKGROUND

An urgent/emergency care center (UECC) may provide three major services:[1]

1. Care of critically ill or injured patients;
2. Offices where physicians can examine their own patients; and
3. Care for individuals who do not use other ambulatory care services.

Urgent care centers function like physicians' offices with extended hours. Regardless of services provided, patients at UECCs undergo various procedures and may have infectious diseases. In fact, community-acquired infections in both children and adults are evaluated primarily in the UECC. Thus, UECC patients and practitioners have a high potential for exposure to a number of communicable diseases. The management of major trauma also places personnel at high risk for exposure to blood and body fluids.[2]

Any procedure performed in the UECC has the potential to lead to complications for patients, including infection of an access site or of the bloodstream, eye infections, or wound infections.[3,4] Communicable diseases of issue to both patients and staff are bloodborne pathogens (e.g., hepatitis and human immunodeficiency virus [HIV]), tuberculosis (TB), and influenza. In a study at an inner-city emergency department, consecutive adult patients were evaluated for bloodborne pathogens over a six-week period. Twenty-four percent of 2,523 patients were positive for HIV, hepatitis B virus (HBV), or hepatitis C virus (HCV).[5] UECC

staff may develop infections due to patient exposures. In one study, 30% of 30 emergency nurses were positive for HBV markers.[6] Patients with TB are often evaluated initially in UECCs, and there may be a prolonged time until patients are isolated.[7–10]

DEVICES

Any procedure performed in the UECC may place a patient at risk for infection, including placement of intravenous and urinary catheters, lumbar puncture, and suturing. Staff is at risk from sharp objects used on patients, splashing during procedures, and various types of procedural tasks performed. Needle-stick injuries are the most likely source of percutaneous exposure for personnel. Resuscitation of traumatized patients also poses a risk for staff.[11]

RISKS

Infection risks to patients are related to the patient's underlying condition and procedures performed.[1] In addition, patients risk exposure to communicable diseases due to extended time in open waiting areas. For example, children who visited an emergency department were more likely to develop measles than control patients who did not.[12–13]

UECC personnel are at risk for exposure to blood and body fluids.[14–16] Risk factors include the emergent, unpredictable nature of patient care, prolonged contact with patients' blood or body fluids, and high numbers of trauma cases.[15,17] In one study, 92% of procedures performed in one emergency department involved exposure to blood or body fluids.[18] Blood contact per 100 procedures was estimated at 11.2 instances for ungloved workers and 1.3 for gloved workers.[19]

Compliance with Standard Precautions practices in UECCs is reported to be poor. In one study only 55% of staff were compliant during major procedures and 56% during interventions on patients who were bleeding profusely.[20] In another study, the authors noted that glove use was high for trauma procedures.[21] However, use of eye protection, gowns, and masks was low for intubation, central line placement, and lumbar puncture. During trauma cases only 62% of staff reported the use of gowns, masks, and eye protection during most or all cases. The authors concluded that emergency healthcare workers underestimate the risk of occupational exposure to bloodborne pathogens.[17] Hand hygiene activities were also generally not in compliance with recommendations.[22–23]

PREVENTION

Patient-focused prevention techniques include aseptic procedures (e.g., urinary or intravascular [IV] catheterization, lumbar puncture, dressing changes, and blood drawing), care of the IV access site, and evaluation and management of communicable diseases. Employee-focused prevention techniques include use of barriers, vaccination, and education.

Use of Barrier Precautions and Hand Hygiene

- Use Standard Precautions for all patients (see Chapter 6).
- Hands must be washed routinely before and after patient care, especially if visibly soiled. If hands are not visibly soiled, use of an alcohol-based hand rub can be substituted for handwashing.[24]
- Gloves are required whenever there is potential exposure to blood or body fluids.[18,25]
- Gloves are required for vascular access procedures, including starting IVs and drawing blood.[25]
- Gloves may be clean or sterile depending on the procedure.
- Gloves must be changed between patients.

- Care must be taken to avoid touching surfaces with gloved hands that will later be touched with ungloved hands.
- Healthcare workers must wear gowns and face/eye protection when performing procedures during which spurting or spattering of blood or other potentially infectious material (OPIM) might occur.[25] These procedures include chest tube insertion, lumbar puncture, wound irrigation, and intubation.[18]
- Appropriate barriers should be worn during invasive procedures, resuscitation, and wound care. These barriers include personal protective equipment to protect staff from blood or OPIM, as well as sterile barriers appropriate to the procedure to protect patients. See Chapter 4 for information on personal protective equipment.

Patient-Care Equipment

- If a common cart is used for supplies, it should not be taken into patient treatment areas. Remove needed supplies (e.g., gauze, tape) for individual patients.
- Disposable airway equipment or resuscitation devices should be readily available and used.
- Multiple-use patient care items (e.g., blood pressure cuffs) must be cleaned and disinfected between each patient use.

Intravascular Devices[26]

- Wash hands before and after inserting or dressing any intravascular device.
- Wear gloves when inserting an intravascular device.[25, 27]
- Cleanse the IV site with an antiseptic (e.g., 2% chlorhexidine, 70% alcohol, or povidone iodine, or 2% tincture of iodine) before insertion. Allow the antiseptic to remain on the insertion site for an appropriate length of time before inserting the catheter.
- Use either sterile gauze or a transparent dressing to cover the catheter site.
- Minimize manipulation of the catheter.

Use of Medications and Multiple-Dose Vials (MDVs)

- When MDVs are used, individual patient doses should be prepared in a clean area.
- The access diaphragm of MDVs should be wiped with alcohol prior to puncture.[26]
- Use a new sterile device for any access into the medication vial.[26]
- MDVs should not be carried from station to station.
- Store vaccines according to the manufacturer's recommendations.

Cleaning Environmental Surfaces

- Medical equipment (e.g., hemostats, clamps, stethoscopes) should be cleaned and a low-level disinfectant should be applied between uses.
- If an item is visibly contaminated with blood, a low-level disinfectant should be used (see Chapter 3).
- Blood spills should be cleaned immediately with a cloth soaked in a low-level disinfectant. After all visible blood is cleaned, a new cloth or towel should be used to apply disinfectant a second time (see Chapter 3).
- Use a barrier (e.g., a sheet) for each patient on examination tables. Clean the table/area when wet or soiled and at regular intervals (e.g., daily).

Physical Space

Sinks must be conveniently available for healthcare staff. They can be placed in or adjacent to work areas.[28] All areas must have surfaces that can be easily cleaned.

Containers for sharp items must be placed at locations that allow users to discard items easily and safely. Needles must never be recapped using two hands. Safety devices (e.g., protected IV catheters, safety needles/syringes, and safety scapels) should be used to prevent potential percutaneous injuries.[29]

Waste Management

- Environmental services staff members should promptly remove trash and medical waste, and

should maintain an environment that enhances patient care.
- Any waste contaminated with blood, hazardous substances, and sharp items must be discarded according to local and state regulations.

Evaluation and Management of Communicable Diseases

General: Communicable Diseases

Chicken pox, measles, mumps, respiratory syncytial virus, and meningitis are communicable diseases that may occur in an UECC patient population. A large number of individuals can be exposed in a busy center.[30]

Patients should be assessed for signs and symptoms of communicable diseases, such as rash, open skin lesions, or productive cough. A triage screening protocol is important to identify potentially contagious patients and outline appropriate actions to minimize spread (see Appendix C). Promptly triage patients with febrile exanthems and suspected communicable diseases. Mask the patient and separate him or her appropriately according to the area's isolation precautions procedures (see Chapter 6).

Tuberculosis

Screen for TB in the triage area.[31] UECCs should develop a TB protocol to identify patients at triage and promptly separate patients who may have active TB. The protocol should target persons from groups at high risk for TB who present with symptoms of active disease. Patients with risk factors and suspicious symptoms should be provided with a mask and have a chest radiograph. Patients with risk factors and an abnormal chest radiograph, regardless of clinical presentation, should be targeted for immediate intensive infection prevention and control measures.[8,32–33]

Each UECC should have an isolation room, treatment room, or other area available that is capable of preventing the escape of droplet nuclei generated by patients with active TB. The ventilation system should provide a minimum of six air exchanges per hour with negative room pressure to draw air in, which is then vented to the outside. Airborne Precautions signs must be posted on a closed door to the room. Risky procedures (e.g., sputum induction) should not be performed without adequate facilities, such as booths or other enclosures that meet appropriate ventilation requirements.[33]

All persons entering the room of a patient with suspected or known TB should wear properly fitting personal respirator devices. Patients suspected of having TB should remain in the separation room with the door closed, except when being taken to areas for procedures. When being moved outside the room, the patient should wear a standard surgical mask. There should also be protocols that facilitate admission to hospital isolation beds, if appropriate, and communication with local public health facilities for rapid disposition of outpatient care and follow-up[34] (see Appendix C).

Staff should have a tuberculin skin test annually, at a minimum. Determine the frequency based on the facility's risk assessment. All healthcare workers should receive TB education that is appropriate for their risk of exposure and occupation.

Antibiotic-Resistant Microorganisms

If a patient has a record of colonization with an antibiotic-resistant microbe (e.g., vancomycin-resistant enterococcus) the following specific practices are appropriate:[35]

1. Place the patient in a private room, if available.
2. Wash hands whenever anything in the vicinity of the patient was touched (including environmental surfaces).
3. Use gloves for *any* patient contact.
4. If the patient's skin integrity is intact (no open, draining wounds) and his or her clothes are clean, a gown is not required for staff. However, if contact with moist body substances is anticipated, then a fluid-resistant gown must be worn to protect clothing and all areas of exposed skin (following Standard Precautions).
5. Bedside equipment (stethoscope, sphygmomanometer, and thermometer) must remain in the patient's area. If such devices must be used on

other patients, they must be cleaned and disinfected first.
6. Other reusable patient care equipment (e.g., scales, monitoring devices) that has contact with the patient or that may have been contaminated by the HCW must be cleaned and disinfected before being used by another patient.
7. No special precautions are required for laboratory specimens.

Employee-Focused Prevention Techniques

Immunize staff for communicable diseases such as measles, rubella, and pertussis.[36] All emergency health care workers with any potential for blood exposure should receive hepatitis B vaccine unless medically contraindicated and should be tested for immunity after vaccination.[37] Appropriate annual infection prevention and control training is required for staff.

SURVEILLANCE AND PUBLIC HEALTH

An active surveillance system can assist with early detection of infectious complications due to UECC practices. See Chapter 20 for information on surveillance for health care-associated infections. The Centers for Disease Control and Prevention issued a strategic plan to address the threat of emerging infections in the United States.[38] Practitioners in UECCs are also an important component of this strategy.

The UECC is a major link to the community and other healthcare facilities. Each state has a list of diseases that are required by law to be reported to the local health department. The UECC must have protocols outlining responsibility for this function. Protocols should include emergency contact telephone numbers for infection prevention and control and public health resources.

Personnel must be educated in issues related to biological and chemical threat agents.[39] UECCs are the most likely area where individuals will go to seek treatment for exposures or actual disease. It is important for each UECC to include biological disaster response information as part of its emergency preparedness plan[40] (see Chapter 23).

References

1. Jackson, M. M., and Lynch, P. Ambulatory Care Settings. In: *Hospital Infections*. 4th Ed. Bennett, J. V., and Brachman, P. S., eds. Philadelphia: Lippincott-Raven Publishers; 1998: 431–444.

2. Talan, D. A. Infectious disease issues in the emergency department. *Clin Infect Dis*. 1996; 23:1–14.

3. Smith, D., Gottsch, J., Froggatt, J., Dwyer, D., Karanfil, L., and Groves, C. Performance improvement process to control epidemic keratoconjunctivitis transmission. *Infect Control Hosp Epidemiol*. 1996; 17(Suppl):P36, Abstract S52.

4. Richmond, S., Burman, R., Crosdale, E., Cropper, L., and Longson, D. A large outbreak of keratoconjunctivitis due to adenovirus type 8. *J Hyg Camb*. 1984; 93:285–291.

5. Kelen, G. D., Green, G. B., Purcell, R. H., Chan, D. W., Qaqish, B. F., and Sivertson, K. T., et al. Hepatitis B and hepatitis C in emergency department patients. *N Engl J Med*. 1992; 326:1399–1404.

6. Dienstag, J. L., and Ryan, D. M. Occupational exposure to hepatitis B virus in hospital personnel: Infection or immunization? *Am J Epidemiol*. 1982; 115:26–39.

7. Moran, G. J., McCabe, F., Morgan, M. T., and Talan, D. A. Delayed recognition and infection control for tuberculosis patients in the emergency department. *Ann Emerg Med*. 1995; 26:290–295.

8. Haley, C. E., McDonald, R. C., Rossi, L., Jones, W. D., Haley, R. W., and Luby, J. P. Tuberculosis epidemic among hospital personnel. *Infect Control Hosp Epidemiol*. 1989; 10:204–210.

9. Griffith, D. E., Hardeman, J. L., Zhang, Y., Wallance, R. J., and Mazurek, G. H. Tuberculosis outbreak among healthcare workers in a community hospital. *Am J Respir Crit Care Med*. 1995; 152:808–811.

10. Moran, G. J., Fuchs, M. A., Jarvis, W. R., and Talan, D. A. Tuberculosis infection-control practices in United States emergency departments. *Ann Emerg Med*. 1995; 26:283–289.

11. Berk, W. A., and Todd, K. Infection control for health care workers caring for critically injured patients: A national survey. *Am J Emerg Med*. 1994; 12:60–63.

12. Miranda, A. C., Falcao, J. M., Dias, J. A., Nobrega, S. D., Rebelo, M. J., and Pimeta, Z. P., et al. Measles transmission in health facilities during outbreaks. *Int J Epidemiol*. 1994; 23:843–848.

13. Farizo, K. M., Stehr-Green, P. A., Simpson, D. M., and Markowitz, L. E. Pediatric emergency room visits: A risk factor for acquiring measles. *Pediatrics*. 1991; 87:74–79.

14. Henderson, D. K. Risks for exposures to and infection with HIV among health care providers in the emergency department. *Emerg Med Clin N Am*. 1995; 13:199–211.

15. Jagger, J., Powers, R. D., Day, J. S., Detmer, D. E., Blackwell, B., and Pearson, R. D. Epidemiology and prevention of blood and body fluid exposures among emergency department Staff. *J Emerg Med*. 1994; 12:753–765.

16. Kelen, G. D., DiGiovanna, T., Bisson, L., Kalainov, D., Sivertson, K. T., and Quinn, T. C. Human immunodeficiency virus infection in emergency department Patients. *JAMA*. 1989; 262:516–522.

17. Kim, L. E., Evanoff, B. A., Parks, R. L., Jeffe, D. B., Mutha, S., Haase, C., and Fraser, V. J. Compliance with Universal Precautions among emergency department personnel: Implications for prevention programs. *Am J Infect Control*. 1999; 27:453–455.

18. Kelen, G. D., Hansen, K. N., Green, G. B., Tang, N., and Ganguli, C. Determinants of emergency department procedure- and condition-specific Universal (barrier) Precaution requirements for optimal provider protection. *Ann Emerg Med*. 1995; 25:743–750.

19. Marcus, R., Culver, D. H., Bell, D. M., Srivastava, P. U., Mendelson, M. H., and Zalenski, R. J., et al. Risk of human immunodeficiency virus infection among emergency department workers. *Am J Med*. 1993; 94:363–370.

20. Kelen, G. D., Green, G. B., and Hexter, D. A., et al. Substantial improvement in compliance with Universal Precautions in an emergency department following institution of policy. *Arch Intern Med*. 1991; 151:2051–2056.

21. Madan, A. K., Rentz, D. E., Wahle, M. J., and Flint, L. M. Noncompliance of health care workers with universal precautions during trauma resuscitations. *South Med J*. 2001; 94:277–280.

22. Dorsey, S. T., Cydulka, R. K., and Emerman, C. L. Is handwashing teachable?: Failure to improve handwashing behavior in an urban emergency department. *Acad Emerg Med*. 1996; 3:360–365.

23. Meengs, M. R., Giles, B. K., Chisholm, C. D., Cordell, W. H., and Nelson, D. R. Hand washing frequency in an emergency department. *Ann Emerg Med*. 1994; 23:1307–1312.

24. Centers for Disease Control and Prevention. Guideline for hand hygiene in health-care settings: Recommendations of the Healthcare Infection Control Practices Advisory Committee and the HICPAC/SHEA/APIC/IDSA Hand Hygiene Task Force. *MMWR*. 2002; 51 (No. RR-16):1–44.

25. Department of Labor, OSHA. Occupational Exposure to Bloodborne Pathogens: Final Rule. *Fed Reg*. 1991; 56:64175–64182.

26. Centers for Disease Control and Prevention. Guidelines for the prevention of intravascular catheter-related infections, 2002. *MMWR*. 2002: 51(RR-10):1–32, *http://www.cdc.gov/ncidod/hip/ IV/Iv.htm*.

27. Centers for Disease Control and Prevention. Update: Universal precautions for prevention of transmission of HIV, Hepatitis B, and other bloodborne pathogens in healthcare settings. *MMWR*. 1988; 24:377–382, 387–388.

28. AIA. *Guidelines for Design and Construction of Hospitals and Health Care Facilities*. Washington, DC: The American Institute of Architects and the Facilities Guidelines Institute; 2001.

29. Occupational Exposure to Bloodborne Pathogens: Needlestick and Other Sharps Injuries: Final Rule. *Fed Reg*. 2001; 66:5317–5325.

30. Schoolfield, M. B., and Peters, S. J. Infectious disease screening and isolation for pediatric patients in an emergency department. *J Emerg Nurs*. 1995; 21:33–36.

31. Curry, J. L. Identifying the patient with tuberculosis and protecting the emergency department staff. *J Emerg Nurs*. 1994; 20:293–304.

32. Mathias, S., and Hodgdon, A. K. Resurgence of tuberculosis: Implications for emergency nurses. *J Emerg Nurs*. 1997; 23:425–428.

33. Guidelines for preventing the transmission of *Mycobacterium tuberculosis* in health-care facilities, 1994. *MMWR*. 1994; 43:1–132.

34. ENA, *Position Statement Tuberculosis Exposure in the Emergency Department*. Des Plaines, IL: Emergency Nurses Association; 2000, *http://www.ena.org/about/position/tuberculosisexposure.asp*.

35. Garner, J. S. The Hospital Infection Control Practices Advisory Committee. Guidelines for isolation precautions in hospitals. *Am J Infect Control.* 1996; 24:24–52.

36. Wright, S. W., Edwards, K. M., Decker, M. D., and Lamberth, M. M. Pertussis seroprevalence in emergency department staff. *Ann Emerg Med.* 1994; 24:413–417.

37. Bloodborne Infections in Emergency Medicine, Policy number 400293. Irving, TX: American College of Emergency Physicians; 2000, *http://www.acep.org/2,2394,0.html.*

38. Centers for Disease Control and Prevention. *Addressing Infectious Disease Threats: A Prevention Strategy for the United States.* Atlanta: US DHHS, Public Health Service; 1994.

39. Keim, M., and Kaufmann, A. F. Principles for emergency response to bioterrorism. *Ann Emerg Med.* 1999; 34:177–182.

40. Richards, C. F., Burstein, J. L., Waeckerle, J. F., and Hutson, H. R. Emergency physicians and biological terrorism. *Ann Emerg Med.* 1999; 34:183–190.

CHAPTER 18

Laboratory Practices

A laboratory is defined as any facility that performs laboratory testing on specimens derived from humans for the purpose of providing information for the diagnosis, prevention, and treatment of disease or assessment of health. Eighty-four percent of pediatric office practices in Illinois performed laboratory tests in a survey completed during 1996. Typical tests included urine dipstick, streptococcal antigen, hemoglobin or hematocrit, blood count, and stool occult blood.[1] Certain tests are considered waived; that is, some laboratory examinations and procedures have been approved for home use or, as determined by the Food and Drug Administration (FDA), are simple laboratory examinations and procedures with an insignificant risk of an erroneous result. See Table 18.1 for a listing of waived tests. To ensure accuracy and reliability of test results and protect staff and the public, various governmental, professional, and accreditation requirements are applicable to laboratories.

CLINICAL LABORATORY IMPROVEMENT AMENDMENTS

The Clinical Laboratory Improvement Amendments (CLIA) (*http://www.cms.hhs.gov/clia/*) established quality standards for all laboratory testing to ensure the accuracy, reliability, and timeliness of patient test results regardless of where the test was performed. In 1988 Congress passed changes (CLIA'88, 42CFR493) to the CLIA of 1967. In 1992, the Centers for Medi-

care & Medicaid Services [CMS] (formerly known as the Health Care Financing Administration) issued final regulations to implement CLIA. CMS has primary responsibility for financial management operations of the CLIA program.

CLIA covers all laboratory testing, including physician office laboratories and clinics. It mandates specific personnel, proficiency testing, quality control, patient test management, and computer system activities.[2] CLIA regulations require that a laboratory enroll in an approved proficiency testing program for all regulated tests performed. States typically enforce CLIA through licensing and certification divisions of state health departments.

U.S. FOOD AND DRUG ADMINISTRATION

The minimum framework on which standards are constructed for blood use comes under the FDA and is published in the Code of Federal Regulations (*http://www.access.gpo.gov/nara/cfr/*). The FDA requires that establishments that transport blood products across state lines be licensed.

COMMISSION ON OFFICE LABORATORY ACCREDITATION

The Commission on Office Laboratory Accreditation (COLA) (*http://www.cola.org/default.asp*) accredits a variety of laboratories including physician office

Table 18.1   Waived Tests Used in Laboratory Systems*

Alanine aminotransferase (ALT) (SGPT)	Ketone, Blood
Albumin, urinary	Ketone, Urine
Alcohol, saliva	Lactic Acid (Lactate)
Amines	Luteinizing Hormone (LH)
Amphetamines	Lyme Disease Antibodies (*Borrelia burgdorferi* ABS)
Bladder tumor associated antigen	Methamphetamine/Amphetamine
Cannabinoids (THC)	Methamphetamines
Catalase, urine	Microalbumin
Cholesterol	Morphine
Cocaine metabolites	Nicotine and/or Metabolites
Collagen Type I Crosslink, N-Telopeptides (NTX)	Opiates
Creatinine	Ovulation Test (LH) By Visual Color Comparison
Erythrocyte Sedimentation Rate, nonautomated waived	PH
Estrone-3 Glucuronide	Phencyclidine (PCP)
Ethanol (Alcohol)	Prothrombin Time (PT)
Fecal Occult Blood	Semen
Fern Test, Saliva	Spun Microhematocrit
Follicle Stimulating Hormone (FSH)	Streptococcus, Group A
Fructosamine	Triglyceride
Gastric Occult Blood	Urine Dipstick or Tablet Analytes, Nonautomated
Gastric PH	Urine Hcg By Visual Color Comparison Tests
Glucose	Urine Qualitative Dipstick Ascorbic Acid
Glucose Monitoring Devices (FDA Cleared/Home Use)	Urine Qualitative Dipstick Bilirubin
Glucose, Fluid (Approved by FDA for Prescription Home Use)	Urine Qualitative Dipstick Blood
	Urine Qualitative Dipstick Chemistries
Glycosylated Hemoglobin (HGB A1C)	Urine Qualitative Dipstick Creatinine
HCG, Urine	Urine Qualitative Dipstick Glucose
HDL Cholesterol	Urine Qualitative Dipstick Ketone
Helicobacter pylori	Urine Qualitative Dipstick Leukocytes
Helicobacter pylori Antibodies	Urine Qualitative Dipstick Nitrite
Hematocrit	Urine Qualitative Dipstick Ph
Hemoglobin by Copper Sulfate, Nonautomated	Urine Qualitative Dipstick Protein
HGB, Single Analyte Inst. w/Self-Cont.	Urine Qualitative Dipstick Specific Gravity
Infectious Mononucleosis Antibodies (Mono)	Urine Qualitative Dipstick Urobilinogen
Influenza A/B	Vaginal Ph

*From U.S. FDA, Center for Devices and Radiological Health, *http://www.accessdata.fda.gov/scripts/cdrh/cfdocs/cfClia/analyteswaived.cfm.*

laboratories, ambulatory surgical centers, community clinics, and student health services. COLA is a nonprofit organization that uses a voluntary peer-review and educational process to ensure quality in laboratories. The laboratory accreditation program meets CLIA, Joint Commission on Accreditation of Healthcare Organizations (JCAHO), and many state requirements.

AMERICAN ASSOCIATION OF BLOOD BANKS (AABB)

Blood centers and transfusion services must meet general requirements for healthcare facilities that are contained in the American Association of Blood Bank's *Standards for Blood Banks and Transfusion Services.*[3]

COLLEGE OF AMERICAN PATHOLOGISTS

The College of American Pathologists (CAP) (*www.cap.org*) uses standards for laboratory inspections set by the College's Commission of Laboratory Accreditation. This is a voluntary process to improve the quality of laboratory services.

Both COLA and CAP have requirements for meeting basic laboratory safety and infection prevention and control practices. These include use of Standard Precautions, aseptic practices, and proper medical waste handling.

NCCLS

The NCCLS (*http://www.nccls.org*) used to be known as the National Committee for Clinical Laboratory Standards; however, it is now known only by its acronym. This organization is comprised of more than 2000 member organizations from government, industry, and professional and clinical societies. It develops testing standards and guidelines through consensus. NCCLS is nonregulatory; however, it outlines a voluntary framework for laboratories to follow to ensure quality.

JOINT COMMISSION ON ACCREDITATION OF HEALTHCARE ORGANIZATIONS

The JCAHO has specific standards for laboratories in its accreditation manual.[4] These standards are:

PE.1.10 Pathology and clinical laboratory services and consultation are readily available to meet patients' needs.

PE.1.10.1 The organization provides for prompt performance of adequate examinations in anatomic pathology, hematology, chemistry, microbiology, clinical microscopy, parasitology, immunohematology, serology, virology, and nuclear medicine related to pathology and clinical laboratory services.

PE.1.10.1.1 While the patient is under the organization's care, all laboratory testing is done in the organization's laboratories or approved reference laboratories.

PE.1.10.2 When organized central pathology and clinical laboratory services are not offered, the organization identifies acceptable reference or contract laboratory services.

PE.1.10.2.1 Reference and contract laboratory services meet applicable federal standards for clinical laboratories.

PE.1.11 The organization defines the extent to which the test results are used in an individual's care (definitive or used only as a screen).

PE.1.12 The organization identifies the staff responsible for performing and supervising waived testing.

PE.1.13 Staff performing tests have adequate, specific training and orientation to perform the tests and demonstrate satisfactory levels of competence.

PE.1.14 Policies and procedures governing specific testing-related processes are current and readily available.

PE.1.15 Quality control checks are conducted on each procedure as identified by the organization.

PE.1.15.1 At a minimum, manufacturers' instructions are followed.

PE.1.15.2 Appropriate quality control and test records are maintained.

The JCAHO standards evaluate policies and procedures, infection control and safety practices, preventive maintenance and quality control, and proficiency testing. The surveyors review various types of documents, for example, administrative, technical, safety, and infection prevention and control policies and procedures; proficiency testing records; and related information. The JCAHO recognizes CAP and COLA accreditation as "deemed status."

OCCUPATIONAL SAFETY AND HEALTH ADMINISTRATION

The Occupational Safety and Health Administration (OSHA) has rules for protecting healthcare personnel from exposure to bloodborne pathogens.[5] OSHA defines a clinical laboratory as a workplace where diagnostic or other screening procedures are performed on blood or other potentially infectious materials. These laboratories must follow applicable OSHA rules (see Chapter 22).

DEPARTMENT OF TRANSPORTATION

The Department of Transportation (DOT) (*www.dot.gov*) has responsibility for safe transport of goods. It has stringent packaging requirements related to transport of laboratory cultures, specimens, or biological products (*http://63.141.231.101/cgi-bin/om_isapi. dll?infobase=netdot&softpage=Doc_Frame_Pg42*).

GENERAL LABORATORY PRACTICES

Hepatitis B infection was historically the most commonly reported laboratory-associated infection.[6] The risk of hepatitis C is a current concern. Also, many cases of occupationally acquired human immunodeficiency virus (HIV) infections identified in healthcare workers are associated with phlebotomy.[7] Practices performed in laboratories must ensure accurate results and protect staff from potential exposure to blood or body fluids.

Standard Precautions

The use of Standard Precautions is designed for the care of all patients and their body substances, regardless of their diagnosis. It includes the concept of universal precautions used with bloodborne pathogens (see Chapter 6). Specific laboratory activities include:

- Wear gloves when obtaining and handling blood or body fluid specimens and when coming in contact with blood or body fluids.
- Change gloves between patient contacts.
- Wash hands if contaminated, after removing gloves, and before leaving the laboratory.
- Handle sharp items safely. Needles should never be recapped, bent, broken, or manipulated by hand. Discard sharp items into sharps containers.

- Minimize droplets or aerosols during procedures (e.g., properly balancing centrifuges and using a "wrap and snap" technique to remove stoppers when processing blood in vacuum-sealed tubes).
- Use mechanical pipetting devices for manipulating liquids. Do not pipette by mouth.
- Protective garb (e.g., lab coats) must be available and used if splashing is likely.
- Place a biohazard label on any container used to transport specimens and waste.
- Discard all potentially contaminated materials under the facility's medical waste protocol. Consult specific state laws for requirements of medical waste handling.
- Clean blood and body fluid spills, and then disinfect the area.
- Disinfect all laboratory surfaces at the end of each shift.
- Do not eat or drink in the laboratory.
- Offer hepatitis B vaccination to laboratory workers.

Specimens

Appropriate specimen collection, transport, and handling are crucial to ensure valid results. Specimens could be rejected because of drying out, insufficient amount, not in proper transport medium, not received in sterile container, or excessive delay in transport. Specific activities include:

- Make sure appropriate specimen collection container/tube is used.
- Ensure that specimen containers are not cracked or have poorly fitting lids (i.e., to prevent leakage).
- Prevent contamination of specimens (e.g., blood, urine, and wound) through proper skin cleansing of the patient prior to specimen collection.
- Label the specimen appropriately.
- Avoid contamination of the outside of the specimen container.
- Deliver specimens to the laboratory as soon as possible. For microbiology procedures, an unrefrigerated specimen needs to be plated within one-half hour of collection.[8]
- Transport specimens outside the facility safely according to DOT and state regulations. Special mailing containers are required.

- Label specimen refrigerators/freezers with a bio-hazard symbol. Only store specimens in these refrigerators/freezers. Ensure proper temperatures by checking them routinely.

Blood Collection

Accidental needlestick injury and contamination of a blood specimen pose significant risks during phlebotomy.[9] Therefore, safe practices include:

- Safety devices should be used whenever possible, including winged ("butterfly") safety needles, blunt collection needles, disposable blood collection multi-sample luer adapters, collection needles with recapping sheath, and hinged recapping sheath needles.[6]
- Sharps disposal containers must be provided in convenient locations near the point of use.
- Discard all needles and sharp items into sharps containers.
- For routine blood draws: Cleanse skin with alcohol, and do not palpate site after skin preparation.
- For blood cultures: Cleanse culture bottle stoppers with alcohol, cleanse skin with alcohol and iodophor, allow iodophor to dry before performing venipuncture, and do not palpate site after skin preparation.[10]

- For blood donors: Prepare the skin with an antimicrobial scrub solution (e.g., iodophor). Prepare at least a 3 cm area around the phlebotomy site. Do not palpate the site after skin preparation.[11] Allow the solution to dry completely.

Blood Banks

Blood banking practices must ensure the safety of the blood donor, protect the integrity of the blood components, ensure the safety of the recipient, and ensure the safety of medical and other staff.[11] Donors are screened to determine whether they have an increased risk of being infected. In addition, a sample of blood is tested to look for evidence of infection. Blood is collected in a sterile, closed system. Requirements for preparation of components, storage, and discard of blood are outlined by the AABB.[3]

Quality Control

Adequate quality control is essential for a laboratory. There should be a comprehensive procedure manual that outlines standards for performance, administrative responsibilities, and employee safety activities. A model for a quality system for laboratories is available.[12]

References

1. Binns, H. J., LeBailly, S., and Gardner, G. The physicians' office laboratory. *Arch Pediatr Adolesc Med.* 1998; 152:585–592.

2. MacDonald, L. L., and Pugliese, G. Regulatory, Accreditation, and Professional Agencies Influencing Infection Control Programs. In: Wenzel, R. P., ed., *Prevention and Control of Nosocomial Infections.* 3rd Ed. Baltimore: Williams & Wilkins; 1997: 63–68.

3. *Standards for Blood Banks and Transfusion Services.* 21st Ed. Bethesda, MD: American Association of Blood Banks; 2002.

4. *2000–2001 Standards for Ambulatory Care.* Oakbrook Terrace, IL: Joint Commission on Accreditation of Healthcare Organizations; 2000: 83–84.

5. Occupational Exposure to Bloodborne Pathogens: Final Rule. *Fed Reg.* 1991; 56 (Dec. 6):64175–64182.

6. Evans, M. R., Henderson, D. K., and Bennett, J. E. Potential for laboratory exposures to biohazardous agents found in blood. *Am J Pub Health.* 1990; 80:423–427.

7. Centers for Disease Control and Prevention. Evaluation of safety devices for preventing percutaneous injuries among healthcare workers during phlebotomy procedures—Minneapolis, St. Paul, New York City, San Francisco, 1993–1995. *MMWR.* 1997; 46:21–25.

8. Presswood, G. M. Collection, Transport, and Interpretation of Microbiologic Specimens. In: *Infection Control and Critical Care.* Rockville, MD: Aspen Systems Corporation; 1983: 13–29.

9. Dale, J. C., Pruett, S. K., and Maher, M. D. Accidental needlesticks in the phlebotomy service of the Department of Laboratory Medicine and Pathology at May Clinic Rochester. *Mayo Clin Proc.* 1998; 73:611–615.

10. Parini, S. How to collect specimens. *Nursing.* 2000; 30:66–67.

11. Dodd, R. Y. Transfusion Services. In: Abrutyn, E., Goldmann, D. A., and Scheckler, W. E., eds., *Saunders Infection Control Reference Service.* 2nd Ed. Philadelphia: W.B. Saunders Co.; 2001: 705–712.

12. Berte, L. M. New quality guidelines for laboratories. *MLO: Medical Laboratory Observer.* 2000; 32:46–50.

CHAPTER 19

Occupational Health

Contributing authors:
Susan G. Blitz, M.D.
Clinical Assistant Professor
Division of General Medicine
Department of Internal Medicine
University of Michigan Health System
Ann Arbor, MI

Mary Carol Fromes, M.D.
Research Fellow
Environmental Health Sciences
University of Michigan
Ann Arbor, MI

The authors want to acknowledge Christine Pionk, M.S.N., for comments and assistance.

Comprehensive occupational health services are essential to an effective infection prevention and control program. The occupational health provider supplies the clinical services that protect the health of both employees and patients. Healthcare workers (HCW) are exposed to a myriad of biological, chemical, and physical hazards; a thorough knowledge of the types and extent of exposures and possible controls is critical.

Despite the hazardous nature of health care, the industry has only lately received scrutiny by regulatory agencies. The Occupational Safety and Health Administration (OSHA) promulgated standards applying to healthcare settings, the Bloodborne Pathogens Standard.[1] The National Institute for Occupational Safety and Health (NIOSH), a branch of the Centers for Disease Control and Prevention (CDC), advanced policies and procedures for protecting workers when a case of occupational human immunodeficiency virus (HIV) transmission to a HCW was first documented.[2]

The CDC guidelines for infection control in healthcare personnel were published in 1998.[3] These guidelines, as well as a consensus report on the requirements for an effective infection prevention and control program,[4] underscore the importance of collaboration between the infection control and employee occupational health programs. In addition, they identify essential components of employee health services relating to clinical, educational, and administrative functions. The infection control functions of an occupational health service are as follows:

- Policies and procedures to support infection prevention and control
- Pre-placement health assessments and periodic health assessments
- Immunization programs
- Management of employees with infectious diseases
- Management of work-related illnesses and exposures, including bloodborne pathogens
- Health and safety education
- Data management and recordkeeping
- Data analysis for trends in infectious exposures and diseases

The organization and staffing of an occupational health service should take into account the size of the organization, the scope of services, number of employees, the types of patients seen, and the specific hazards encountered.[5] Accessibility, continuity of care, and availability of services for all shifts of employees is essential. Occupational health services for ambulatory care facilities may be provided on-site, through a hospital-based employee-health department, or through emergency departments. Personnel charged with protecting the health of employees must be familiar with the types of hazards in the specific environment, effective control measures, and must keep abreast of changes in recommendations and technologic developments.

RECORDKEEPING

Accurate recordkeeping is essential for complying with regulatory agency requirements, providing data necessary for quality improvement, and analyzing trends of infections and exposures. The OSHA standard for recording and reporting occupational incidents was revised in January 2001.[6] Sections relevant to the infection prevention and control program include the requirement for recording all contaminated needle-stick and other sharps exposures on the OSHA 300 log of occupational injuries and illnesses, regardless of whether prophylaxis was provided or infection was transmitted. To protect the employee's privacy, the name of the exposed employee is not entered on the log. Splashes and other non-sharps exposures are entered as illnesses on the log only if they result in a bloodborne illness or the incident meets one or more of the recording criteria, such as restrictions or absence from work, medical care beyond "first aid," or loss of consciousness. An employer must establish and maintain a sharps injury log for recording exposures that includes the type and brand of device involved in the incident, the department or work area where the exposure occurred, and the circumstances of the incident.[7]

Tuberculosis (TB) skin test conversions and TB following occupational exposure to active TB must be recorded on the OSHA 300 log unless it can be determined that the infection was not related to an occupational exposure.

The employee medical record must be compiled and maintained by a physician, registered nurse, or other healthcare professional and must include medical and occupational history; medical complaints; evaluation; diagnostic tests; treatment, including immunizations;

and recommendations regarding exposure incidents. Employee exposure records must be maintained for the duration of employment plus 30 years.[5]

The occupational health service's database is a valuable tool for documenting compliance with the Joint Commission on Accreditation of Healthcare Organizations' requirements and for demonstrating commitment to process improvement. Using aggregate data to identify areas or aspects of patient care that should be targeted for implementation of control measures is encouraged.

Medical information included in the employee medical record should be maintained in a confidential manner. Employees may be wary of discussing medical issues with the employer's representative, such as occupational health personnel, for fear that their supervisors or coworkers will have access to that information. The employee health service's confidentiality policies and procedures must be sufficiently rigorous that employees are reassured that their privacy will be guarded. Records should be under the authority of a medical department and kept separate from personnel records. If employee health information is kept in the employee's institutional medical record, access should be monitored and controlled.

HEALTH ASSESSMENTS

Pre-placement health assessments are an important component of an occupational health service. Their purpose is to determine whether the employee is able to perform the essential functions of the job with or without accommodations, establish baseline data for medical surveillance, and document any limitations in the use of recommended personal protective equipment, such as respirators and latex gloves. They also provide an excellent opportunity for educating employees about safe practices and ensuring that they are familiar with the procedure for reporting occupational exposures or communicable diseases.

The essential components include an infectious disease history, review of immunizations record, assessment of any health conditions that may increase the employee's risk of acquiring or transmitting an infectious disease, physical examination relevant to job performance, and baseline medical surveillance including tuberculin skin testing. An immunization inventory completed by the employee prior to the pre-placement visit can simplify the procedure (see Appendix J).

If the employee will be exposed to reproductive toxins, a reproductive history should also be completed. Employees should be informed that the visit is designed to gather specific job-related information and is not a substitute for a examination by their personal healthcare provider.

Periodic health assessments are recommended for employees exposed to biological, chemical, or physical hazards in order to document any changes in health that might be attributable to exposure. Employees returning to work following treatment for a nonoccupational illness should be evaluated for changes in job duties or job placement to protect their health.

IMMUNIZATION

The likelihood of exposure to vaccine-preventable diseases and the safety and effectiveness of the vaccines should assist in the design of a healthcare organization's immunization program. State, federal, and accreditation regulatory bodies may require specific vaccinations for healthcare workers. The most recent publications from the CDC regarding immunization programs for healthcare workers provide detailed rationale and recommendations.[3,8] In addition to the specific vaccine recommendations, general principles of immunization storage, administration, contraindications, and adverse events are also available.[9,10] A list of vaccinations that should be provided or offered to HCWs follows:[8]

- Hepatitis B vaccine
- Measles, Mumps, Rubella (MMR) live vaccine
- Influenza vaccine
- Varicella zoster live vaccine
- Hepatitis B immune globulin (post exposure)
- Varicella-zoster immune globulin (post exposure)

The decision to prescreen for serologic immunity prior to vaccination should take into account the likelihood of immunity, the relative cost of laboratory tests and vaccine, and the feasibility of multiple visits by staff. Recommendations for vaccinating pregnant and immunocompromised individuals are included in the CDC references. In general, the risk of vaccination during pregnancy is largely theoretical; the decision to vaccinate a pregnant woman should take into account

the benefit of immunization for mother and fetus and the risk of toxicity. Although pregnancy is a contraindication for measles, mumps, and rubella vaccines, no cases of congenital rubella syndrome or abnormalities attributable to the rubella vaccine have been observed in pregnant women inadvertently vaccinated with rubella vaccine.[9]

Hepatitis B Virus

In the pre-vaccine era, the prevalence of hepatitis B virus (HBV) infection in HCWs was more than twice that of individuals without occupational exposure.[11] Due to the acceptance of vaccination and adoption of Standard Precautions, the number of HBV infections in HCWs declined by 93%, from 12,000 cases in 1985 to 800 cases a decade later.[12]

Hepatitis B recombinant vaccine is provided as a series of three injections over a six-month period. The usual schedule is for the second dose to be given one month after the first dose and the third dose at six months. If the vaccination series is interrupted after the first dose, the second dose should be administered as soon as possible. The second and third doses should be separated by an interval of at least two months. If only the third dose is delayed, it should be administered when convenient.[13]

After proper administration of the series into the deltoid muscle, over 90% of healthy adults will develop protective immunity to HBV.[14] Protection has been documented to persist for at least 11 years. Antibody titer declines over time and may decrease to nondetectable levels. However, an anamnestic response to the antigen is proposed as the basis for long-term protection. Therefore, booster doses are not recommended for adults who respond to the initial series.[8,15]

Although universal testing for antibody after hepatitis B vaccination is not recommended, HCWs who are at ongoing risk of exposure to blood or body fluids should be tested for antibody one to two months after completion of the third dose. HCWs who do not respond to an initial three-dose series should be evaluated for HBV antigenemia. If negative, a second series should be started. Individuals who do not achieve a positive antibody response after a second series should be considered nonresponders and should be counseled regarding their susceptibility to HBV and the importance of prompt reporting of exposures so that appropriate treatment can be provided.[8]

The OSHA Bloodborne Pathogens Standard mandates that hepatitis B vaccination be offered free of charge within 10 working days of initial assignment to employees with potential exposure to blood and body fluids, unless the employee has previously received the vaccine or is immune. If the employee does not wish to receive the vaccine, a declination form using text outlined in the Standard must be signed[1] (see Appendix J). An employee who declines the vaccine initially may receive the vaccine at a later date.

Measles, Mumps, and Rubella

All HCWs should be immune to measles, mumps, and rubella (MMR). Therefore, if vaccination is provided to an adult HCW, the preferred vaccine is the combined MMR vaccine rather than the individual components.[16] In healthcare workers, evidence for immunity to these diseases is defined as:

1. Documented administration of one dose of measles, mumps, and rubella vaccines on or after the first birthday and an additional dose of measles (or MMR) vaccine at least one month after the first;
2. For measles and mumps, documentation of physician-diagnosed disease; or
3. Serologic evidence of immunity.

Because these illnesses used to be so prevalent, birth before 1957 has been accepted as evidence of immunity to measles, mumps, and rubella; however, surveillance studies have demonstrated gaps in immunity in HCWs born before 1957. Therefore, one dose of MMR vaccine is recommended if documented physician-diagnosed disease or serologic proof of immunity is not available, particularly if the HCW will be exposed to pediatric patients.

Although pre-vaccination serologic screening for measles, mumps, and rubella immunity may be cost-effective, it should not replace vaccination at the new employee visit unless the occupational health provider is confident that the employee will return for vaccination if found to be susceptible.

Influenza

Influenza vaccine should be offered annually to all HCWs. Vaccination prevents transmission of infection from caregiver to patient and decreases absences from work.[17] Several categories of high-risk individuals present as outpatients; therefore, ambulatory care workers should be immunized for their patients' protection. Occupational health providers should diligently educate HCWs about the importance of vaccination and the rarity of adverse reactions to the vaccine.[18] In addition, providing convenient access to vaccination in proximity to employees' worksites and during work hours will increase the rate of vaccination, which is especially important if a centralized occupational health department provides services to off-site locations.

Varicella

HCWs should be immune to varicella, either through past infection or vaccination. Unlike other infectious diseases, a history of chicken pox is considered adequate evidence of immunity. When adults with a history of chicken pox have been tested for serologic immunity, over 95% are seropositive, and even adults with an uncertain or negative history of disease are likely to be seropositive.[8] Therefore, pre-vaccination screening for varicella immunity in employees without a clear history of chicken pox is recommended.

For susceptible individuals, the vaccine should be given in a two-dose schedule, four to eight weeks apart. Pregnant women or women who plan to conceive within one month should not be vaccinated with varicella vaccine. The vaccine is 70% to 90% effective against infection and significant protection is long lasting.[19] Vaccinated individuals exposed to varicella infrequently develop breakthrough infections with mild disease.[8] In view of the imperfect efficacy of the vaccine and the possibility of breakthrough infections, vaccinated HCWs should avoid exposure to varicella and, if exposed, consideration should be given to avoiding contact with immunocompromised or other patients who are at greater risk for complications of varicella.

A vesicular rash occurring within two weeks after vaccination may be associated with wild-type virus. In the presence of a rash, secondary transmission of the virus can occur, although it is exceedingly rare.[20] If a rash develops after vaccination, the HCW should be removed from patient contact until the lesions are crusted.

Other Vaccine-Preventable Diseases

Pneumococcal vaccination may be offered to HCWs with risk factors, such as chronic cardiovascular or respiratory disease, asplenia, diabetes, or immunocompromised status. In the United States, HCWs are not at increased risk of diphtheria or tetanus; however, all adults should complete a diphtheria and tetanus primary series and receive booster doses of the toxoids every 10 years. HCWs have not been found to be at increased risk for hepatitis A infection if proper infection prevention and control practices are maintained. However, the vaccine is recommended for travel to most foreign countries and should be provided in the event of job-related travel. Vaccination against TB with Bacille-Calmette-Guerin vaccine (BCG) should be considered only for HCWs in areas where multidrug–resistant tuberculosis is prevalent and a strong likelihood of infection exists from close or prolonged contact.[8] Responding to recent concerns regarding bioterrorism and the possibility of an intentional release of variola (smallpox) virus, the CDC has published guidelines for the use of vaccinia vaccine in the event of increased risk or actual release of variola virus. Healthcare workers who might be at occupational risk of exposure may be one of the priority groups for vaccination[21] (see Chapter 23).

TUBERCULOSIS ASSESSMENT AND CONTROL

TB Skin Testing

Identification of latent tuberculosis infection (LTBI), indicated by a positive TB skin test, is an important part of a pre-placement health assessment. HCWs with a reliable history of a positive skin test should not be retested but should undergo symptom review and chest radiography to rule out active disease. Information about past exposure to TB, the year that the skin test became positive, results of prior chest X-rays, and a general health history should be recorded. LTBI is not infectious, and treatment for LTBI should not be a requirement for employment. The HCW should be reminded of the signs and symptoms of active TB and should be instructed to report any change in health status that might indicate active disease to occupational health staff. Employees with active disease are restricted from working until treatment has been initiated and three daily negative sputum collections are documented.

New employees without a history of a positive skin test or with an unknown history should undergo tuberculin skin testing to establish a baseline test and to identify LTBI. Infected persons develop a delayed-type hypersensitivity reaction to antigenic components of the mycobacterium (tuberculin) manifested as a palpably raised hardened area (induration) at the injection site. The Mantoux method is the standard for identifying infection with *M. tuberculosis*. The induration caused by the delayed hypersensitivity reaction peaks between 48 and 72 hours after injection and should be read during that time frame.

Previous vaccination with BCG should not preclude TB skin testing.[22] Because the protective effect of BCG is highly variable and BCG is administered in areas where TB is prevalent, it is important to identify LTBI in individuals who have received BCG. The tuberculin reaction to BCG vaccination is variable, and there is no reliable way to distinguish a reaction to BCG from infection. Therefore, recipients of BCG without a history of a positive skin test should undergo testing, and their tests should be classified as positive or negative using the criteria listed in Table 19.1.

The TB skin test should be administered and read by a trained HCW familiar with proper technique for placing and reading the test and knowledgeable in the epidemiology and clinical features of TB. An occupational health service may not be proximate to the ambulatory care setting, so mandating that placement and reading of skin tests take place in the occupational health clinic may result in hardship on employees and decreased compliance. To increase access while ensuring quality, staff at ambulatory care sites may be trained in proper skin testing procedures, if not prohibited by local regulations. The CDC has a number of training resources, including the Core Curriculum on Tuberculosis and a free skin testing videotape.[23]

If the baseline skin test is positive, the employee is evaluated for the presence of active TB disease with a symptom review, directed physical examination, and chest radiography. If active disease is found, the employee must undergo treatment and be considered

Table 19.1 Classification of Positive TB Skin Tests by Degree of Induration*

Induration ≥5 mm	Induration ≥10 mm	Induration ≥15 mm
HIV-positive person. Recent contacts of TB case. Fibrotic changes on chest radiograph consistent with old TB. Persons with organ transplants and immunosuppression.	Immigration from high-prevalence country in the past 5 years. Employees of high-risk settings (including healthcare facilities and mycobacterial labs). Persons with medical conditions associated with increased risk of tuberculosis.	Persons without risk factors for TB, including new employees of healthcare facilities without other risks.

*Adapted from *Core Curriculum on Tuberculosis. What the Clinician Should Know.* 4th Ed. Atlanta, GA: Centers for Disease Control and Prevention; 2000, http://www.cdc.gov/nchstp/tb/pubs/corecurr/default.htm.

noinfectious prior to beginning employment or returning to work.

Two-Step Skin Testing

For employees who will undergo periodic skin testing, a two-step method is preferred upon initial employment. Two-step testing reduces the risk of misclassifying an old positive reaction as a new conversion, an error that can occur due to the "booster phenomenon." Although infection with TB should result in a persistently positive skin test reaction, the delayed hypersensitivity response can wane over time, resulting in a falsely negative reaction to a skin test. However, this initial test "boosts" the immunologic memory and subsequent tests will be markedly positive. These positive tests will be misconstrued as a new positive rather than prior infection. Boosting is most common in individuals older than 50 years of age and in persons who have been vaccinated with BCG.

In two-step testing, an initial skin test is placed and, if negative, a second test is placed one to three weeks later. If the second test is positive, this is clearly a "boosted" test and not a recent infection. If the second test is negative, the person is considered uninfected and can be retested annually. Although two-step testing is very useful in establishing rates of true skin test conversions, it is cumbersome, and compliance with two-step testing may be difficult to achieve. The most efficient approach is to have the initial skin test placed at the new employee health assessment and, rather than have the employee return in 48 to 72 hours for the reading, instruct the employee to return for the initial reading in seven days. A skin test cannot accurately be interpreted as negative past 72 hours, but if it is still positive seven days later, the test can be considered a valid positive and the second step is unnecessary. If the test is negative, the second step is placed at the one-week visit and is read 48 to 72 hours after placement. This schedule requires three, rather than four, visits, so it is less burdensome for the employee and occupational health provider.[24] If a new employee had a skin test within the preceding 12 months, it can serve as the first step, and only one skin test is needed for employment.

Periodic Testing

The frequency of testing staff is determined by the likelihood of TB exposure. The CDC guidelines[25] determine the periodicity of ongoing skin test surveillance by assigning a risk category based on the number of TB patients admitted to a facility or area of the facility, the types of procedures performed, and the rate of employee skin test conversion. Ambulatory care facilities that care for a large number of patients with high-risk characteristics (HIV, recent immigrants from high-prevalence areas, and the homeless) may fall into the intermediate or high-risk categories. The intermediate and high-risk categories require skin testing every three or six months; facilities in the other categories can test annually. The annual skin test visit should include reinforcement of proper risk reduction practices and review of the signs and symptoms of active TB. In addition to annual testing, employees who have experienced an exposure to *M. tuberculosis* should be tested at baseline and 12 weeks after exposure to assess for infection. If performed within several months of the exposure, the annual test can serve as the baseline. Treatment of LTBI should be strongly considered for post-exposure conversions.

Employees with a positive skin test are not retested and should not undergo chest radiographs unless symptoms of active TB are reported. Skin test-positive employees should be reminded of the signs and symptoms of TB and should be aware of the need for prompt reporting should they develop any suspicious symptoms. Some facilities choose to administer an annual symptom questionnaire to these employees.

Skin Test Conversions and Treatment for LTBI

A skin test conversion is defined as an increase of ≥10 mm of induration within a two-year period, regardless of the person's age.[26] Individuals with recent TB infection are at higher risk of developing active TB. Therefore, all new skin test converters should be considered for treatment of LTBI. The decision to treat should consider the likelihood of developing active disease and the potential risks of treatment. Recommendations for specific treatment regimens should consider the efficacy of the treatment as well as the risk of toxicity and the likelihood of adherence to a medication schedule. The most recent recommendation for first line therapy of LTBI is nine months of daily isoniazid therapy; however, alternative regimens may be preferable in specific cases.[26] Because LTBI is not infectious, treatment should not be a condition of employment.

Medical Evaluation for TB Respirator Use

Respiratory protection is a component of TB control in all healthcare facilities. Although early identification and isolation of patients with infectious TB will minimize exposure, HCWs must be protected from airborne exposure when caring for patients with active disease. The respirators approved by OSHA for protection against *M. tuberculosis* include the disposable N-95 mask, the disposable high-efficiency particulate air (HEPA) respirator, and the powered air purifying respirator (PAPR) hood fitted with a HEPA filter.[27] The N-95 type respirator is easier to use and less expensive than the HEPA respirator. The PAPR must be used in employees with facial hair or other conditions that preclude proper fitting of the N-95 respirator.

OSHA requires that individuals who will wear respiratory protection undergo a medical evaluation to ensure that there are no physical or mental conditions that would contraindicate respiratory protection. This requirement can be fulfilled with a questionnaire, using face-to-face follow-up for those employees who indicate possible difficulties on the questionnaire. After medical clearance, fit testing for the N-95 type respirator must be performed. The PAPR hood does not require fit testing and is well suited for use in situations where the need for respiratory protection is infrequent or unexpected.

EXPOSURE TO BLOODBORNE PATHOGENS

The OSHA Bloodborne Pathogens (BBP) Standard[1] mandates offering vaccination against bloodborne pathogens (currently only feasible against hepatitis B), prevention of exposure through Standard Precautions, education and training on the risks of exposure and prevention, evaluation for post-exposure prophylaxis (PEP), and monitoring and record-keeping requirements to track infection resulting from exposure.

Post Exposure Evaluation and Management

Protocols for the evaluation and management of BBP exposures should be outlined. The protocols should be reviewed periodically and revised as new recommendations become available. Employee confidentiality should be protected by limiting access to baseline and follow-up blood tests or coding specimens without use of names. In addition, an effective BBP management program includes counseling for emotional concerns following exposure, monitoring for adverse effects of PEP, prompt reporting of source blood test results to the employee, and an active system for reminding employees when follow-up blood testing is due. Reviewing the circumstances involved in exposure incidents with the employee and the employee's supervisor can identify opportunities for safety training and hazard reduction. The infection prevention and control program should review aggregate exposure data at least annually.

The definition of an exposure should be clearly stated and applied consistently. The BBP standard defines an exposure incident as "a specific eye, mouth, other mucous membrane, non-intact skin, or parenteral contact with blood or other potentially infectious materials that results from the performance of an employee's duties." Other potentially infectious materials (OPIM) refer to body substances that theoretically could or have been documented to transmit BBP. Feces, nasal secretions, saliva (except in dental settings), sputum, sweat, tears, urine, and vomitus are not considered infectious unless they contain blood.[28]

If an exposure occurs, the site should be washed with soap and water; mucous membranes should be flushed with water. If the source of the exposure is known, blood should be obtained for hepatitis B surface antigen (HBsAg), hepatitis C antibody, and HIV antibody testing in accordance with local regulations of informed consent and confidentiality. A rapid HIV antibody test is available and can be useful for making timely, appropriate decisions regarding prophylaxis and for reassuring employees if the source patient proves to be negative for HIV. If the source patient is negative for all bloodborne pathogens, baseline and follow-up testing of the exposed person are not necessary but may be offered for employee reassurance.

If the source of exposure is unknown or cannot be tested, the risk of exposure to bloodborne pathogens should be assessed from information on risk factors of the particular source and the prevalence of BBP in the patient population. Generally, the CDC does not recommend HIV PEP for exposure to an unknown source unless exposure to an HIV-infected person is likely (e.g., in an HIV treatment clinic).[29]

Management of HBV exposure takes into consideration the antigen status of the source patient and the antibody status of the exposed person. A HCW who has a documented adequate titer of hepatitis B antibody is considered immune and does not have to be retested or treated. If the response to vaccination is unknown, the exposed person should be tested at the time and treated according to the result of the test. If the exposed person has inadequate titer of antibody after one vaccine series, treatment with hepatitis B immune globulin (HBIG) is indicated, followed by a second dose of HBIG one month later or initiation of a second vaccine series. If the person has received two hepatitis B vaccine series and has not demonstrated an adequate antibody titer, a second dose of HBIG at one-month post-exposure is indicated.

HBIG is administered at a dose of 0.06 ml/kg in the deltoid muscle and should be given as soon as possible after exposure, preferably within 24 hours. The effectiveness of two doses of HBIG in preventing transmission of HBV infection is approximately 75%; the effectiveness of HBIG given seven or more days after exposure is unknown. Susceptible HCWs exposed to HBV should have follow-up testing for HBsAg at three and six months post-exposure. Table 19.2 summarizes the recommendations for treatment of HBV exposures.

Table 19.2   Post-Exposure Prophylaxis for HBV*

Vaccination and Immune Status of Exposed Person	Treatment If Source Is HbsAg+	Treatment If Source Is HbsAg–	Source Unknown or Cannot Be Tested
Unvaccinated	HBIG x 1 dose and initiate vaccination	Initiate vaccination	Initiate vaccination
Previously vaccinated—adequate response by titer	No treatment	No treatment	No treatment
Previously vaccinated—inadequate response by titer	HBIG x 1 dose; dose #2 in 1 month or initiate 2nd series	No treatment	If known high-risk source, treat as if HbsAg+
Vaccinated; antibody response unknown	Test for antibody titer: If adequate, treat as responder; if inadequate, HBIG x 1 dose and vaccine booster	No treatment	Test for antibody titer: If adequate, treat as responder; if inadequate, administer vaccine booster and recheck titer in 1 month

*Adapted from Centers for Disease Control and Prevention. Updated U.S. Public Health Service guidelines for the management of occupational exposures to HBV, HCV, and HIV and recommendations for postexposure prophylaxis. *MMWR*. 2001; 50(RR-11):1–52.

Persons exposed to HBV do not need to refrain from pregnancy or breastfeeding or modify their sexual practices; however, they should be counseled to refrain from donating blood, plasma, organs, tissue, or semen.[29]

Management of HCV exposures focuses on testing for transmission of infection because there is no effective PEP. The commonly used screening test for HCV infection, anti-HCV antibody by enzyme immunoassay, is sensitive but is associated with a high false-positive rate in low-prevalence populations. All positive enzyme immunoassay results should be confirmed using a more specific supplemental test, such as a recombinant immunoblot assay (RIBA).

Persons exposed to an HCV-infected source patient should undergo baseline testing for hepatitis C and liver function. Follow-up testing for anti-HCV and liver function tests should be performed at three and/or six months. HCV ribonucleic acid (RNA) can be demonstrated as early as several weeks after infection. Testing the exposed person for HCV RNA at four weeks following exposure is an option that should be considered in light of recent evidence that early treatment of HCV infection may result in better outcomes than treatment of chronic disease.[30] If HCV infection is identified, the employee should be referred to a specialist knowledgeable in the management of HCV. Persons exposed to HCV do not need to refrain from pregnancy or breastfeeding or modify their sexual practices; however, they should be counseled to refrain from donating blood, plasma, organs, tissue, or semen.[29]

Although PEP for occupational HIV exposures has been widely prescribed since 1990, human studies demonstrating evidence of effectiveness of PEP were not published until 1997. In a retrospective case-control study conducted by the CDC, administration of PEP with zidovudine was associated with an 81% reduction in seroconversion.[31] Animal studies suggest that efficacy is greatest when PEP is administered within one hour after exposure. Although that time frame often is not feasible in the occupational setting, vigorous efforts to initiate PEP within two hours after exposure are advised. PEP regimens should be continued for 28 days. If PEP is initiated prior to source HIV test results becoming available, reevaluation should occur as soon as test results are known. If the source is HIV-negative, PEP should be discontinued. Because toxicity of the antiviral agents commonly employed in PEP is not trivial, PEP should be administered only by

health professionals familiar with the risk of transmission, the recommended treatment regimens, and monitoring for PEP toxicity.

Resources for expert consultation for HIV exposures include the National Clinicians' Post-Exposure Prophylaxis Hotline (PEPline, 1 (888) HIV-4911) and the NEEDLESTICK! Interactive Web site administered through the University of California, Los Angeles, *www.needlestick.mednet. ucla.edu.*

The current recommendations for HIV PEP, as well as management of HBV and HCV exposures, were published in 2001.[29] A combination drug of zidovudine and lamivudine taken for four weeks is recommended as the basic regimen; a protease inhibitor is added for higher-risk exposures. If the source HIV patient is known to be resistant to zidovudine and lamivudine or there are other reasons to choose an alternate regimen, expert consultation is advised. An algorithm incorporating information from the CDC guideline is detailed in Appendix J. HCWs receiving PEP should be monitored closely for toxicity with a symptom review and blood testing. Baseline, two-, and four-week testing with a complete blood count and renal and hepatic function tests is recommended.[32]

Any HCW with exposure to HIV, regardless of whether PEP is used, should be counseled regarding safer sex practices; avoidance of pregnancy; and refraining from blood, organ, or semen donation during at least the first three months of follow-up. Women who are breastfeeding should be counseled regarding the possibility of transmission and the risk to the child of PEP drugs in breast milk.[29] HCWs exposed to HIV should have baseline HIV antibody testing and follow-up testing at six weeks, three months, and six months. An optional 12-month follow-up can be offered, particularly if the HCW was exposed to HIV and HCV simultaneously, as delayed seroconversion has been noted in that situation.[33]

EXPOSURES TO OTHER INFECTIOUS DISEASES

In the ambulatory care environment, the most important airborne transmitted infections are TB, measles, and varicella. Droplet-spread diseases encountered in ambulatory settings include pertussis, mumps, rubella, influenza, and many other respiratory infections. Common diseases transmitted by contact include viral conjunctivitis and impetigo. Enforcing vaccination requirements is the most effective method of controlling the vaccine-preventable diseases.

WORK RESTRICTIONS

Ambulatory care centers should have written policies and procedures mandating all employees to report infectious diseases or exposures. The initial report will often be to supervisory staff who, depending on the disease or exposure, should initiate a referral to the occupational health service and a report to infection control. The infection control staff can determine whether other employees or patients were exposed, investigate the cause of the exposure, and make recommendations to prevent future exposures. The occupational health professionals should:

- Evaluate the employee;
- Recommend treatment, including relevant immunizations;
- Assess the need for work restrictions during incubation or active disease; and
- Reinforce proper infection prevention and control and hygiene practices that prevent transmission.

The HCW's job duties should be taken into consideration when determining whether work restrictions are necessary. Restrictions for certain skin, upper respiratory, or gastrointestinal infections may apply only to employees with direct patient care activities or to food handlers. However, some infections, such as TB, measles, and varicella, are so infectious that even employees with no patient contact should not enter the workplace. Occupational health professionals should be familiar with state and local public health department regulations that may impose certain restrictions on HCWs and food handlers. Table 19.3 summarizes restriction recommendations for common infectious diseases and exposures encountered in ambulatory care settings.

HCWs with bloodborne pathogen infections do not pose a significant risk of transmission if they observe Standard Precautions and do not perform "exposure-prone procedures." The risk of transmission from HCW to patient is considerably lower than the reverse situation; however, spread of all three infections from infected surgeons and dentists has been demonstrated.[34–36] HCWs with HIV and HBV infection should refrain from performing exposure-prone procedures—procedures in which percutaneous injury of the HCW is likely with subsequent contamination of the patient's wound, body cavity, or mucous membrane with HCW blood. Each healthcare institution should define applicable exposure-prone procedures, establish an expert panel to deal with the issue of work restrictions, and encourage HCWs who perform exposure-prone procedures to know their HIV and HBsAg status.[35] Hepatitis B e-antigen–positive HCWs should not perform procedures identified as a risk for HCW-to-patient HBV transmission. HCV- and HIV-infected HCWs should not be excluded from any aspect of patient care unless future evidence links those procedures to transmission despite adequate precautions.[36–37] Any provider with bloodborne pathogen infections performing exposure-prone procedures should double-glove.

OCCUPATIONAL HEALTH CONCERNS OF PREGNANT HCWS

Although there are very few specific work restrictions that are advised for pregnant HCWs, the risk of exposure and the consequences of infection in the fetus can be a major concern for staff. Infection prevention and control policies should include provisions for educating employees regarding infections during pregnancy and for evaluating and managing potential exposures in pregnant HCWs. Most immunizations are considered safe during pregnancy; however, the data regarding safety may be limited, so the risks and benefits of the specific circumstance should be weighed.[38]

The CDC guideline for healthcare personnel does not specifically preclude pregnant women from caring for patients infected with rubella or varicella.[3] However, because of the highly infectious nature of the diseases and severe fetal effects that may occur, many healthcare facilities choose to restrict susceptible HCWs from contact with patients with those diseases. Pregnant HCWs may also be restricted from contact with patients with significant shedding of parvovirus B19 (Fifth disease). HCWs should strictly observe isolation precautions and hygiene recommendations and, if properly practiced, the risk of infection from most pathogens is remote (see Chapter 6).

Table 19.3   Suggested Work Restrictions for HCWs Exposed to or Infected with Infectious Diseases*

Disease	Restriction	Duration	Comments
Conjunctivitis	No contact with patients or patients' environment	Until discharge ceases	Adenovirus keratoconjunctivitis is particularly infectious; bacterial conjunctivitis occurs less frequently in adults but can be treated with antibacterials.
Cytomegalovirus	None		
Diarrheal illness	No contact with patients or patients' environment; no food handling	Until symptoms resolve	Salmonella species may be subject to more stringent requirements.
Enteroviral infections	No contact with infants, neonates, and immunocompromised patients or their environments	Until symptoms resolve	
Hepatitis A	No contact with patients or patients' environment; no food handling	Until 7 days after onset of jaundice	Transmission from patient to HCW can be minimized by proper hygiene; travelers and persons at high risk should be vaccinated; immune globulin and vaccine can be used in outbreak situations.
Herpes simplex virus (HSV)—herpetic whitlow	No contact with patients or patients' environment	Until lesions heal	HSV infections of the hands should be evaluated for secondary bacterial infection.
Herpes simplex—orofacial	No contact with high-risk patients should be considered	Until lesions heal	Risk is small and can be reduced by avoiding contact with the orofacial lesion.
Measles—active disease	Exclude from duty	Until 4 days after rash appears	
Measles—post exposure	Exclude from duty (if non-immune)	From fifth day after 1st exposure through 21st day after last exposure and/or 4 days after rash appears	Pre-exposure vaccination is mandatory.
Meningococcal infections	Exclude from duty	Until 24 hrs. after start of effective therapy	HCWs having close contact with respiratory secretions should receive prophylaxis; asymptomtic carriers do not require restrictions.
Mumps—active disease	Exclude from duty	Until 9 days after onset of parotitis	
Mumps—post exposure	Exclude from duty (if non-immune)	From 12th day after 1st exposure to 26th day after last exposure and/or 9 days after onset of parotitis	Pre-exposure vaccination should be mandatory.

(continued)

Table 19.3   (continued)

Disease	Restriction	Duration	Comments
Parvovirus B19 (Fifth disease)	Consider restricting contact with high-risk patients	During acute illness	Pregnant women should be advised of risk to fetus, but risk of infection is minimal.
Pertussis—active disease	Exclude from duty	From beginning of catarrhal stage through 3rd week after onset of paroxysmal cough or until 5 days after effective antimicrobial therapy	Many cases of pertussis in adults are misdiagnosed.
Pertussis—post exposure	None		Post-exposure prophylaxis recommended for HCWs exposed to respiratory secretion.
Rubella—active	Exclude from duty	Until 5 days after rash appears	
Rubella—post exposure	Exclude from duty (if non-immune)	From 7th day after 1st exposure through 21st day after last exposure and/or until 5 days after rash appears	Pre-exposure vaccination is mandatory. Susceptible HCWs who are pregnant should not care for patients with rubella.
Staphylococcal skin infections	No contact with patients or patients' environment; no food handling	Until effective treatment administered and lesions have healed	No work restrictions necessary for asymptomatic carriers unless epidemiologically linked to heath care-associated infection transmission.
Streptococcal infection, group A	No contact with patients or patients' environment; no food handling	Until 24 hrs. after effective treatment	No restrictions necessary for asymptomatic carriers unless epidemiologically linked to heath care-associated infection transmission.
Varicella—active	Exclude from duty	Until lesions crusted	
Varicella—post exposure	Exclude from duty (if non-immune)	From 10th day after 1st exposure through 21st day after last exposure and/or all lesions crusted	Consider post-exposure prophylaxis with VZIG for high-risk HCWs; if VZIG given, restrict from duty through 28th day. Consider vaccine for post-exposure prophylaxis.
Varicella Zoster—localized	Cover lesions; no contact with high-risk patients	Until lesions crusted	
Varicella Zoster—in immuno-suppressed HCW	No patient contact	Until lesions crusted	

(continued)

Table 19.3   (continued)

Disease	Restriction	Duration	Comments
Varicella Zoster—post exposure	Exclude from duty (if non-immune)	From 10th day after 1st exposure through 21st day after last exposure and/or all lesions crusted	Consider post-exposure prophylaxis for high-risk HCWs as per varicella.
Viral respiratory infections, if febrile	Consider limiting patient contact with high-risk patients	Until acute symptoms resolve	Immunize HCWs against influenza.

HCW: Health care worker

VZIG: Varicella zoster immune globulin

*Adapted from Bolyard, E. A., Tablan, O. C., Williams, W. W., Pearson, M. L., Shapiro, C. N., and Deitchman, S. D., et al. Guideline for infection control in health care personnel, 1998. *Am J Infect Control.*1998; 26:289–354.

Other infections of interest during pregnancy include:

- Rubella infection during pregnancy is associated with a significant risk of perinatal transmission (90% in first 12 weeks of gestation) and the congenital syndrome that develops can be severe. Susceptible pregnant women are likely to be extremely anxious if asked to care for a patient who is infectious for rubella. Therefore, restricting them from care of the patient is appropriate.
- Measles is not associated with a particular congenital syndrome; however, perinatal infection can cause abortion and prematurity.
- Perinatal varicella is associated with congenital malformations.
- Hepatitis B infection in pregnancy may result in chronic infection in the fetus.
- In the event of an inadvertent exposure to measles, varicella, or hepatitis B, susceptible pregnant women may be given immune globulin (IG), varicella-zoster IG, or HBIG, respectively.
- Parvovirus B19 (Fifth disease) infection in pregnancy can cause fetal death; however, the risk of death has been estimated at less than 10%.[39] Patient care does not pose a significant risk of exposure because viral shedding in secretions is low once the rash appears, the time when the majority of patients present for treatment. However, patients with sickle cell and other chronic hemolytic anemias can develop a transient aplastic crisis with the infection and viral shedding may be prolonged. Viral shedding may also be prolonged in immunocompromised patients who develop chronic anemia with parvovirus B19 infection. Although the risk should be low if Droplet Pre-

cautions are maintained, consideration may be given to restricting pregnant HCWs from caring for patients who may have chronic shedding.
- Cytomegalovirus (CMV) infection of the fetus can cause hearing loss, hepatosplenomegaly, and mental retardation. CMV is transmitted through intimate contact or contact with body substances, particularly saliva and urine. If handwashing and Standard Precautions are applied, the risk of occupational infection in the healthcare setting is not significant.[40]
- Influenza infection in the second and third trimester of pregnancy has been associated with maternal complications. All HCWs who will be in the second and third trimester during the influenza season should be vaccinated. The CDC considers influenza vaccine to be safe throughout pregnancy; however, women in their first trimester should consult with their physicians regarding the risks and benefits of vaccination.[41]

CHEMICAL HAZARDS

Latex Allergy and Hand Dermatitis

The introduction of Standard Precautions ushered in an explosion of latex use in the healthcare environment, primarily through increased use of gloves. Glove use is associated with the development of dermatitis, especially if worn frequently and for long periods of time. The incidence of hand dermatitis in HCWs has increased dramatically in the past decade. Although most hand dermatitis is not caused by latex allergy, the manifestations of latex allergy can be systemic and serious and are a concern for many HCWs.

In the workplace, exposure to latex can occur through contact with gloves, goggles, and other items or, if latex proteins are present in the air, through inhalation. If the latex proteins adsorb onto cornstarch or other glove powder, the allergens can become aerosolized when the gloves are donned and removed. There is wide variation in the allergenic protein content of gloves made by different manufacturers. Levels of latex proteins in the air can be markedly reduced by using only nonpowdered latex gloves.[42]

Employees who will have frequent contact with latex, particularly gloves, should be screened for latex allergy. This should be done at the new employee health assessment by taking a history and/or using a standardized questionnaire (see Appendix J). Individuals with positive responses and employees who develop symptoms compatible with latex allergy should undergo further diagnostic testing with blood tests that measure specific immunoglobulins (IgE) to latex proteins (RAST) or skin-prick testing. Skin-prick testing should be performed under the supervision of a physician familiar with the technique and the possible adverse reactions that may occur.

Manifestations of latex allergy include localized reactions such as contact urticaria and systemic reactions such as rhinoconjunctivitis, asthma, generalized urticaria, and anaphylaxis. Local reactions generally occur within minutes of skin contact. The lesions are usually confined to the area of contact and resolve fairly quickly once the gloves are removed.

Persons with Type I hypersensitivity reactions to latex should avoid contact with latex at work and home and should wear a medical alert bracelet to prevent inadvertent exposure during emergency treatment. Besides the Type I latex allergy, there are two other major types of hand dermatitis caused by gloves: irritant dermatitis and Type IV delayed-type allergic contact dermatitis. Although true latex allergy may not be the culprit in the majority of glove-related skin diseases, any form of dermatitis may increase the absorption of latex proteins beyond the skin barrier and predispose to development of latex sensitization.

The most common form of skin disease caused by gloves is nonspecific irritant contact dermatitis. This is a nonallergic response that may be caused by sweating or rubbing under the gloves or from soaps/cleansers used before and after gloving. Irritant dermatitis appears as dry, cracking, erythematous skin. Wearing cotton glove liners and applying moisturizing lotion can alleviate irritant dermatitis. HCWs who must wash their hands frequently should be careful not to irritate the skin further while drying hands and should apply moisturizing lotion as necessary. Glutaraldehyde, chlorhexidine, povidone-iodine, and alcohol can be irritating and have been implicated in causing allergic dermatitis.[43]

Ambulatory care sites, regardless of size, should address the issue of latex allergy in patients and staff. A comprehensive latex allergy program should include the following elements:[44–45]

- An educational program for employees
- Identification and documentation of latex allergy in patients and staff
- Accessibility of latex-free alternative medical supplies
- Use of powder-free, low-allergen gloves when latex gloves are used
- Availability of alternative gloves for employees and patients with latex allergy
- Provisions for reassignment of latex-sensitive employees to non-high-risk areas

Disinfectants

Several compounds routinely used in disinfection procedures can be hazardous to some HCWs. In addition to being irritating to mucous membranes, formaldehyde is a suspect human carcinogen and is a potent sensitizer that can cause allergic dermatitis and occupational asthma. OSHA regulates exposure to formaldehyde, and employees with significant exposure must be provided with respiratory protection and must undergo medical surveillance.[46] Glutaraldehyde is commonly used to disinfect equipment; ambulatory-care employees may be exposed to high levels of vapor if used in improperly ventilated areas or open soak containers. Glutaraldehyde can irritate the mucous membranes and skin and can cause allergic contact dermatitis, rhinitis, and asthma.[47] Adequate ventilation and personal protective equipment, such as goggles, impervious gloves, and gowns, will decrease exposure.[48] Employees with asthma or chronic headaches may be particularly sensitive to the odor properties of certain disinfectants and cleansers that might not be considered hazardous or unacceptable to most individuals.

Collaboration between supervisory, infection control staff, and occupational health personnel is crucial for limiting exposure to and spread of infection. Generally, infection control or supervisory staff in small ambulatory sites bear the primary responsibility for identifying potentially infectious patients, developing and implementing isolation precautions practices, and educating employees regarding transmission of infection from patient to employee and vice versa. The primary functions of occupational health include clinical evaluation of employees with exposures and infections, providing post-exposure prophylaxis, and, when necessary, recommending work restrictions.

References

1. Occupational Safety and Health Administration. Occupational exposure to bloodborne pathogens: Final rule. CFR part 1910.1030. *Fed Reg.* 1991; 56:64004–64182.

2. Lipscomb, J., and Rosenstock, L. Healthcare workers: Protecting those who protect our health. *Infect Control Hosp Epidemiol.* 1997; 18:397–399.

3. Bolyard, E. A., Tablan, O. C., Williams, W. W., Pearson, M. L., Shapiro, C. N., and Deitchman, S. D., et al. Guideline for infection control in health care personnel. *Am J Infect Control.* 1998; 26:289–354.

4. Friedman, C., Barnette, M., Buck, A. S., Ham, R., Harris, J., and Hoffman, P., et al. Requirements for infrastructure and essential activities of infection control and epidemiology in out-of-hospital settings: A Consensus Panel report. *Am J Infect Control.* 1999; 27:418–430.

5. U.S. Department of Labor. Occupational Safety and Health Administration. *Framework for a Comprehensive Health and Safety Program in the Hospital Environment.* Washington, DC: U.S. Government Printing Office; 1993.

6. Recording and reporting occupational injuries and illnesses. 29 CFR Part 1904. *Fed Reg.* 2001; 66:6122–6135.

7. Occupational exposure to bloodborne pathogens; needlestick and other sharps injuries: Final Rule. 29 CFR Part 1910. *Fed Reg.* 2001; 66:5317–5325, *http://www.osha-slc.gov/FedReg_osha_pdf/FED2001 0118A.pdf.*

8. Centers for Disease Control and Prevention. Immunization of healthcare workers: Recommendations of the Advisory Committee on Immunization Practices (ACIP) and the Hospital Infection Control Practices Advisory Committee (HICPAC). *MMWR.* 1997; 46(RR-18):1–42.

9. Centers for Disease Control and Prevention. General recommendation on immunization: Recommendations of the Advisory Committee on Immunization Practice (ACIP) and the American Academy of Family Physicians (AAFP). *MMWR.* 2002; 51(RR-02):1–36.

10. Centers for Disease Control and Prevention. Update: Vaccine side effects, adverse reactions, contraindications and precautions recommendations of the Advisory Committee on Immunization Practices (ACIP) *MMWR.* 1996; 45(RR-12);1–35.

11. Gibas, A., Blewett, D. R., Schoenfeld, D. A., and Dienstag, J. L. Prevalence and incidence of viral hepatitis in health workers in the pre-hepatitis B vaccination era. *Am J Epidemiol.* 1992; 136:603–610.

12. DHHS (NIOSH). Publication #2000-127. *Worker Health Chartbook.* Washington, DC: National Institute for Occupational Safety and Health; 2000, *http://www2.cdc.gov/chartbook/CDplem/Chartbk0. htm.*

13. Centers for Disease Control and Prevention. Hepatitis B virus: A comprehensive strategy for limiting transmission in the United States through universal childhood vaccination. *MMWR.* 1991; 40 (RR-13):1–25.

14. Recombivax HB drug insert. West Point, PA: Merck & Co.; Issued 2/2000.

15. Mahoney, F. J., Steward, K., Hu, H., Coleman, P., and Alter, M. J. Progress toward the elimination of hepatitis B virus transmission among health care workers in the United States. *Arch Intern Med.* 1997; 157:2601–2605.

16. Centers for Disease Control and Prevention. Measles, Mumps, and Rubella—vaccine use and strategies for elimination of measles, rubella and congenital rubella syndrome and control of mumps: Recommendations of the Advisory Committee on Immunization Practices (ACIP). *MMWR.* 1998; 47(RR-8):1–57.

17. Nichol, K. L., Lind, A., Margolis, K. L., Murdoch, M., McFadden, R., and Hauge, M., et al. The effectiveness of vaccination against influenza in healthy, working adults. *N Engl J Med.* 1995; 333:889–893.

18. Bradley, S. F., and Long Term-Care Committee of the Society of Healthcare Epidemiology of America. Prevention of influenza in long-termcare facilities. *Infect Control Hosp Epidemiol.* 1999; 20:629–637.

19. Lim, S., Rogers, M., Odishoo, A., Eagan, J., Armstrong, D., and Sepkowitz, K., et al. Seroconversion rates among HCWs post varicella virus vaccine. *Am J Infect Control.* 1998; 26:175, Abstract.

20. Centers for Disease Control and Prevention. Prevention of Varicella: Update recommendations of the Advisory Committee on Immunization Practices (ACIP). *MMWR.* 1999; 48(RR-6):1–5.

21. Centers for Disease Control and Prevention. Vaccinia (smallpox) vaccine: Recommendations of the Advisory Committee on Immunization Practices (ACIP). 2001. *MMWR.* 2001; 50(RR-10):1–25.

22. Diagnostic standards and classification of tuberculosis in adults and children: Official statement of the American Thoracic Society and the Centers for Disease Control and Prevention. *Am J Respir Crit Care Med.* 2000; 161:1376–1395.

23. *Core Curriculum on Tuberculosis: What the Clinician Should Know.* 4th Ed. Atlanta, GA: Centers for Disease Control and Prevention; 2000, *http://www.cdc.gov/nchstp/tb/pubs/corecurr/default.htm.*

24. Pugliese, G. Screening for tuberculous infection: An update. *Am J Infect Control.* 1992; 20:1:37–40.

25. Centers for Disease Control and Prevention. Guidelines for preventing the transmission of *Mycobacterium tuberculosis* in health-care facilities. *MMWR.* 1994; 43(RR-13):1–132.

26. Centers for Disease Control and Prevention. Targeted tuberculin testing and treatment of latent tuberculosis infection. *MMWR*. 2000; 49(RR-6):1–54.

27. U.S. Department of Labor, Occupational Safety and Health Administration (OSHA). Respiratory protection for *M. tuberculosis*. 1998. 29 CFR 1910.139, *http://www.osha-slc.gov/html/respirator.html*.

28. Centers for Disease Control and Prevention. Perspectives in disease prevention and health promotion: Universal precautions for prevention of transmission of HIV, HBV and other bloodborne pathogens in health-care settings. *MMWR*. 1988; 37:377–388.

29. Centers for Disease Control and Prevention. Updated U.S. Public Health Service guidelines for the management of occupational exposures to HBV, HCV, and HIV and recommendations for postexposure prophylaxis. *MMWR*. 2001; 50 (RR-11):1–42.

30. Jaeckel, E., Cornberg, M., Wedemyer, H., Santantonio, T., Mayer, J., and Zankel, M., et al. Treatment of acute hepatitis C with interferon alpha-2b. *N Engl J Med*. 2001; 345:1452–1457.

31. Cardo, D. M., Culver, D. H., Ciesielski, C. A., Srivastava, P. U., Marcus, R., and Abiteboul, D., et al. A case-control study of HIV seroconversion in health care workers after a percutaneous exposure. *N Engl J Med*. 1997; 337:1485–1490.

32. Henderson, D. K. HIV prophylaxis in the 21st century. *Emerg Infect Dis*. 2001; 7:254–258.

33. Ridzon, R., Gallagher, K., Cieseilski, C., Ginsberg, M. B., Robertson, B. J., and Luo, C. C., et al. Simultaneous transmission of human immunodeficiency virus and hepatitis C virus from a needle-stick injury. *N Engl J Med*. 1997; 336:919–922.

34. Esteban, J. I., Gomez, J., Martell, M., Cabot, B., Quer, J., and Camps, J., et al. Transmission of hepatitis C virus by a cardiac surgeon. *N Engl J Med*. 1996; 334:555–560.

35. Centers for Disease Control and Prevention. Recommendations for preventing transmission of human immunodeficiency virus and hepatitis B virus during exposure-prone procedures. *MMWR*. 1991; 40(RR-8):1–9.

36. AIDS/TB Committee of the Society for Healthcare Epidemiology of America. Management of healthcare workers infected with hepatitis B virus, hepatitis C virus, human immunodeficiency virus, or other bloodborne pathogens. *Infect Control Hosp Epidemiol*. 1997; 18:349–363.

37. Centers for Disease Control and Prevention. Recommendations for prevention and control of hepatitis C virus (HCV) infection and HCV-related chronic disease. *MMWR*. 1998; 47(RR-19):1–39.

38. Centers for Disease Control and Prevention. Recommendations of the Advisory Committee on Immunization Practices (ACIP). *Guidelines for Vaccinating Pregnant Women*. Atlanta, GA: Centers for Disease Control and Prevention; 2002 *http://www.cdc.gov/nip/publications/preg-guide.htm*.

39. Centers for Disease Control and Prevention. Current trends: Risks associated with human Parvovirus B19 infection. *MMWR*. 1989; 38:81–88, 93–97.

40. Balcarek, K. B., Bagley, R., Cloud, G., and Pass, R. F. Cytomegalovirus infection among employees of a children's hospital: No evidence for increased risk associated with patient care. *JAMA*. 1990; 263:840–844.

41. Centers for Disease Control and Prevention. Prevention and control of influenza: Recommendations of the Advisory Committee on Immunization Practice (ACIP). *MMWR*. 2001; 50(RR-4):1–44.

42. Sussman, G. L., and Beezhold, D. K. Allergy to latex rubber. *Ann Intern Med*. 1995; 122:43–46.

43. Fisher, A. A. Allergic contact reactions in health personnel. *J Allergy Clin Immunol*. 1992; 90:729–738.

44. Latex Hypersensitivity Committee. Position statement, American Academy of Asthma, Allergy and Immunology. Latex allergy: An emerging healthcare problem. *Ann Asthma Allergy Immunol*. 1995: 75:19–21.

45. Cohen, D. E., Scheman, A., Stewart, L., Taylor, J., Pratt, M., and Trotter, K., et al. American Academy of Dermatology's position paper on latex allergy. *J Am Acad Dermatol*. 1998; 39:98–106.

46. Occupational Safety and Health Administration. Final rule on occupational exposure to formaldehyde. 29 CFR 1910.1048. *Fed Reg*. 1992; 57:22290.

47. Rutala, W. A. APIC Guideline for selection and use of disinfectants. *Am J Infect Control*. 1996; 24:313–342.

48. DHHS (NIOSH). Publication #2001-115. *Glutaraldehyde: Occupational hazards in hospitals*. Washington, DC: National Institute for Occupational Safety and Health; 2001, *http://www.cdc.gov/niosh/2001-115.html*.

CHAPTER 20

Data Management

BACKGROUND

One of the major functions of an infection prevention and control (IPC) program is to obtain and manage critical data and information. The major component of data management activities is surveillance for infections, tailoring the methods used to the setting. Activities include developing and implementing surveillance (data management) plans, monitoring these plans, and internal and external reporting of infection information and data.[1,2]

Surveillance is an active method of detecting, collecting, disseminating, and analyzing information on the occurrence of health care-associated infections that might be a consequence of a diagnostic or therapeutic procedure. The surveillance data are collected in order to monitor outcomes and processes, describe risk factors and methods of transmission, identify and evaluate problems, and develop improvement initiatives.[3]

Surveillance has long been identified as an essential component of an effective IPC program in hospitals.[4] Ongoing surveillance of nosocomial infections within U.S. hospitals became increasingly common in the 1960s. By 1970, on the basis of pilot studies, the Centers for Disease Control and Prevention (CDC) recommended that surveillance be performed routinely in all hospitals. Currently, some type of surveillance activities is performed in all acute care settings.

These monitoring activities are not routinely practiced in ambulatory care settings. However, there have been reports in the literature of clusters of infections associated with ambulatory care visits and practices illustrating that the performance of routine surveillance

activities is important in certain ambulatory care settings.[5,6] Health care-associated infections in ambulatory care have been defined as those associated temporally with an ambulatory care visit or with the care provided during the visit.[7]

Patients seen in ambulatory care settings most often leave the site after the visit and are not readily available for follow-up. In addition, it is often difficult to obtain appropriate denominator data in these settings. Therefore, performing surveillance on this population is a challenge and requires innovative surveillance methods.[8]

SURVEILLANCE OR DATA MANAGEMENT PLAN

A surveillance plan should be developed to outline data management objectives for an ambulatory care facility/setting. It should include the rationale for choosing which patients are to be monitored for infections and how the data will be disseminated (see examples in Appendix G). Any surveillance plan must be focused on those infections that have the potential to be prevented. The plan must also contain some mechanism for follow-up of patients in order to identify the occurrence of an infection. Implementing the surveillance plan requires multidisciplinary collaboration between individuals responsible for data collection and clinical and support staff.[9]

157

The steps in developing a surveillance plan include:[1,2,9]

1. Assessment of the population
2. Definition of the population at risk
3. Identification and description of the outcome or process to be studied
4. Use of standard definitions
5. Identification and description of data sources and case-finding methods
6. Determination of data collection methods
7. Selection of appropriate methods of measurement, including statistical tools and performance of data analysis
8. Application of risk stratification methodology
9. Reporting and using surveillance information

The main objective of the surveillance plan is to determine the frequency and types of endemic health care-associated infections, identify those that have a potential for prevention, and gather data about the selected infection and the associated risk factors to make recommendations to reduce the infection risk and rate in future patients.[3,4] To be successful, a surveillance plan needs to be clear and specific. It should be evaluated routinely and modified as necessary.

Surveillance activities must be specific to each facility because the data can help identify the underlying risk of the population and the effectiveness of the IPC program.[10–11] Surveillance, therefore, assists in monitoring the effectiveness of prevention and control strategies that are consistent with the organization's goals and objectives.[2]

Assessment of the Population

An assessment of the population covered in a particular ambulatory care setting must be made in order to determine what type of surveillance should be performed and how the monitoring should occur. The following evaluations will assist with this determination:[10]

- types of practice (e.g., endoscopy, dialysis, etc.) and care provided
- patient case mix (e.g., most common diagnoses, elderly, or immunocompromised patients)
- patient volume (i.e., visits per day, per month)
- types of surgical or invasive procedures performed
- types of medical services or treatments provided

- types of instruments or equipment used
- previous surveillance data, if available

Activities that increase the risk for health care-associated infections include the use of invasive devices, surgical procedures, and therapeutic interventions.[12] Thus, ambulatory care areas of special importance for routine surveillance, with regard to potential risk of infection, are dialysis, infusion therapy, and surgical procedure areas. Indicators for these areas might include access site infections, bloodstream infections, and surgical site infections, respectively. Other areas for surveillance include diagnostic and treatment settings where a plan could involve process surveillance, for example, reviewing the care of instruments and equipment (see Appendix G).

When assessing a population seen in a physician's office, also keep in mind the potential of patients being exposed to others with infection. For example, if patients visiting a pediatrician's office are exposed to children with measles (or another communicable disease), there is concern that they might acquire the infection also. This, then, might be an appropriate indicator to monitor.[13]

Definition of the Population at Risk

The decision as to which outcome or process to study as part of the surveillance plan is based on determining which patient populations are at highest risk for infection. For example, if bloodstream infections are high risk for infusion patients, this infection should be monitored in this population. If surgical procedures are performed, certain types of procedures (those with a high risk) should be monitored for the development of surgical site infections. Defining these populations in the surveillance plan ensures that these risks were considered when developing the plan.

Identification and Description of the Outcome or Process to Be Studied

Because it is not realistic to perform organization-wide surveillance for all events, the plan should allocate resources appropriately and focus on areas of highest risk, highest cost, or problem-prone procedures. Therefore, outcomes and processes included in the surveillance plan should be those that have the most important impact on the population served. The impact can be increased risk to patients or the most common practices in a population. Decisions may be based on morbidity, cost, potential to contribute to prevention activities, organizational goals, or other parameters.[9] These areas of surveillance focus are often called quality or performance indicators.[14–15] The plan should be evaluated routinely to ensure that the indicators remain appropriate over time.

Use of Standard Definitions

Use specific, consistent case definitions relevant to the setting to distinguish health care-associated infections from community infections. There are no specific definitions for ambulatory care-related infections. However, many institutions adapt acute care definitions from the CDC's National Nosocomial Infections Surveillance (NNIS) System.[16] This is especially true for surgical site infections.[17] Definitions ensure reproducibility and provide a basis for comparison both internally and externally. It is important to use the same definitions over time to ensure valid comparisons.

Identification and Description of Data Sources and Case-Finding Methods

Case finding and data collection to identify health care-associated infections present unique challenges in ambulatory care because patients leave the area after a procedure or treatment and might not return to that provider.[10] In addition, microbiologic cultures that might indicate an infection are often not performed on this population. However, there are a variety of sources to use to identify patients with infections. These include direct patient examination, medical records, information services, quality/utilization management, ancillary service reports (e.g., laboratory, radiology, pharmacy), surgical databases, administrative/management reports,[18] risk management databases, and communication with staff. A method to collect required information then would be developed using the most appropriate source.

Finding data sources to determine the number of patients seen might be more difficult (for denominator data). Areas to investigate include coded procedure databases, infusion, surgery or dialysis records, and financial data.

Determination of Data Collection Methods

Various methods can be used for data collection. Once a decision is made regarding which high-risk or problem-prone areas to focus on and where to obtain the information, the appropriate approach to surveillance can be determined for the setting. The types of surveillance methods that might be suitable for ambulatory care include:[19]

- Comprehensive (institution-wide): The objective is to detect all health care-associated infections occurring in all patients at all times. This process is very resource-intensive and time-consuming. It likely will produce more data than are needed, making interpretation of the information difficult. This type of monitoring generally is not recommended for any setting.
- Periodic: The focus is placed on evaluating all infections periodically (e.g., one month out of each quarter) or shifting focus from one area to another at different time periods (e.g., dialysis one month, infusion therapy another month). This procedure helps save resources and can still provide valuable data; however, one may miss problems when not monitoring an area.
- Laboratory-based: This method is designed to detect outbreaks of infections by charting the frequency of isolation of particular microorganisms. Review of actual patient charts would be performed only if the number of isolates exceeds a set baseline. This system is not useful in situations where microbiologic cultures are not routinely performed.
- Targeted: This process concentrates resources on high-risk areas and those with a potential to reduce risks, for example, specific sites or procedures (i.e., catheter-related bloodstream infections, dialysis-associated infections, and surgical procedure-related infections). One targets the highest-risk or highest-morbidity procedures or those with the greatest potential for improvement. It is flexible and efficient; however, it may miss outbreaks in nontargeted areas.
- Ambulatory surgery and post-discharge surveillance: This method is used primarily for surgical-site infection (SSI) surveillance. Many surgical procedures are performed on an ambulatory basis;

therefore, there is often a need to focus surveillance activity on this population.

The CDC's Study on the Effectiveness of Nosocomial Infection Control[20] revealed that an important activity in decreasing SSIs is to report surgeon-specific SSI rates back to surgeons. Various authors recommend providing this information to ambulatory care surgeons.[21–22] When reporting SSI rate information to surgeons, include the clean SSI rate for the entire department for comparison.[22]

One issue in ambulatory care settings is how to determine who has developed an SSI. There are a variety of methods outlined in the literature for acquiring SSI information. These methods include surgeon self-reporting, surveys, phone calls to patients, patient mail-back questionnaires, use of microbiology data, and direct wound examination. One study reviewed every patient's chart 30 days after surgery.[23]

In ambulatory settings, the most efficient and reliable method is active surgeon follow-up.[24–25] In one study of 515 patients undergoing primarily orthopedic procedures, 19 SSIs were identified by the surgeon while only seven were identified by calling patients.[26] Manian et al. determined that patient phone surveys do not add any information to a monthly physician questionnaire.[27]

One system for obtaining SSI information involves sending a list of patients to surgeons monthly or quarterly. The surgeon then is asked to note whether the patient developed a health care-associated infection based on specific criteria provided. This method could be used as an adjunct to other means of identifying SSIs, such as microbiology laboratory reports.[28–29]

Approximately 10 to 50% of SSIs are identified after discharge from an acute-care hospital.[30–31] Because of this, monitoring patients through ambulatory care sites is critical to ensure accurate hospital data. There should be a system in place to notify hospital-based infection control professionals regarding infections identified in ambulatory care patients that are likely to be nosocomial.[1]

Persons performing surveillance activities must have access to all required data and vital information.[1] This includes access to computerized databases that are needed for accurate and complete identification of infectious complications.

Regardless of methodology, a data collection worksheet or tool is critical when collecting surveillance data. The form can be computerized or paper, designating space for each piece of desired information (see Appendix G). All data elements to be collected must be clearly defined. Having a worksheet ensures that the data collected will be limited to only what is needed. (Information can be overwhelming, so don't collect what you don't need!) Potential information to incorporate on a data collection form includes:

- Basic demographics (name, record number, age, gender, date of visit)
- Infection information (date of onset, site of infection, microorganisms)
- Clinical information (relevant information for the specific infection)
- Laboratory information (date of culture, results)
- Antibiotic therapy (preoperative, therapeutic)
- Surgery information (date of procedure, start and stop times of procedure, surgeons, American College of Surgeons' wound classification, severity of illness score [e.g., American Society for Anesthesiology, or ASA, score])[32]
- Procedure information (type, date)
- Predisposing factors (diabetes, steroids)

Selection of Appropriate Methods of Measurement and Performance of Data Analysis

An important component of the surveillance process is how to organize data and then its subsequent analysis. There are software packages available for management of surveillance data. However, they are often expensive and primarily focused on hospital systems. A simpler and more economical system can be developed in a database management or spreadsheet application or by using the CDC's free Epi Info application, *http://www. cdc.gov/epiinfo/index.htm*. These systems can be used for individual patient-level data collection and will allow for easier analysis of data.

Besides knowing which patients develop which type of infection, it is important to be able to generate rates to make comparisons over time or with benchmark data (see Appendix G). To develop a rate, an appropriate numerator and denominator must be chosen for each outcome or process indicator. Numerator data are the patients with the outcome or process indicator of interest—for example, the number of patients with bloodstream infections who are receiving infusion therapy. Denominator data are the patient population affected—for example, number of patients who are receiving infusion therapy or number of infusion days for a specific time period.

Infections that develop after an ambulatory care visit pose difficulties in the selection of appropriate and readily obtainable denominators. However, often they can be linked to a particular procedure or therapy, such as wound infection per surgical procedure or bloodstream infection per infusion therapy days.[33] Once data have been collected for a period of time, a baseline rate can be determined from which future comparisons can be made.[19]

Data can be analyzed using various methods, including line listings, rate development, and use of statistical measures (see Appendix G for examples).

- Line listing: This method allows for the organization of the data collected in a meaningful manner.
- Rates/ratios: A major form of data analysis includes ratios, proportions, and rates that can be used in measuring outcomes and processes. The numerator is the event being monitored (e.g., number of bloodstream infections in January) and the denominator is a measurement of the population in which the event may occur (e.g., number of infusion patients during January or number of infusion days in January). The denominator should reflect the appropriate population at risk. Rates can be calculated by site, by procedure, by month, and so forth.
- Statistics: Simple statistical measures can be used in an analysis of the data. These include reviewing average rates over time and comparisons of rates using statistical tests.

The time frame to be analyzed will depend on the activity of the indicator. That is, if many procedures are performed, the data might be analyzed monthly. However, if few procedures are performed, the data analysis might be performed quarterly.

Application of Risk Stratification Methodology

Within a population under study there are frequently differences, such as age and severity of underlying illnesses. Such differences require that the population be subdivided into groups with like characteristics. This adjustment is called **risk stratification**. Without risk stratification, comparisons of rates over time or with other facilities may be misleading.[14]

Thus it is important to use risk adjustment techniques when appropriate. The most prevalent use of risk stratification relates to surgical site infections. Patients undergoing the same procedure may have varied risks of infection. Therefore, it is important to control for variations in the patient's risk and identify specific procedure- and process-related issues that may be contributing to increased rates of health care-associated infections.[34]

The CDC's SSI risk stratification system involves a score assigned to a patient based on a combination of risk factors. These are: 1) wound class III or IV (the American College of Surgeons' wound classification of contaminated or dirty), 2) procedure >t hours (a cut point for the length of surgery), and 3) ASA score ≥3 (the ASA score reflects the patient's overall preoperative physical status). One point is assigned to each factor, resulting in a range from 0 to 3.[32] Risk adjustment can assist in presenting more useful information to surgeons.

Reporting and Using Surveillance Information

Once data are collected and analyzed, it is important to prepare and distribute reports to appropriate groups and individuals that can impact on and improve care. Information should be reported to the Infection Control Committee (if there is one), to the facility's leadership, and to clinical staff.

These reports should be distributed periodically, perhaps every three to six months, and annually. The report should outline appropriate actions that have been taken or can be taken based on the data. Because the main reason for performing surveillance is to monitor and improve outcomes, reporting epidemiologically significant findings to appropriate staff can result in these improvements.

When reporting data, use graphs, charts, and tables to display the information. These methods help to present a pictorial view of trends in the data that can be evaluated quickly (see examples in Appendix G).

INDICATORS: OUTCOMES AND PROCESSES

Most ambulatory care IPC programs will incorporate both measures of outcome and measures of process into the surveillance plan design. Outcome measures focus on the results of an activity, such as a surgical procedure or a specific therapy. Health care-associated infections are examples of adverse outcomes that may occur after a procedure.

Process surveillance involves monitoring of practices that directly or indirectly contribute to a health outcome. Then information collected is used to improve outcomes. Process surveillance focuses on observations and analysis of practices and environmental conditions. It can be used to observe, describe, and measure implementation and compliance with IPC policies.[35] Most methods of process surveillance involve a survey tool for collection of information—either observational or written—to ensure a uniform review (see site review form in Appendix G). The tool can be divided into procedures performed, environment, therapy provided, and other sections.[36–37] Assessment techniques can include interviews and observations. Then documentation of compliance or noncompliance is recorded. Identified issues may be resolved during the site review itself or followed up as necessary. Process measures may be particularly valuable when an outcome is rare or collection of outcome data is difficult or not feasible.[38]

The data collected during a process survey can be compiled into a summary format for analysis. The quality of overall adherence to IPC practices can be assessed and stated objectively. In addition, specific policies or regulations can be cited as references. This can be used as an ongoing system for reviewing and verifying the implementation of IPC practices. It is important to send summary reports to administrators and clinical staff. They are the individuals who need to make changes, enforce practices, and monitor improvements.

Suggestions for outcome and process indicators for surveillance in ambulatory care settings include healthcare associated infections, operating room traffic, tuberculin skin test conversions, immunization rates (in staff or patients), biological indicators (sterilizer monitoring), surgical antibiotic prophylaxis, and antibiotic timing.[12]

Attempts to compare infection rates, or benchmark, with other ambulatory care facilities require careful evaluation of variations in patient characteristics and definitions of infection to ensure comparability.

The Joint Commission on Accreditation of Healthcare Organizations has an initiative that integrates outcomes and other performance measurement data into the accreditation process. The National Committee on Quality Assurance's (NCQA) Health Plan Employer Data and Information Set (HEDIS) contains over 50 measures of performance, including immunization status (*http://www.ncqa.org/pages/programs/hedis/00measures.htm*). There is also a national surveillance system focusing on dialysis patients.[39]

Currently there is no national benchmark for most ambulatory care infection rates. Therefore, a facility must compare its current rate of infection with its historical rates for the same infection, looking for trends.[3] A facility's data management activities for infection prevention and control are an important component of its patient safety program.[40]

References

1. Friedman, C., Barnette, M., Buck, A. S., Ham, R., Harris, J., and Hoffman, P., et al. Requirements for infrastructure and essential activities of infection control and epidemiology in out-of-hospital settings: A Consensus Panel report. *Am J Infect Control.* 1999; 27:418–430.

2. Horan-Murphy, E., Barnard, B., Chenoweth, C., Friedman, C., Hazuka, B., and Russell, B., et al. APIC/CHICA-Canada infection control and epidemiology: Professional and practice standards. *Am J Infect Control.* 1999; 27:47–51.

3. Lynch, P., and Jackson, M. M. Monitoring: Surveillance for nosocomial infections and uses for assessing quality of care. *Am J Infect Control.* 1985; 13:161–173.

4. Haley, R. W. Surveillance by objective: A new priority-directed approach to the control of nosocomial infections. *Am J Infect Control.* 1985; 13:78–89.

5. Goodman, R. A., and Solomon, S. L. Transmission of infectious diseases in outpatient health care settings. *JAMA.* 1991; 265:2377–2381.

6. Hugar, D. W., Newman, P. S., Hugar, R. W., Spencer, R. B., and Salvino, K. Incidence of postoperative infection in a free-standing ambulatory surgery center. *J Foot Surg.* 1990; 29:265–267.

7. Jackson, M. M., and Lynch, P. Ambulatory Care Settings. In: Bennett, J. V., and Brachman, P. S., eds., *Hospital Infections.* 4th Ed. Philadelphia: Lippincott-Raven Publishers; 1998: 431–444.

8. Jarvis, W. R. Infection Control and changing health care delivery systems. *Emerg Infect Dis.* 2001; 7:170–173.

9. Lee, T. B., Baker, O. G., Lee, J. T., Scheckler, W. E., Steele, L., and Laxton, C. Recommended practices for surveillance. *Am J Infect Control.* 1998; 26:277–288.

10. Jennings, J., Thibeault, M., Olmsted, R., and Craig, C. In: *APIC Text of Infection Control and Epidemiology.* Washington, DC: Association for Professionals in Infection Control and Epidemiology; 2000: 38:1–29.

11. Roth, R. A., and Verbridge, N. Surgical wound surveillance. *AORN J.* 1988; 47:722–729.

12. Lee, T. B. Surveillance in acute care and nonacute care settings: Current issues and concepts. *Am J Infect Control.* 1997; 25:121–124.

13. Lobovits, A. M., Freeman, J., Goldmann, D. A., and McIntosh, K. Risk of illness after exposure to a pediatric office. *N Engl J Med.* 1985; 313:425–428.

14. Decker, M. D. The development of indicators. *Infect Control Hosp Epidemiol.* 1991; 12:490–492.

15. Crede, W. B., and Hierholzer, W. J. Surveillance for quality assessment: III. The critical assessment of quality indicators. *Infect Control Hosp Epidemiol.* 1990; 11:197–201.

16. Garner, J. S., Jarvis, W. R., Emori, T. G., Horan, T. C., and Hughes, J. M. CDC definitions for nosocomial infections, 1988. *Am J Infect Control.* 1988; 16:128–140.

17. Horan, T. C., Gaynes, R. P., Martone, W. J., Jarvis, W. R., and Emori, T. G. CDC definitions of nosocomial surgical site infections, 1992: A modification of CDC definitions of surgical wound infections. *Am J Infect Control.* 1992; 20:271–274.

18. Massanari, R. M., Joshua, A. P., Jain, R., and Wells, C. Screening for adverse outcomes following ambulatory surgery using administrative data sets. SHEA abstract #S50. *Infect Control Hosp Epidemiol.* 1996; 17:P35.

19. Pottinger, J. M., Herwaldt, L. A., and Perl, T. M. Basics of surveillance—an overview. *Infect Control Hosp Epidemiol.* 1997; 18:513–527.

20. Haley, R. W., Culver, D. H., White, J. W., Morgan, W. M., Emori, T. G., and Munn, V. P., et al. The efficacy of infection surveillance and control programs in preventing nosocomial infections in U.S. hospitals. *Am J Epid.* 1985; 121:182–205.

21. Manian, F. A. Surveillance of surgical site infections in alternative settings: Exploring the current options. *Am J Infect Control.* 1997; 25:102–105.

22. Flanders, E., and Hinnant, J. R. Ambulatory surgery postoperative wound surveillance. *Am J Infect Control.* 1990; 18:336–339.

23. Vilar-Compte, D., Roldán, R., Sandoval, S., Corominas, R., de la Rosa, M., Gordillo, P., and Volkow, P. Surgical site infections in ambulatory surgery: A 5-year experience. *Am J Infect Control.* 2001; 29:99–103.

24. Fanning, C., Johnston, B. L., MacDonald, S., LeFort-Jost, S., and Dockerty, E. Postdischarge surgical site infection surveillance. *Can J Infect Control.* 1995; 10:75–79.

25. Yozzo, J. C. Is it feasible to track infections in an ambulatory surgery center? *J Post Anes Nursing.* 1989; 4:255–258.

26. Zoutman, D., Pearce, P., McKenzie, M., and Taylor, G. Surgical wound infections occurring in day surgery patients. *Am J Infect Control.* 1990; 18:277–282.

27. Manian, F. A., and Meyer, L. Comparison of patient telephone survey with traditional surveillance and monthly physician questionnaires in monitoring surgical wound infections. *Infect Control Hosp Epidemiol.* 1993; 14:216–218.

28. Roth, R. A., and Verbridge, N. Surgical wound surveillance. *AORN J.* 1988; 47:722–729.

29. Manian, F. A., and Meyer, L. Adjunctive use of monthly physician questionnaires for surveillance of surgical site infections after hospital discharge and in ambulatory surgical patients: Report of a seven-year experience. *Am J Infect Control.* 1997; 25:390–394.

30. Topal, J., Reagan-Cirincione, P., Mazon, D., Guidetti, D., Veiga, F., and Ahmad, I., et al. Validation of a post-discharge surveillance (PDS) system for surgical site infections (SSI's) in cardiothoracic Surgery. *Eleventh Annual Meeting of the Society for Healthcare Epidemiology of America.* Abstract 246, April 1–3, 2001.

31. Livingston, J., and Platt, R. Postdischarge surgical site infections in patients undergoing coronary artery bypass grafting: Relationship to time of discharge. *Eleventh Annual Meeting of the Society for Healthcare Epidemiology of America.* Abstract 247, April 1–3, 2001.

32. Culver, D. H., Horan, T. C., Gaynes, R. P., Martone, W. J., Jarvis, W. R., and Emori, T. G., et al. Surgical wound infection rates by wound class, operative procedure, and patient risk index. *Am J Med.* 1991; 91(suppl 3B):152S–157S.

33. Rhame, F. S. Surveillance objectives: Descriptive epidemiology. *Infect Control.* 1987; 8:454–458.

34. Gaynes, R. P., and Solomon, S. Improving hospital-acquired infection rates: The CDC experience. *J Quality Improvement.* 1996; 22:457–467.

35. Friedman, C., Richter, D., Skylis, T., and Brown, D. Process surveillance: Auditing infection control policies and procedures. *Am J Infect Control.* 1984; 12:228–232.

36. Bradford, M., and Flynn, N. M. Ambulatory care infection control quality assurance monitoring. *Am J Infect Control.* 1988; 16:21A–28A.

37. Infection control practitioner qudit form for patient/resident service units. *Can J Infect Control.* 2002; 17:23–26.

38. Baker, O. G. Process surveillance: An epidemiologic challenge for all health care organizations. *Am J Infect Control.* 1997; 25:96–101.

39. Tokars, J. I. Description of a new surveillance system for bloodstream and vascular access infections in outpatient hemodialysis centers. *Semin Dial.* 2000; 13:97–100.

40. Leape, L. L., Berwick, D. M., and Bates, D. W. What practices will most improve safety? *JAMA.* 2002; 288:501–513.

CHAPTER 21

Outbreak Investigation

Outbreaks of infections usually involve a specific population, often with some risk or exposure, in a particular geographic location. As healthcare services move to outpatient facilities, it is anticipated that outbreaks will occur more frequently in ambulatory care settings.[1] Surveillance activities will assist in the recognition of outbreaks or unusual disease clusters.[2] Whenever there is a cluster of infections greater than expected or the occurrence of an unusual infection, regardless of the number, an outbreak investigation should be performed. There must be adequate resources to ensure a comprehensive and timely investigation so that appropriate control measures can be implemented.[3]

The goal of an outbreak investigation is to control and prevent further disease and to identify factors that contributed to the outbreak in order to develop and implement measures to prevent future similar outbreaks.[4] Investigations may need to be performed when there is an occurrence of unusual microorganisms, when there is an increase in infections, or when highly resistant bacteria increase in the population. Staff unfamiliar with outbreak investigation may find it helpful to consult with infection control professionals from an institution that performs similar procedures to those implicated in the investigation.

The steps to take when conducting an outbreak investigation include:

1. Confirm that an outbreak exists.
2. Characterize the cases by person, place, and time.
3. Formulate tentative hypotheses.
4. Test the hypotheses.
5. Institute appropriate control measures.
6. Evaluate the control measures.
7. Communicate findings.

STEP 1: CONFIRM THAT AN OUTBREAK EXISTS

First, it is important to determine whether an outbreak actually exists and, if so, the magnitude of the problem. To assist with this determination, develop a **case definition**. This statement outlines which type of patient will be classified as a case, that is, an individual who has the infection under investigation. A case definition helps to focus the investigation and should include:

- Who: Which patients are involved in the outbreak
- When: The time under consideration (period from first to last suspected case)
- Where: The place involved (e.g., surgery, infusion or dialysis center, or clinic where cases may have been exposed to an infectious agent)

Next, review previous experience with the illness under investigation (e.g., infection rates or number of cases) and compare it with the numbers or rate calculated for the outbreak period. If a background rate is not available, the outbreak data can be compared to information obtained from articles in the literature. Review the literature to obtain information on similar situations that have been investigated by others.

It is also important to establish or verify the diagnosis and to identify the microbiologic agent involved.

Obtain appropriate laboratory specimens or microbiologic cultures from suspect cases if necessary. Any appropriate microorganisms should be saved in the laboratory in case they are needed for subsequent testing.[5]

Once an outbreak is confirmed, it is important to determine whether further investigation is warranted. Heightening awareness of infection prevention and control recommendations to staff is often enough to terminate an outbreak.[6] It may also be enough to implement appropriate **control measures** to stop transmission. Control measures may include:

- Ensure that basic infection control procedures are followed.
- Use appropriate isolation precautions for cases and suspect cases.
- Dedicate certain equipment to be used for cases only.
- Geographically separate cases from other patients (i.e., cohort cases together) and/or provide separate staff dedicated to caring for cases.
- Discontinue certain procedures or use of certain devices or products that may be linked to transmission.

For any suspected or confirmed outbreak or cluster, notify those responsible for infection prevention and control—including medical directors, administrative staff, those staff members directly involved in the care of the patients, and other affected departments—regarding the investigation. It may also be appropriate to notify the local health department. Check state regulations to determine specific requirements.

Looking for additional cases not initially identified can be performed after a case definition is developed. This **case finding** is usually conducted by reviewing laboratory and medical records for the pertinent time period, performing interviews with clinicians, and reviewing procedure records. Staff should be encouraged to report any suspected new case. Conducting culture surveys of patients to determine the extent of colonization or infection if a particular microbe is involved may also be important.

A data collection form to organize the information can be developed once there is a case definition. It will ensure that the same information is obtained for each case in an organized manner. Data collection forms can include:

- Demographic information (e.g., name, service, date and location of procedure or visit)
- Clinical information (e.g., signs, symptoms, onset date)
- Risk factors (e.g., procedures performed, devices used, caregiver information)
- Microbiologic and other pertinent diagnostic test results

STEP 2: CHARACTERIZE THE CASES BY PERSON, PLACE, AND TIME

A **line listing** of cases will assist in evaluating case information. The line list provides a quick method to examine what factors are common to all or most cases; therefore, only important information should be included on it. This list can be used to describe cases by person, place, and time. Outline who acquires the disease, where the disease occurs, and when it occurs.[6] (see Table 21.1). Examination of the line list can provide the first evidence to suggest a possible cause of an outbreak.

Describing the outbreak over time can be performed by graphing the cases according to onset of illness. Typically, this is performed using a graph called an **epidemic curve** (see Figure 21.1). An epidemic curve can provide useful information about an outbreak, because the type of outbreak will often dictate the shape of the curve. A peak in case numbers will usually indicate a common-source outbreak (e.g., contaminated equipment or medications). When there is no clear peak in the curve, it is likely that infections are spread in a propagated manner. Cases then will occur over a relatively long time period.

Place may refer to a location where devices are used or procedures are performed; therefore, maps may be useful for outlining the location of cases if infections occur at various sites.

STEP 3: FORMULATE TENTATIVE HYPOTHESES

Initial review of the collected information will assist in developing conclusions or forming a hypothesis. This hypothesis is a "best guess" as to the likely cause of the outbreak. It will help explain most of the cases.

Table 21.1   Line Listing of Cases: Mt. Sinai Eye Center—Epidemic Keratoconjunctivitis (EKC) Infections

Name	Number	Age	Sex	Visit Date	Onset Date	Procedure	Medications	Physician
Robert	45238	69	M	7/10	7/17	Tonometry	Drops	JA
Kaplan	48263	51	F	7/12	7/20	Tonometry	Drops	LS
Heinauer	46255	56	F	7/14	7/19	Tonometry	Abx	CC
Simpson	48333	70	M	7/15	7/21	Tonometry	Drops	KV
Paul	47901	65	M	7/15	7/24	Tonometry	Dye	KV
James	46822	67	M	7/16	7/24	Tonometry	Dye	AH
Leah	48845	45	F	7/16	7/25	Tonometry	Drops	JS
Berg	46768	37	M	7/16	7/21	Tonometry	Dye	GJ
Alexander	45882	26	M	7/17	7/25	Tonometry	Abx	CC
Murphy	47792	40	F	7/17	7/24	Tonometry	Dye	JS
Forman	48196	50	F	7/17	7/22	Tonometry	Drops	LS
Benjamin	46833	43	M	7/17	7/24	Tonometry	Drops	CC
Jordan	45671	73	F	7/18	7/22	Tonometry	Drops	JA
Milgrom	48263	55	M	7/18	7/25	Tonometry	Dye	AH
Spink	47555	49	F	7/18	7/24	Tonometry	Abx	CC
Sweet	48241	47	F	7/19	7/29	Tonometry	Drops	JA
Frederick	46895	35	M	7/19	7/25	Tonometry	Drops	CC
Saman	47253	57	M	7/20	7/27	Tonometry	Abx	CC
Peters	45654	74	F	7/21	7/30	Tonometry	Dye	LS

Figure 21.1   Cases of EKC by Visit Date

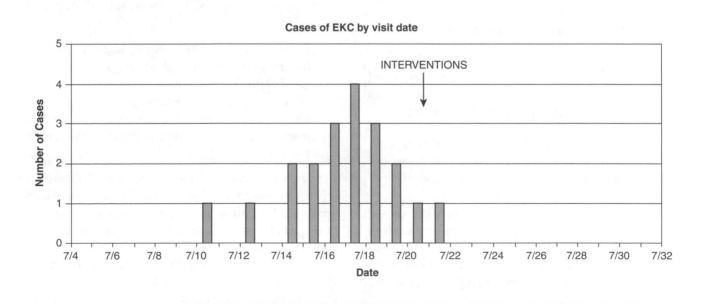

At this point in the investigation additional data collection may also be indicated. For example, if an environmental source is implicated, environmental culturing may be useful. If epidemiologic data implicate a specific healthcare worker (HCW), cultures from that HCW may provide useful information. Direct observations of patient care practices, such as surgery, catheter insertion, or dialysis procedures, may also provide useful information in the investigation.

STEP 4: TEST THE HYPOTHESES

Many investigations will not reach this step and the problem may end without additional interventions.[4] However, the hypothesis or "best guess" can be tested by applying it to all the cases and determining whether it explains their development. Once data analysis is complete, findings from the investigation can be interpreted.[7] These results then form the basis for control measures. Sometimes additional information is needed and the hypothesis must be tested through further epidemiologic studies. Epidemiologic studies for hypothesis testing include a case-control or a cohort study. The case-control approach is the most common methodology used to investigate outbreaks of health care-associated infection.[8–9] These references provide detailed information on performing a case-control study.

STEP 5: INSTITUTE APPROPRIATE CONTROL MEASURES

More specific control measures should be developed and implemented based on results of an investigation and the assumed cause. Control measures may be:[10]

- Directed against the reservoir of infection (e.g., removal of a contaminated product or device, or screening of patients with subsequent cohorting of infected or colonized patients).
- Measures that interrupt the transmission of the pathogen (e.g., changes in techniques for handling needleless devices for outbreaks related to needleless intravenous systems, improvements in disinfection or sterilization of equipment, or improving hand hygiene).
- Measures that reduce susceptibility of the host (e.g., active immunization of patients or staff, or improvements in timing of antibiotic prophylaxis for surgical procedures).

STEP 6: EVALUATE THE CONTROL MEASURES

Ongoing evaluation of control measures should be conducted throughout the investigation. Once control measures are effective, the outbreak should cease or infections should return to pre-outbreak levels. Continued surveillance should be conducted following the outbreak to determine that no new cases develop.

If new cases are identified, it is important to determine whether control measures were initiated before these cases developed. If they occur afterward, a reevaluation of the findings from the investigation is necessary. Perhaps a factor was overlooked that might lead to a different conclusion.

STEP 7: COMMUNICATE FINDINGS

At the end of the investigation, prepare a report and distribute it to individuals who oversee infection prevention and control activities and pertinent involved staff, including medical directors and administrative staff. This report will serve as a formal document to help demonstrate actions taken to outside agencies and accrediting organizations, and will help if there is a similar problem in the future. It is important to also keep any internal notes. The report should include the following:

- Description of circumstances leading to the outbreak
- Summary of the outbreak investigation
- Case definition and data analysis
- Outline of control measures
- Plan for continued surveillance and ongoing maintenance of infection prevention and control measures.

A standing protocol should be developed to assist in any investigation. Design the protocol to include background information, hypotheses, methods, interventions, analyses, and evaluation components[2] (see Appendix H).

It is important to note that although a formal outbreak investigation may be performed, a specific cause may not always be identified. However, the outbreak may end anyway. Many outbreaks are due to multiple factors, and changing one or two activities may lead to an end of the cases. Attention to the problem may cause staff to make changes such as wash their hands more frequently, spend more time on cleaning items, or review disinfection protocols. These changes may halt the outbreak.

SUMMARY OF PATIENT OUTBREAKS IDENTIFIED IN AMBULATORY CARE SETTINGS

In general, half of the outbreaks in ambulatory care settings are associated with a common source. The remainder is due to person-to-person or airborne spread.[11] Outbreaks in ambulatory care settings can be divided into five types:[1]

1. Inadequate sterilization or disinfection
2. Absent or inappropriate use of barrier precautions
3. Absent or inappropriate work restrictions for infected healthcare workers
4. Inadequate hand hygiene
5. Miscellaneous causes

Even though numerous outbreaks in outpatient settings have been reported, there are no accurate estimates of the frequency of these problems.[11] Table 21.2 outlines some of these investigations. Findings from these investigations can assist with identification of prevention and control measures.[12]

Table 21.2 Outbreaks Identified in Ambulatory Care Settings

Type	Area/Cause	Reference
Due to inadequate sterilization or disinfection	Dialysis	Humar,[13] Hindman,[14] Gordon,[15] Egwari,[16] Flaherty,[17] Danzig,[18] Beck-Sague,[19] CDC,[20] Wang,[21] Jochimsen,[22] Jackson,[23] Rudnick,[24] Longfield,[25] Arnow,[26] Bolan,[27] CDC,[28]
	Multidose vials/medications	Nakashima,[29] Alter,[30] Stetler,[31] Greaves,[32] Kothari,[33] Pegues,[34] Kantor,[35] CDC,[36] Borghans,[37] Inman,[38] Edell,[39] D'Angelo,[40] Grohskopf,[41] Simon,[42] Huang,[43] Kidd-Ljunggren[44]
	Jet injectors	Canter,[45] Wenger[46]
	Acupuncture needles	Kent,[47] Stryker[48]
	Endoscopy	Schembre,[49] Beecham,[50] Umphrey,[51] Hoffmann,[52] Wheeler,[53] Dwyer,[54] Kressel,[55] Sorin,[56] Rossetti,[57] Ramsey[58]
	Peritoneal dialysis	Goetz[59]
	Reprocessing techniques	Velandia,[60] Koo,[61] Jernigan,[62] Istre,[63] Rutala,[64] Lowry,[65] Keenlyside,[66] Murrah,[67] Martin,[68] Wegman,[69] Meyers[70]
Due to absent or inappropriate use of barrier precautions		Hlady,[71] Niu,[72] Welbel[73]
Due to absent or inappropriate work restrictions for infected health care workers		Wenzel[74]
Due to inadequate hand hygiene		Severo,[75] Jorm,[76] Buehler[77]
Due to miscellaneous causes	Social contact in clinics	Govan[78]
	General infection control practice	Warren,[79] Montessori,[80] Martin,[81] Weems,[82] Fridkin[83]

References

1. Herwaldt, L. A., Smith, S. D., and Carter, C. D. Infection control in the outpatient setting. *Infect Control Hosp Epidemiol.* 1998; 19:41–74.

2. Davis, J., MacKenzie, W. R., and Addiss, D. G. Recognition, investigation, and control of communicable-disease outbreaks in child day-care settings. *Pediatrics.* 1994; 94(6 Pt 2):1004–1006.

3. Friedman, C., Barnette, M., Buck, A. S., Ham, R., Harris, J., and Hoffman, P., et al. Requirements for infrastructure and essential activities of infection control and epidemiology in out-of-hospital settings: A Consensus Panel report. *Am J Infect Control.* 1999; 27:418–430.

4. Checko, P. J. Outbreak Investigation. In: *APIC Text of Infection Control and Epidemiology.* Washington, DC: Association for Professionals in Infection Control and Epidemiology, 2000: 15:1–9.

5. Weber, S., Pfaller, M. A., and Herwaldt, L. A. Role of molecular epidemiology in infection control. *Infect Dis Clin North Am.* 1997; 11:257–278.

6. Sinkowitz-Cochran, R. L., and Jarvis, W. R. Epidemiologic approach to outbreak investigation. *Semin Infect Control.* 2001; 1:85–90.

7. Phillips, D. Y., and Arias, K. M. Statistical Methods Used in Outbreak Investigations. In: Arias, K. M., ed., *Quick Reference to Outbreak Investigation and Control in Health Care Facilities.* Gaithersburg, MD: Aspen Publishers, Inc., 2000: 191–209.

8. Friedman, G. D. *Primer of Epidemiology.* 4th Ed. New York: McGraw-Hill; 1994.

9. Koziol, D. E. Research Study Design. In: *APIC Text of Infection Control and Epidemiology.* Washington, DC: Association for Professionals in Infection Control and Epidemiology; 2000: 8:1–6.

10. Mausner, J. S., and Kramer, S. *Mausner & Bahn: Epidemiology - An Introductory Text.* 2nd Ed. Philadelphia, PA: WB Saunders Co.; 1985: 292–294.

11. Goodman, R. A., and Solomon, S. L. Transmission of infectious diseases in outpatient health care settings. *JAMA.* 1991; 265:2377–2381.

12. Arias, K. M. Outbreaks Reported in the Ambulatory Care Setting. In: Arias, K. M., ed., *Quick Reference to Outbreak Investigation and Control in Health Care Facilities.* Gaithersburg, MD: Aspen Publishers, Inc.; 2000:105–118.

13. Humar, A., Oxley, C., Sample, M. L., and Garber, G. Elimination of an outbreak of gram-negative bacteremia in a hemodialysis unit. *Am J Infect Control.* 1996; 24:359–363.

14. Hindman, S. H., Favero, M. S., Carson, L. A., Petersen, N. J., Schonberger, L. B., and Solano, J. T. Pyrogenic reactions during haemodialysis caused by extramural endotoxin. *Lancet.* 1975; 2:732–734.

15. Gordon, S. M., Tipple, M., Bland, L. A., and Jarvis, W. R. Pyrogenic reactions associated with the reuse of disposable hollow-fiber hemodialyzers. *JAMA.* 1988; 260:2077–2081.

16. Egwari, L. O., and Mendie, U. E. Incidence of pyrexia in patients undergoing haemodialysis. *West African J Med.* 1996; 15:101–106.

17. Flaherty, J. P., Garcia-Houchins, S., Chudy, R., and Arnow, P. M. An outbreak of gram-negative bacteremia traced to contaminated O-rings and reprocessed dialyzers. *Ann Intern Med.* 1993; 119:1072–1078.

18. Danzig, L. E., Tormey, M. P., Sinha, S. D., Robertson, B. J., Lambert, S., and Itano, A., et al. Common source transmission of hepatitis B virus infection in a hemodialysis unit. *Infect Control Hosp Epidemiol.* 1995; 16(S):P19, Abstract 24.

19. Beck-Sague, C. M., Jarvis, W. R., Bland, L. A., Arduino, M. J., Aguero, S. M., and Verosic, G. Outbreak of gram-negative bacteremia and pyrogenic reactions in a hemodialysis center. *Am J Nephrol.* 1990; 10:397–403.

20. CDC. Outbreaks of hepatitis B virus infection among hemodialysis patients—California, Nebraska, and Texas, 1994. *MMWR.* 1996; 45:285–288.

21. Wang, S. A., Levine, R. B., Carson, L. A., Arduino, M. J., Killar, T., and Grillo, F. G., et al. An outbreak of gram-negative bacteremia in hemodialysis patients traced to hemodialysis machine waste drain ports. *Infect Control Hosp Epidemiol.* 1999; 20:746–751.

22. Jochimsen, E. M., Frenette, C., Delorme, M., Arduino, M., Aguero, S., and Carson, L., et al. A cluster of bloodstream infections and pyrogenic reactions among hemodialysis patients traced to dialysis machine waste-handling option units. *Am J Nephrol.* 1998; 18:485–489.

23. Jackson, B. M., Beck-Sague, C. M., Bland, L. A., Arduino, M. J., Meyer, L., and Jarvis, W. R. Outbreak of pyrogenic reactions and gram-negative bacteremia in a hemodialysis center. *Am J Nephrol.* 1994; 14:85–89.

24. Rudnick, J. R., Arduino, M. J., Bland, L. A., Cusick, L., McAllister, S. K., and Aguero, S. M., et al. An outbreak of pyrogenic reactions in chronic hemodialysis patients associated with hemodialyzer reuse. *Artificial Organs.* 1995; 19:289–294.

25. Longfield, R. N., Wortham, W. G., Fletcher, L. L., and Nauscheutz, W. F. Clustered bacteremias in a hemodialysis unit: Cross-contamination of blood tubing from ultrafiltrate waste. *Infect Control Hosp Epidemiol.* 1992; 13:160–164.

26. Arnow, P. M., Garcia-Houchins, S., Neagle, M. B., Bova, J. L., Dillon, J. J., and Chou, T. An outbreak of bloodstream infections arising from hemodialysis equipment. *J Infect Dis.* 1998; 178:783–791.

27. Bolan, G., Reingold, A. L., Carson, L. A., Silcox, V. A., Woodley, C. L., and Hayes, P. S., et al. Infections with *Mycobacterium chelonei* in patients receiving dialysis and using processed hemodialyzers. *J Infect Dis.* 1985; 152:1013–1019.

28. CDC. Outbreaks of gram-negative bacterial bloodstream infections traced to probable contamination of hemodialysis machines—Canada, 1995; United States, 1997; and Israel, 1997. *MMWR.* 1998; 47:55–58.

29. Nakashima, A. K., McCarthy, M. A., Martone, W. J., and Anderson, R. L. Epidemic septic arthritis caused by *Serratia marcescens* and associated with a benzalkonium chloride antiseptic. *J Clin Microbiol.* 1987; 25:1014–1018.

30. Alter, M. J., Ahtone, J., and Maynard, J. E. Hepatitis B virus transmission associated with a multiple-dose vial in a hemodialysis unit. *Ann Int Med.* 1983; 99:330–333.

31. Stetler, H. C., Garbe, P. L., Dwyer, D. M., Facklam, R. R., Orenstein, W. A., and West, G. R., et al. Outbreaks of group A streptococcal abscesses following diphtheria-tetanus toxoid-pertussis vaccination. *Pediatrics.* 1985; 75:299–303.

32. Greaves, W. L., Hinman, A. R., Facklam, R. R., Allman, K. C., Barrett, C. L., and Stetler, H. C. Streptococcal abscesses following diph-

theria-tetanus toxoid-pertussis vaccination. *Ped Infect Dis J.* 1982; 1:388–390.

33. Kothari, T., Reyes, M. P., Brooks, N., Brown, W. J., and Lerner, A. M. *Pseudomonas cepacia* septic arthritis due to intra-articular injections of methylprednisolone. *Can Med Assoc J.* 1977; 116:1230–1232.

34. Pegues, D. A., Carson, L. A., Anderson, R. I., Norgard, M. J., Argent, T. A., and Jarvis, W. R., et al. Outbreak of *Pseudomonas cepacia* bacteremia in oncology patients. *Clin Infect Dis.* 1993; 16:407–411.

35. Kantor, R. J., Carson, L. A., Graham, D. R., Petersen, N. J., and Favero, M. S. Outbreak of pyrogenic reactions at a dialysis center: Association with infusion of heparinized saline solution. *Am J Med.* 1983; 74:449–456.

36. Centers for Disease Control and Prevention. Infection with *Mycobacterium abscessus* associated with intramuscular injection of adrenal cortex extract—Colorado and Wyoming, 1995–1996. *MMWR.* 1996; 45:713–715.

37. Borghans, J. G., and Stanford, J. L. *Mycobacterium chelonei* in abscesses after injection of diphtheria-pertussis-tetanus-polio vaccine. *Am Rev Respir Dis.* 1973; 107:1–8.

38. Inman, P. M., Beck, A., Brown, A. E., and Stanford, J. L. Outbreak of injection abscesses due to *Mycobacterium abscessus*. *Arch Dermatol.* 1969; 100:141–147.

39. Edell, T. A. *Serratia marcescens* abscesses in soft tissue associated with intramuscular methylprednisolone injections. In: *Program and abstracts of the 28th Annual Epidemic Intelligence Service Conference;* Atlanta, GA: Centers for Disease Control; April 2–6, 1979.

40. D'Angelo, L. J., Hierholzer, J. C., Holman, R. C., and Smith, J. D. Epidemic keratoconjuctivitis caused by adenovirus type 8: Epidemiologic and laboratory aspects of a large outbreak. *Am J Epidemiol.* 1981; 113:44–49.

41. Grohskopf, L. A., Roth, V. R., Feikin, D. R., Arduino, M. J., Carson, L. A., and Tokars, J. I., et al. *Serratia liquefaciens* bloodstream infections from contamination of epoetin alfa at a hemodialysis center. *N Engl J Med.* 2001; 344:1491–1497.

42. Simon, P. A., Chen, R. T., Elliott, J. A., and Schwartz, B. Outbreak of pyogenic abscesses after diphtheria and tetanus toxoids and pertussis vaccination. *Ped Infect Dis J.* 1993; 12:368–371.

43. Huang, A., Stamler, D., Edelstein, P., Skalina, D., and Brennan, P. J. Isolation of *Pseudomonas pickettii* in a sinus clinic. *Infect Control Hosp Epidemiol.* 1993; 14:432, Abstract M18.

44. Kidd-Ljunggren, K., Broman, E., Ekvall, H., and Gustavsson, O. Nosocomial transmission of hepatitis B virus infection through multiple-dose vials. *J Hosp Infect.* 1999; 43:57–62.

45. Canter, J., Mackey, K., Good, L. S., Roberto, R. R., Chin, J., and Bond, W. W., et al. An outbreak of hepatitis B associated with jet injections in a weight reduction clinic. *Arch Int Med.* 1990; 150:1923–1927.

46. Wenger, J. D., Spika, J. S., Smithwick, R. W., Pryor, V., Dodson, D. W., and Carden, G. A., et al. Outbreak of *Mycobacterium chelonae* infection associated with use of jet injectors, *JAMA.* 1990; 264:373–376.

47. Kent, G. P., Brondum, J., Keenlyside, R. A., LaFazia, L. M., and Scott, H. D. A large outbreak of acupuncture-associated hepatitis B. *Am J Epidemiol.* 1988; 127:591–598.

48. Stryker, W. S., Gunn, R. A., and Francis, D. P. Outbreak of hepatitis B associated with acupuncture. *J Fam Pract.* 1986; 22:155–158.

49. Schembre, D. B. Infectious complications associated with gastrointestinal endoscopy. *Gastro Endoscopy Clin North Am.* 2000; 10:215–232.

50. Beecham, H. J., 3rd, Cohen, M. L., and Parkin, W. E. *Salmonella typhimurium.* Transmission by fiberoptic upper gastrointestinal endoscopy. *JAMA.* 1979; 241:1013–1015.

51. Umphrey, J., Raad, I., Tarrand, J., and Hill, L. A. Bronchoscopes as a contamination source of *Pseudomonas putida*. *Infect Control Hosp Epidemiol.* 1996; 17(S):P42, Abstract M2.

52. Hoffmann, K. K., Weber, D. J., and Rutala, W. A. Pseudo-outbreak of *Rhodotorula rubra* in patients undergoing fiberoptic bronchoscopy. *Am J Infect Control.* 1989; 17:99, Abstract.

53. Wheeler, P. W., Lancaster, D., and Kaiser, A. B. Bronchopulmonary cross-colonization and infection related to mycobacterial contamination of suction valves of bronchoscopes. *J Infect Dis.* 1989; 159:954–958.

54. Dwyer, D. M., Klein, E. G., Istre, G. R., Robinson, M. G., Neumann, D. A., and McCoy, G. A. *Salmonella newport* infections transmitted by fiberoptic colonoscopy. *Gastrointes Endoscopy.* 1987; 33:84–87.

55. Kressel, A. B., and Kidd, F. Pseudo-outbreak of *Mycobacterium chelonae* and *Methylobacterium mesophilicum* caused by contamination of an automated endoscopy washer. *Infect Control Hosp Epidemiol.* 2001; 22:414–418.

56. Sorin, M., Segal-Maurer, S., Mariano, N., Urban, C., Combest, A., and Rahal, J. J. Nosocomial transmission of imipenem-resistant *Pseudomonas aeruginosa* following bronchoscopy associated with improper connection to the Steris System 1 processor. *Infect Control Hosp Epidemiol.* 2001; 22:409–413.

57. Rossetti, R., Lencioni, P., Innocenti, F., and Tortoli, E. Pseudoepidemic from *Mycobacterium gordonae* due to a contaminated automatic bronchoscope washing machine. *Am J Infect Control.* 2002; 30:196–197.

58. Ramsey, A. H., Oemig, T. V., Davis, J. P., Massey, J. P., and Török, T. J. An outbreak of bronchoscopy-related *Mycobacterium tuberculosis* infections due to lack of bronchoscope leak testing. *Chest.* 2002; 121:976–981.

59. Goetz, A., and Muder, R. R. *Pseudomonas aeruginosa* infections associated with use of povidone-iodine in patients receiving continuous ambulatory peritoneal dialysis. *Infect Control Hosp Epidemiol.* 1989; 10:447–450.

60. Velandia, M., Fridkin, S. K., Cardenas, V., Boshell, J., Ramirez, G., and Bland, L., et al. Transmission of HIV in dialysis centre. *Lancet.* 1995; 345:1417–1422.

61. Koo, D., Bouvier, B., Wesley, M., Courtright, P., and Reingold, A. Epidemic keratoconjunctivitis in a university medical center ophthalmology clinic: Need for re-evaluation of the design and disinfection of instruments. *Infect Control Hosp Epidemiol.* 1989; 10:547–552.

62. Jernigan, J. A., Lowry, B. S., Hayden, F. G., Kyger, S. A., Conway, B. P., and Groschel, D. H., et al. Adenovirus type 8 epidemic keratoconjunctivitis in an eye clinic: Risk factors and control. *J Infect Dis.* 1993; 167:1307–1313.

63. Istre, G. R., Kreiss, K., Hopkins, R. S., Healy, G. R., Benziger, M., and Canfield, T. M., et al. An outbreak of amebiasis spread by colonic irrigation at a chiropractic clinic. *N Engl J Med.* 1982; 307:339–342.

64. Rutala, W. A., Weber, D. J., and Thomann, C. A. Outbreak of wound infections following outpatient podiatric surgery due to contaminated bone drills. *Foot Ankle Int.* 1987; 7:350–354.

65. Lowry, P. W., Jarvis, W. R., Oberle, A. D., Bland, L. A., Silberman, R., and Bocchini, J. A., Jr., et al. *Mycobacterium chelonae* causing otitis media in an ear-nose-and-throat practice. *New Engl J Med.* 1988; 319:978–982.

66. Keenlyside, R. A., Hierholzer, J. C., and D'Angelo, L. J. Keratoconjuctivitis associated with adenovirus type 37: An extended outbreak in an ophthalmologist's office. *J Infect Dis.* 1983; 147:191–198.

67. Murrah, W. F. Epidemic keratoconjuctivitis. *Am J Ophthalmol.* 1998; 20:36–38.

68. Martin, M. V. The significance of the bacterial contamination of dental unit water systems. *Br Dent J.* 1987; 183:152–154.

69. Wegman, D. H., Guinee, V. F., and Millian, S. J. Epidemic keratoconjuctivitis. *Am J Public Health.* 1970; 60:1230–1237.

70. Meyers, H., Brown-Elliott, B. A., Moore, D., Curry, J., Truong, C., and Zhang, Y., et al. An outbreak of *Mycobacterium chelonae* infection following liposuction. *Clin Infect Dis.* 2002; 34:1500–1507.

71. Hlady, W. G., Hopkins, R. S., Ogilby, T. E., and Allen, S. T. Patient-to-patient transmission of hepatitis B in a dermatology practice. *Am J Public Health.* 1993; 83:1689–1693.

72. Niu, M. T., Alter, M. J., Kristensen, C., and Margolis, H. S. Outbreak of hemodialysis-associated non-A, non-B hepatitis and correlation with antibody to hepatitis C virus. *Am J Kidney Dis.* 1992; 19:345–352.

73. Welbel, S. F., Schoendorf, K., Bland, L. A., Arduino, M. J., Groves, C., and Schable, B., et al. An outbreak of gram-negative bloodstream infections in chronic hemodialysis patients. *Am J Nephrol.* 1995; 15:1–4.

74. Wenzel, R. P., and Perl, T. M. The significance of nasal carriage of *Staphylococcus aureus* and the incidence of postoperative wound infections. *J Hosp Infect.* 1995; 31:13–24.

75. Severo, C. A., Abensur, P., Buisson, Y., Lafuma, A., Detournay, B., and Pechevis, M. An outbreak of hepatitis A in a French day-care center and efforts to combat it. *Euro J Epidemiol.* 1997; 13:139–144.

76. Jorm, L. R., and Capon, A. G. Communicable disease outbreaks in long day care centres in western Sydney: Occurrence and risk factors. *J Peds Child Health.* 1994; 30:151–154.

77. Buehler, J. W., Finton, R. J., Goodman, R. A., Choi, K., Hierholzer, J. C., and Sikes, R. K., et al. Epidemic keratoconjunctivitis: Report of an outbreak in an ophthalmology practice and recommendations for prevention. *Infect Control.* 1984; 5:390–394.

78. Govan, J. R. W., Brown, P. H., Maddison, J., Doherty, C. J., Nelson, J. W., and Dodd, M., et al. Evidence for transmission of *Pseudomonas cepacia* by social contact in cystic fibrosis. *Lancet.* 1993; 342:15–19.

79. Warren, D., Nelson, K. E., Farrar, J. A., Hurwitz, E., Hierholzer, J., and Ford, E., et al. A large outbreak of epidemic keratoconjunctivitis: Problems in controlling nosocomial spread. *J Inf Dis.* 1989; 160:938–943.

80. Montessori, V., Scharf, S., Holland, S., Werker, D. H., Roberts, F. J., and Bryce, E. Epidemic keratoconjunctivitis outbreak at a tertiary referral eye care clinic. *Am J Infect Control.* 1998; 26:399–405.

81. Martin, M. V. The significance of the bacterial contamination of dental unit water systems. *Br Dent J.* 1987; 163:152–153.

82. Weems, J. J., Jr., Usry, G., and Schwab, U. Infection due to rapidly-growing mycobacteria associated with ultrasound directed prostate biopsy. *Infect Control Hosp Epidemiol.* 1996; 17(S):P50, Abstract M67.

83. Fridkin, S. K., Kremer, F. B., Bland, L. A., Paghye, A., McNeil, M. M., and Jarvis, W. R. *Acremonium kiliense* endophthalmitis that occurred after cataract extraction in an ambulatory surgical center and was traced to an environmental reservoir. *Clin Infect Dis.* 1996; 22:222–227.

CHAPTER 22

Public Health, Accrediting, & Regulatory Agencies

Understanding the role of public health, regulatory, and accrediting agencies will assist a facility with both performance improvement activities and compliance. Various agencies are important to infection prevention and control in ambulatory care facilities; a few of the most important are outlined in this chapter.[1]

STATE HEALTH DEPARTMENTS

Communicable Diseases

Reportable disease requirements are administered by states through local health departments. Reporting is required, as it enables public health officials to follow up on significant cases and assists in identifying outbreaks or other public health concerns.

As of January 1, 1999, a total of 58 infectious diseases were designated as notifiable at the national level. A notifiable disease is one for which regular, frequent, and timely information regarding individual cases is considered necessary for the prevention and control of the disease. Data for nationally notifiable diseases are collated and published weekly in the Morbidity and Mortality Weekly Report (MMWR) (*http://www.cdc.gov/mmwr/*). States specify which diseases are notifiable in each state, including the federally designated diseases.

Healthcare providers are responsible for reporting communicable diseases to local or state health departments. Ambulatory care facilities need a mechanism to ensure that reporting occurs as required by local regulations. (See *http://www.cdc.gov/other.htm#states* for links to state health departments.)

Other Health Department Responsibilities

Immunization

State laws typically mandate that children receive all required vaccinations before entering day care and kindergarten. These immunization programs seek to reduce and eradicate vaccine-preventable diseases.

Waste Disposal

In any given state, the Environmental Protection Agency (EPA) (*http://www.epa.gov/epaoswer/other/medical/*) or a state hazardous waste agency enforces the hazardous waste laws. Most states define regulated, infectious, or medical waste in waste handling rules. The EPA enforces practices related to waste disposal under the Resource Conservation and Recovery Act (RCRA), which was enacted by Congress in 1976. RCRA's primary goals are to protect human health and the environment from the potential hazards of waste disposal, to conserve energy and natural resources, to reduce the amount of waste generated, and to ensure that wastes are managed in an environmentally sound manner.

Medical waste is generally defined as any solid waste that is generated in the diagnosis, treatment, or immunization of human beings or animals, in research, or in the production or testing of biologicals. Table 22.1 outlines the types of medical waste typically generated in an ambulatory care facility.

Table 22.1   Medical Waste in Ambulatory Care Settings

Category	Examples
Sharps	Lancets, needles, scalpels, syringes with needles
Cultures and stocks	Culture dishes and other glassware, swabs used to inoculate cultures
Human pathological wastes	Removed body tissue
Human blood and blood products	Suction canisters, blood-soaked bandages

Licensing

There may be local or state requirements for licensure of ambulatory care facilities, which may include specific requirements for infection prevention and control. Some states also have laws or regulations pertaining to office-based surgery or free-standing outpatient surgery facilities.[2]

Construction/Renovation

Health departments also may have a role in the review and oversight of healthcare construction and modernization projects, participate in surveys and inspections of healthcare facilities, review private sewage systems at healthcare facilities, and serve as consultants on issues related to the physical plant and sewage disposal systems at healthcare facilities.

CENTERS FOR DISEASE CONTROL AND PREVENTION

The Centers for Disease Control and Prevention (CDC) mission is to promote health and quality of life by preventing and controlling disease, injury, and disability. It accomplishes its mission by working with partners to monitor health, detect and investigate health problems, conduct research to enhance prevention, develop and advocate sound public health policies, implement prevention strategies, promote healthy behaviors, foster safe and healthful environments, and provide leadership and training (*http://www.cdc.gov/*). The CDC's Division of Healthcare Quality Promotion will assist healthcare facilities with outbreak investigations upon request.

Healthcare Infection Control Practices Advisory Committee

The Healthcare Infection Control Practices Advisory Committee (HICPAC) provides advice and guidance at a national level regarding the practice of infection control and strategies for surveillance, prevention, control of infections (e.g., nosocomial or health care-associated infections), antimicrobial resistance, and related events in settings where health care is provided (*http://www.cdc.gov/ncidod/hip/HICPAC/Hicpac.htm*). It has promulgated various guidelines and recommendations, including:

- Infection Control in Healthcare Personnel, 1998[3]
- Nosocomial Pneumonia, 1994[4]
- Prevention of Intravascular-Catheter-Related Infections, 2002[5]
- Surgical Site Infections, 1999[6]
- Isolation Precautions, 1996[7]
- Recommendations for Preventing the Spread of Vancomycin Resistance, 1995[8]
- Hand Hygiene in Healthcare Settings, 2002[9]

National Institute for Occupational Safety and Health

The National Institute for Occupational Safety and Health (NIOSH) is the federal agency responsible for conducting research and making recommendations for the prevention of work-related disease and injury. NIOSH provides information on various infection prevention and control topics, including:

- Bloodborne Infectious Diseases—HIV/AIDS, Hepatitis B Virus, and Hepatitis C Virus: Safe Needle Devices, Sharps Containers, Capillary Tubes, Surveillance of Health Care Workers (*http://www.cdc.gov/niosh/topics/bbp/*)

- Occupational Latex Allergies (*http://www.cdc.gov/niosh/latexpg.html*)
- Tuberculosis (*http://www.cdc.gov/niosh/tbifopg.html*)
- West Nile Virus (*http://www.cdc.gov/niosh/topics/westnile/*)

Other CDC Guidelines

- Preventing Transmission of Infections Among Chronic Hemodialysis Patients, 2001 (*http://www.cdc.gov/mmwr/preview/mmwrhtml/rr5005a1.htm*)
- General Infection Control Recommendations— Dialysis, 1996 (*http://www.cdc.gov/ncidod/hip/Dialysis/RECCOMD.HTM*)
- Occupational Health (*http://www.cdc.gov/ncidod/hip/Occhealt/ochealth.htm*)
- Sterilization and Disinfection (*http://www.cdc.gov/ncidod/hip/Sterile/sterile.htm*)
- Multidrug-Resistant Organisms in Non-Hospital Healthcare Settings, 2001 (*http://www.cdc.gov/ncidod/hip/Aresist/nonhosp.htm*)
- Urinary Tract Infections, 1983[10]
- Guidelines for Preventing the Transmission of *Mycobacterium tuberculosis* in Health-Care Facilities, 1994[11]

OCCUPATIONAL SAFETY AND HEALTH ADMINISTRATION

The Occupational Safety and Health Act of 1970 (PL91-596, 1970) established the Occupational Safety and Health Administration (OSHA), a branch of the U.S. Department of Labor. It is charged with conducting research, developing safety standards, monitoring job-related illness, and inspecting workplaces. Specific standards are developed according to identified hazards; then compliance documents are made available that interpret the standards.

States may develop and enforce their own occupational safety and health standards; however, the standards must be at least equivalent to OSHA standards. The OSH Act's general duty clause requires all employers to maintain an environment safe from hazards.[12] OSHA can impose a fine for noncompliance identified through inspections (often a result of employee complaints).[13]

Bloodborne Pathogens

The OSHA rules (OSHA Law 29 CFR part 1910) on occupational exposure to bloodborne pathogens became effective in 1992.[14] The rules are designed to inform workers about possible risks to their health from infections that can be spread by contact with blood and other body fluids. The premise behind the rules is that if body fluids and articles contaminated with blood or body fluids are handled carefully and safely, they are not dangerous in the workplace.

OSHA requires the development of a bloodborne pathogen exposure control plan for health facilities (see example in Appendix I). The written plan must outline how the organization will eliminate or minimize employee exposures. It must include:

1. Exposure determination: The bloodborne rules apply to all workers with occupational exposure to blood or other potentially infectious materials (OPIM). OSHA requires all employers to identify the types of employees whose jobs may expose them to blood or OPIM and identify work practices that will reduce the likelihood that employees will be exposed (i.e., an identification and list of job classifications that have potential occupational exposure).
2. A schedule and method for implementing the plan.
3. A procedure for evaluating exposure incidents (see Chapter 19).

The exposure control plan should outline the following methods for compliance with the OSHA rules:

1. Use of Standard Precautions: See Chapter 6.
2. Engineering controls: Describe methods to be used to reduce hazards in the workplace, such as handwashing facilities, sharps disposal containers near point of use, mechanical devices to reduce handling of contaminated needles, and safety-engineered devices.[15] Employers must provide employees with and ensure that they use equipment and containers that isolate or remove blood, body fluids, and items contaminated with blood or body fluids from the workplace. This includes puncture-resistant sharps containers, mechanical pipetting devices, and biosafety cabinets. Also required are clearly labeled leak-resistant containers or bags for specimens, contaminated linen, and medical waste. Engineering

controls, especially safety devices, must be evaluated annually by staff members.[16–17]

3. Work practice controls: These are techniques to reduce the likelihood of exposure to blood or OPIM by changing the way a task is performed. Examples include handwashing, safety needles, prohibition on recapping needles, and correct use of barriers or personal protective equipment (see Chapter 4). OSHA requires employers to make available to employees who have a potential for exposure to blood or OPIM the following personal protective equipment (PPE): gloves, masks, face shields or eye protection, coats or gowns, caps or hoods, and shoe covers. This equipment must be readily accessible to the employee.

4. Orientation and training: The organization must provide initial and annual training for employees with a potential for exposure to blood or OPIM. OSHA requires that all of these workers receive information and training about bloodborne microorganisms and have access to a copy of the OSHA rules that can be reviewed by the employee, along with an explanation of their contents.

5. Labels and signs: Biohazard warning labels must be placed on all items containing blood or OPIM, including pertinent refrigerators and freezers.

6. Regulated waste: There must be a protocol on the management of regulated waste, using either state regulations or criteria from the EPA.

7. Hepatitis B vaccination: Employees must be offered vaccine if they have the potential for exposure to blood or OPIM. OSHA requires employers to offer prescreening and hepatitis B vaccine free of charge to all employees whose work puts them at risk for exposure to blood or OPIM. Employees who decline vaccination must sign a declination form (see Appendix J).

8. Post-exposure plans: There must be a plan in place if exposures do occur. Employers must make available to all employees who are exposed to blood or OPIM on the job a confidential medical evaluation, treatment, and follow-up. See Chapter 19 for additional information.

Tuberculosis

In 1993 OSHA issued draft guidelines to enforce the protection of healthcare workers from tuberculosis (TB) (*http://www.osha-slc.gov/SLTC/tuberculosis/in-dex.html*). These rules were prompted by increasing numbers of new cases of TB and outbreaks of TB in hospitals[18] and exposures in emergency departments.[19–20] These rules are not final; however, OSHA can enforce the 1994 CDC guidelines[11] under its general duty clause.

A TB control plan should be developed if there is a potential for exposure to TB in an ambulatory care facility, including facilities providing treatment for drug abuse, laboratories that handle specimens that might contain *Mycobacterium tuberculosis*, and settings that perform high-hazard procedures (i.e., cough-inducing or aerosol-generating). States may have specific requirements for ambulatory care facilities.

The following documents should be included in the plan:

1. A risk assessment for the facility.
2. A protocol for the early identification of individuals with active TB.
3. A description of the medical surveillance of employees, including administration and interpretation of TB skin tests.
4. An outline of the evaluation and management of workers with a positive TB skin test, skin test conversion, or who are exhibiting symptoms of TB. Include work restrictions for infectious employees.
5. A description of isolation precautions protocols, including methods of placement of individuals with suspected or confirmed TB (e.g., in an isolation room, if available) (see Chapter 6).
6. Requirements for the use of respiratory protection devices for staff per the facility's risk assessment. Fit-tested N95 masks are the device of choice for staff; see Chapter 6 for additional information. There must also be a written respiratory protection program describing the types of respiratory protection available and fit-testing protocols.
7. An outline of the training and information provided to employees to ensure they are knowledgeable about TB issues.

ACCREDITING AGENCIES

Joint Commission on Accreditation of Healthcare Organizations

The Joint Commission is a national, not-for-profit, voluntary accrediting organization. Its mission is to improve the quality of care through accreditation and related services that support performance improvement. Its standards are developed in cooperation with an advisory committee and professional organizations (*http://www.jcaho.org*). Accreditation by the Joint Commission may be accepted in place of state licensure inspections.

The Joint Commission established the Ambulatory Health Care accreditation program in 1975 to encourage quality patient care in all types of freestanding ambulatory care facilities. More than 1,000 ambulatory care organizations are accredited by the Joint Commission, including:

Ambulatory surgery centers
Community health centers
Group medical practices
Indian health clinics
Military clinics
Mobile services
Multispecialty group practices
Occupational health centers
Office-based surgery offices
Physician offices
Prison health centers
Student health services
Single-specialty providers
   Birthing centers
   Cardiac catheterization centers
   Dental clinics
   Dialysis centers
   Endoscopy centers
   Imaging centers
   Infusion therapy services
   Laser centers
   Lithotripsy services
   MRI centers
Ophthalmology practices
Oral and maxillofacial surgery centers
Pain management centers
Plastic surgery centers
Podiatric clinics
Radiation/oncology clinics
Rehabilitation centers
Sleep centers
Urgent/emergency care centers
Women's health centers

The Joint Commission's standards apply to the full range of ambulatory care providers. To be accredited, organizations must demonstrate compliance with various ambulatory care standards, including the following Surveillance, Prevention, and Control of Infection standards:[21]

IC.1   The organization uses a coordinated process to reduce the risks of endemic and epidemic nosocomial infections in patients and healthcare workers.

IC.2   Case findings and identification of demographically important nosocomial infections provide surveillance data.

IC.3   Infections are reported, when appropriate, within the organization or to public health agencies.

IC.4   The organization takes action to prevent or reduce the risk of nosocomial infections in patients, employees, and visitors.

IC.5   The organization takes action to control outbreaks of nosocomial infections when they are identified.

IC.6   The organization's infection control process is designed to lower the risks and to improve the rates or trends of epidemiologically significant infections.

IC.6.1   Management systems support the infection control process to ensure adequate data analysis, interpretation, and presentation.

The goal of the surveillance, prevention, and control of infection standards is to identify and reduce the risks of acquiring and transmitting infections. Other standards that include infection prevention and control issues are improving organization performance and environment of care. The Joint Commission's Shared Vision—New Pathways strategy will result in some revisions to the standards by 2004.[22] Office-based surgery standards were developed in 2001.[23]

Ambulatory care sites may receive accreditation through various Joint Commission accreditation programs. These include Ambulatory Care (Ambulatory Care accreditation and Office-Based Surgery accreditation), Health Care Networks, or Pathology and Clinical Laboratory Services. Accreditation may also be received as part of the Hospitals accreditation program.

Accreditation Association for Ambulatory Health Care

The Accreditation Association for Ambulatory Health Care's purpose is to operate a peer-based assessment and accreditation program for ambulatory healthcare organizations to assist in providing a high level of care (*http://www.aaahc.org/*). The types of organizations accredited include:

Ambulatory healthcare clinics
Ambulatory surgery centers
Birthing centers
College and university health services
Community health centers
Dental group practices
Diagnostic imaging centers
Endoscopy centers
Health Maintenance Organizations (HMOs)
Independent Physicians Associations (IPAs)
Indian health centers
Managed Care Organizations
Multispecialty group practices
Occupational health services
Office surgery centers and practices
Oral and maxillofacial surgeons' offices
Podiatrists' offices
Radiation oncology centers
Single-specialy group practices
Surgical recovery centers
Urgent or immediate care centers

Important standards related to infection prevention and control of infections include:[24]

Facilities and Environment

- Procedures should be available to minimize the sources and transmission of infections, including adequate surveillance techniques.

Quality Management and Improvement

- The quality improvement program addresses clinical issues . . . as well as actual patient outcomes.
- Improvement problems or concerns in the care of patients are identified. Sources of identifiable problems include . . . unacceptable or unexpected results of ongoing monitoring of care, such as complications . . . and adverse events.

Surgical Services

- A safe environment for treating surgical patients, including adequate safeguards to protect the patient from cross-infection, is ensured through the provision of adequate space, equipment, and personnel.
    i. Provisions have been made for the isolation or immediate transfer of patients with communicable disease.
    ii. All persons entering operating rooms are properly attired.
    iii. Acceptable aseptic techniques are used by all persons in the surgical area.
    iv. Suitable equipment for rapid and routine sterilization is available to ensure that operating room materials are sterile.
    v. Sterilized materials are packaged and labeled in a consistent manner to maintain sterility and identify sterility dates.
    vi. Environmental controls are implemented to ensure a safe and sanitary environment.
    vii. Operating rooms are appropriately cleaned before each operation.

National Committee for Quality Assurance

The National Committee for Quality Assurance (NCQA) is an independent, nonprofit organization whose mission is to evaluate and report on the quality of managed care organizations. NCQA accredits the following types of organizations: managed care organizations, managed behavioral healthcare organizations, preferred provider organizations, and credentials verification organizations.

There are no NCQA standards specific to infection prevention and control; the standards primarily evaluate systems and processes, including quality improvement.

NCQA promotes the Health Plan Employer Data and Information Set (HEDIS). HEDIS is a set of standardized performance measures designed to provide purchasers and consumers with the information they need to compare the performance of managed healthcare plans. Pertinent HEDIS measures are immunization rates and provision of influenza vaccine. (*http://www.ncqa.org/Programs/HEDIS/index.htm*).

REGULATORY AGENCIES

Food and Drug Administration

The Food and Drug Administration (FDA) regulates food, drugs, medical devices, biologics (e.g., vaccines and blood products), animal feed and drugs, cosmetics, and radiation-emitting products. Part of its activities (through the Center for Devices and Radiological Health [*http://www.fda.gov/cdrh/*]) are aimed at the efficacy or safety of specific medical products or devices, including names and classes of specific disinfectants, sterilants, and decontaminants. For medical devices, this includes antiseptics (including those used for handwashing) and chemical germicides used for high-level disinfection or sterilization.

On August 14, 2000, the FDA released a document titled "Enforcement Priorities for Single-Use Devices (SUD) Reprocessed by Third Parties and Hospitals" to provide guidance to third-party and hospital reprocessors about their responsibilities in reprocessing devices labeled for single use (*http://www.fda.gov/cdrh/reuse/index.html*). If a hospital reprocesses a device that was previously marketed as a SUD, the hospital can be considered as the manufacturer of that device and is subject to the same reporting requirements as original equipment manufacturers. The FDA document notes that hospitals are not the only healthcare facilities that reprocess devices labeled for single use. At this time, the agency is limiting its focus to SUDs reprocessed in hospitals. In the future the FDA intends to examine whether other establishments (e.g., ambulatory care facilities) that reprocess SUDs should be included under the enforcement document. Until then, reprocessing of any device marketed or labeled as single-use (e.g., endoscopy accessories or instruments) should be performed with caution using rigorous protocols.

Environmental Protection Agency

Under the Federal Insecticide, Fungicide and Rodenticide Act, the Environmental Protection Agency (EPA) requires companies that register public health antimicrobial pesticide products to ensure the safety and effectiveness of their products before they are sold or distributed. Chemical germicides used in ambulatory care settings for noncritical items, environmental surfaces, or devices fall under these rules (*http://www.epa.gov/oppad001/sciencepolicy.htm*). The EPA also has authority for regulations regarding solid waste, including regulated medical waste.

Clinical Laboratory Improvement Amendments

Congress passed the Clinical Laboratory Improvement Amendments (CLIA) in 1988, establishing quality standards for all laboratory testing to ensure the accuracy, reliability, and timeliness of patient test results, regardless of where the test was performed. In 1992, the then Health Care Financing Administration issued final regulations to implement CLIA. The final regulations extended the scope to all laboratory testing, including physician office laboratories and clinics. CLIA specify the performance requirements that apply to laboratories. States typically enforce CLIA through the licensing and certification division of state health departments (see Chapter 18 for more information).

Centers for Medicare & Medicaid Services

The Centers for Medicare & Medicaid Services (CMS) was established by the U.S. Department of Health and Human Services in 1977 as the Health Care Financing Administration (*http://www.cms.gov*). It is responsible for oversight of Medicare and Medicaid programs. It also monitors healthcare reimbursement under those programs, and implements and enforces quality standards in laboratories, ambulatory care centers, and other healthcare facilities. CMS regulates all laboratory testing (except research) performed on humans in the United States. CMS also has rules overseeing the reuse of dialysis hemodialyzers (42 CFR Part 405, 1990). The Centers for Medicare & Medicaid Services approves of the Joint Commission as a deemed authority for ambulatory surgery centers. In addition, deemed status options are available for Joint Commission-accredited clinical laboratories.

PROFESSIONAL ORGANIZATIONS

Association for Professionals in Infection Control and Epidemiology

The Association for Professionals in Infection Control and Epidemiology (APIC) mission is to improve health care by reducing risks of infection and related adverse outcomes (*http://www.apic.org*). In its role to be a key source of high-quality information, APIC develops guidelines, state-of-the-art reports, position statements, standards, and definitions. APIC also publishes a text, the "APIC Text of Infection Control and Epidemiology," that reflects current infection control and epidemiological practices. Other available documents include:

- APIC guideline for infection prevention and control in flexible endoscopy[25]
- APIC guideline for selection and use of disinfectants[26]

- The role of infection control during construction in healthcare facilities[27]
- The implications of service animals in healthcare settings[28]
- Use of scrubs and related apparel in healthcare facilities[29]
- APIC position paper: Responsibility for interpretation of the PPD tuberculin skin test[30]
- APIC position paper: Hepatitis C exposure in the healthcare setting[31]
- APIC position paper: Immunization[32]
- APIC position paper: Prevention of device-mediated bloodborne infections to healthcare workers[33]
- APIC/CHICA–Canada infection control and epidemiology: Professional and practice standards[34]
- APIC Surveillance Initiative Working Group: Recommended Practices for Surveillance[35]

Society for Healthcare Epidemiology of America

The Society for Healthcare Epidemiology of America (SHEA) was organized in 1980 to foster the development and application of the science of healthcare epidemiology (*http://www.shea-online.org/*). Healthcare epidemiology is defined by the organization as any activity designed to study and/or improve patient care outcomes in any type of healthcare institution or setting. Some of the organization's position papers include:

- How to select and interpret molecular strain typing methods for epidemiological studies of bacterial infections: A review for healthcare epidemiologists[36]
- Management of healthcare workers infected with hepatitis B virus, hepatitis C virus, human immunodeficiency virus, or other bloodborne pathogens[37]
- Medical waste[38]

Society for Gastroenterology Nurses and Associates

The Society for Gastrointestinal Nurses and Associates (SGNA) focuses on the care to patients with known or suspected gastrointestinal problems who are undergoing diagnostic or therapeutic treatment and/or procedures. The organization offers a self-study module on endoscope cleaning and high-level disinfection (*http://www.sgna.org/marketplace/module.cfm*).

Association of periOperative Registered Nurses

The Association of periOperative Registered Nurses (AORN) mission is to promote quality patient care by providing its members with education, standards, services, and representation (*http://www.aorn.org/default.asp*). Official statements of the organization include:

- AORN Revised Statement on Patients and Health Care Workers with Bloodborne Diseases, 2002 (*http://www.aorn.org/about/positions/hiv.htm*)
- Reuse of Single-Use Devices, 2001 (*http://www.aorn.org/about/positions/Reuse.pdf*)
- Latex Guideline, 1998 (*http://www.aorn.org/about/positions/7c-latex-1999rev2.pdf*)

AORN's major reference book, *Standards, Recommended Practices, and Guidelines,*[39] features recommended practices for surgical hazards, packaging systems, and maintaining a sterile field.

American Institute of Architects

The American Institute of Architects (AIA) and the Facilities Guidelines Institute produce a consensus document, *The Guidelines for Design and Construction of Hospital and Health Care Facilities*[40] (*http://www.aia.org/*). This book sets minimum space and equipment needs for clinical and support areas of outpatient, rehabilitation facilities, and other healthcare facilities. The document also establishes minimum engineering design criteria for plumbing, medical gas, electrical, heating, ventilating, and air conditioning systems. Each state may adopt the guidelines or adapt them as a basis for its own state codes.

Association for the Advancement of Medical Instrumentation

The goal of the Association for the Advancement of Medical Instrumentation (AAMI) is to increase the understanding and beneficial use of medical instrumentation (*http://www.aami.org/*). AAMI is a resource for national and international standards on sterilization, biological evaluation, and dialysis. Various documents outlining appropriate practices in these areas are available.

References

1. Yost, A. J., and Serkey, J. M. Rule-makers who establish infection control standards. *Nurs Clin North Am.* 1999; 34:527–533.

2. Franko, F. P. Health policy issues: State laws and regulations for office-based surgery. *AORN J.* 2001; 73:839–840, 843–846.

3. Bolyard, E. A., Tablan, O. C., Williams, W. W., Pearson, M. L., Shapiro, C. N., and Deithman, S. D. HICPAC. Guideline for infection control in health care personnel, 1998. *Am J Infect Control.* 1998; 26(3):289–354, *http://www.cdc.gov/ncidod/hip/guide/infectcont98. htm.*

4. HICPAC. Guideline for prevention of nosocomial pneumonia—1994. *Am J Infect Control.* 1994; 22:247–292, *http://www.cdc.gov/ncidod/ hip/pneumonia/pneu_mmw.htm.*

5. HICPAC. Guidelines for the prevention of intravascular catheter-related infections, 2002. *MMWR Recommendations and Reports.* 2002; 51:1–29, *http://www.cdc.gov/ncidod/hip/IV/IV.HTM.*

6. Mangram, A. J., Horan, T. C., Pearson, M. L., Silver, L. C., and Jarvis, W. R. Guideline for prevention of surgical site infection, 1999. Centers for Disease Control and Prevention (CDC) Hospital Infection Control Practices Advisory Committee. *Am J Infect Control.* 1999; 27(2):97–132, *http://www.cdc.gov/ncidod/hip/SSI/SSI_guideline. htm.*

7. HICPAC. Guideline for isolation precautions in hospitals. *Am J Infect Control.* 1996; 24:24–52, *http://www.cdc.gov/ncidod/hip/isolat/isolat.htm.*

8. HICPAC. Recommendations for preventing the spread of vancomycin resistance: Recommendations of the Hospital Infection Control Practices Advisory Committee (HICPAC). *Am J Infect Control.* 1995; 23:87–94.

9. Centers for Disease Control and Prevention. Guideline for hand hygiene in health-care settings: Recommendations of the Healthcare Infection Control Practices Advisory Committee and the HICPAC/SHEA/APIC/IDSA Hand Hygiene Task Force. *MMWR.* 2002; 51 (No. RR-16):1–44, *http://www.cdc.gov/handhygiene/.*

10. Wong, E. S. Guideline for prevention of catheter-associated urinary tract infections. *Am J Infect Control.* 1983; 11:28–36, *http:// www.cdc.gov/ncidod/hip/guide/uritract.htm.*

11. Guidelines for preventing the transmission of *Mycobacterium tuberculosis* in health-care Facilities, 1994. *MMWR.* 1994; 43(RR-13):1–132, *http://www.cdc.gov/nchstp/tb/pubs/mmwr/rr4313.pdf.*

12. The Role of Regulatory, Accrediting, and Professional Agencies. In: Schaffer, S. D., Garzon, L. S., Heroux, D. L., and Korniewicz, D. M., eds., *Pocket Guide to Infection Prevention and Safe Practice.* St. Louis: Mosby-Year Book, Inc.; 1996:10–14.

13. Favero, M. S., and Sadovsky, R. Office, infection control, OSHA, and you. *Patient Care.* 1993; March 30:117–134.

14. Occupational exposure to bloodborne pathogens: Final rule. *Fed Register.* 1991; 56 (Dec. 6):64175–64182, *http://www.osha-slc.gov/pls/oshaweb/owadisp.show_document?p_table=STANDARDS&p_id=10051&p_text_version=FALSE.*

15. Occupational Exposure to Bloodborne Pathogens: Needlestick and Other Sharps Injuries: Final Rule. *Fed Register.* 2001; 66:5317–5325, *http://www.osha-slc.gov/pls/oshaweb/owadisp.show_document? p_table=FEDERAL_REGISTER&p_id=16265.*

16. Frank, G., and City, E. Nurses welcome standards provided by new needlestick law. *J Emerg Nurs.* 2001; 27:489–491.

17. Murphy, E. Needlestick Safety and Prevention Act. *AORN J.* 2001; 73:458, 461.

18. OSHA enforcement policy and procedures for occupational exposure to Tuberculosis. *Infect Control Hosp Epidemiol.* 1993; 14:694–699.

19. Talan, D. A. Infectious disease issues in the emergency department. *Clin Infect Dis.* 1996; 23:1–14.

20. Sokolove, P. R., Mackey, D., Wiles, J., and Lewis, R. J. Exposure of emergency department personnel to tuberculosis: PPD testing during an epidemic in the community. *Ann Emerg Med.* 1994; 24:418–421.

21. *2000–2001 Standards for Ambulatory Care.* Oakbrook Terrace, IL: Joint Commission on Accreditation of Healthcare Organizations; 2000:227–232.

22. Shared visions—new pathways. *Perspectives.* 2002; 22:1–15.

23. *Accreditation Manual for Office-Based Surgery Practices.* Oakbrook Terrace, IL: Joint Commission on Accreditation of Healthcare Organizations; 2001.

24. *Accreditation Handbook for Ambulatory Health Care.* Wilmette, IL: Accreditation Association for Ambulatory Health Care, Inc.; 2000.

25. Alvarado, C. J., Reichelderfer, M., and the 1997, 1998, 1999 APIC Guidelines Committees. APIC Guideline for infection prevention and control in flexible endoscopy. *Am J Infect Control.* 2000; 28:138–155.

26. Rutala, W. A. APIC guideline for selection and use of disinfectants. *Am J Infect Control.* 1996; 24:313–342.

27. Bartley, J. M., and the 1997, 1998, and 1999 APIC Guidelines Committees. The role of infection control during construction in health care facilities. *Am J Infect Control.* 2000; 28:156–169.

28. Duncan, S. L., and the 1997, 1998, and 1999 APIC Guidelines Committees. The implications of service animals in health care settings. *Am J Infect Control.* 2000; 28:170–180.

29. Belkin, N. L. Use of scrubs and related apparel in health care facilities. *Am J Infect Control.* 1997; 25:401–404.

30. DeCastro, M. G., Denys, G. A., Fauerbach, L. L., Ferranti, J. K., Hawkins, K., and Masters, L. C., et al. APIC position paper: Responsibility for interpretation of the PPD tuberculin skin test. *Am J Infect Control.* 1999; 27:56–58.

31. DeCastro, M. G., Denys, G. A., Fauerbach, L. L., Ferranti, J. K., Hawkins, K., and Masters, L. C., et al. APIC position paper: Hepatitis C exposure in the health care setting. *Am J Infect Control.* 1999; 27:54–55.

32. DeCastro, M. G., Denys, G. A., Fauerbach, L. L., Ferranti, J. K., Hawkins, K., Masters, L. C., Rimland, D., Sharbaugh, R. J., and Zeller, J. APIC position paper: Immunization. *Am J Infect Control.* 1999; 27:52–53.

33. Pirwitz, S., Bertin, M. L., Clark, C. C., DeCastro, M. G., Denys, G. A., and Fauerbach, L. L., et al. APIC position paper: Prevention of device-mediated bloodborne infections to health care workers. *Am J Infect Control.* 1998; 26:578–580.

34. APIC/CHICA—Canada Professional and Practice Standards Task Force. APIC/CHICA—Canada infection control and epidemiology: Professional and practice standards. *Am J Infect Control.* 1999; 27:47–51.

35. Lee, T. B., Baker, O. G., Lee, J. T., Scheckler, W. E., Steele, L., Laxton, C. E., and APIC Surveillance Initiative Working Group. Recommended practices for surveillance. *Am J Infect Control.* 1998; 26:277–288.

36. Tenover, F. C., Arbeit, R. D., and Goering, R. V. How to select and interpret molecular strain typing methods for epidemiological studies of bacterial infections: A review for healthcare epidemiologists. *Infect Control Hosp Epidemiol.* 1997; 18:426–439.

37. AIDS/TB Committee of the Society for Healthcare Epidemiology of America. Management of healthcare workers infected with hepatitis B virus, hepatitis C virus, human immunodeficiency virus, or other bloodborne pathogens. *Infect Control Hosp Epidemiol.* 1997; 18:349–363.

38. Rutala, W. A., and Mayhall, C. G. Medical waste. *Infect Control Hosp Epidemiol.* 1992; 13:38–48.

39. AORN: *2002 Standards, Recommended Practices, and Guidelines.* Denver: Association of Operating Room Nurses, Inc.; 2002.

40. American Institute of Architects. *The Guidelines for Design and Construction of Hospital and Health Care Facilities.* Washington, DC: American Institute of Architects Press; 2001.

CHAPTER 23

Bioterrorism

BACKGROUND

Ambulatory care staff, especially in physician offices and urgent/emergency care centers, may have the first opportunity to recognize and initiate a response to a bioterrorism-related event. Bioterrorism (BT) will likely present in a subtle manner. An incident may be recognized only after a number of victims displaying similar symptoms arrive at the site. Diagnosis may be difficult, and it may be hard to distinguish biological from chemical exposures or the possibility of both immediately after an event like an explosion.[1] Important components of a BT plan in ambulatory care settings are early recognition of unusual diseases/symptoms, prompt notification of infection prevention and control and of public health staff, and communication with internal staff regarding appropriate precautions.[2] Because of the changing nature of this topic, use the Centers for Disease Control and Prevention's (CDC) Web site as a reference, *http://www.bt.cdc.gov/*.

AGENTS

There are potentially many agents that could be used in a BT attack. A **biological agent** is any microorganism or toxin found in nature that can be used to incapacitate, kill, or otherwise impede an adversary.[3]

The CDC groups the agents of greatest threat into categories A, B, and C (see Table 23.1). These agents are categorized based on the following criteria: ease of dissemination/transmission from person to person,

mortality/morbidity probability, potential for public health impact, and potential for public panic and disruption. Category A agents are those that can be easily disseminated or transmitted from person to person, result in high mortality rates, and require special action for public health preparedness. Category B agents are moderately easy to disseminate and result in moderate morbidity rates and low mortality rates. Category C agents include emerging pathogens that could be engineered for mass dissemination in the future. The CDC does not prioritize these agents in any order of importance or likelihood of use.

ISSUES

Early Recognition

Rapid response to a BT-related event requires prompt identification of its onset. Because of the rapid progression to illness and potential for dissemination of some of these agents, it is important to have a high index of suspicion for BT-related disease. It will be necessary to initiate a response (e.g., specific treatment) based on the recognition of high-risk syndromes.

Epidemiologic principles must be used to assess whether a patient's presentation is typical of an endemic disease or is an unusual event that should raise concern. Features that should alert healthcare providers to the possibility of a BT-related outbreak include:[1]

- A rapidly increasing disease incidence (e.g., within hours or days) in a normally healthy population

Table 23.1   Biological Diseases/Agents List*

Category A

Anthrax (*Bacillus anthracis*)
Botulism (*Clostridium botulinum* toxin)
Plague (*Yersinia pestis*)
Smallpox (variola major)
Tularemia (*Francisella tularensis*)
Viral hemorrhagic fevers (filoviruses [e.g., Ebola, Marburg] and arenaviruses [e.g., Lassa, Machupo])

Category B

Brucellosis (*Brucella* species)
Epsilon toxin of *Clostridium perfringens*
Food safety threats (e.g., *Salmonella* species, *Escherichia coli* O157:H7, Shigella)
Glanders (*Burkholderia mallei*)
Melioidosis (*Burkholderia pseudomallei*)
Psittacosis (*Chlamydia psittaci*)
Q fever (*Coxiella burnetii*)
Ricin toxin from *Ricinus communis* (castor beans)
Staphylococcal enterotoxin B
Typhus fever (*Rickettsia prowazekii*)
Viral encephalitis (alphaviruses [e.g., Venezuelan equine encephalitis, eastern equine encephalitis, western equine encephalitis])
Water safety threats (e.g., *Vibrio cholerae, Cryptosporidium parvum*)

Category C

Emerging infectious disease threats such as Nipah virus and hantavirus

*From the Centers for Disease Control and Prevention's Web site, *http://www.bt.cdc.gov/Agent/agentlist.asp.*

- An epidemic curve that rises and falls during a short period of time
- An unusual clinical presentation
- An unusual increase in the number of people seeking care, especially with fever, respiratory, or gastrointestinal complaints
- An endemic disease rapidly emerging at an uncharacteristic time or in an unusual pattern
- Lower attack rates among people who had been indoors, especially in areas with filtered air or closed ventilation systems, compared with people who had been outdoors
- Clusters of patients arriving from a single locale
- Large numbers of rapidly fatal cases

- Any patient presenting with a disease that is relatively uncommon and has BT potential (e.g., pulmonary anthrax, tularemia, or plague)

Historically, physicians report the majority of communicable diseases upon receiving laboratory confirmation of their suspicion, typically days after the patient is seen. In a BT incident, time is critical. Therefore, the local health department should be notified immediately when any unusual syndromes or diseases are noted.

Patient Placement

It may be necessary to cohort patients who present with similar syndromes, that is, to group affected individuals into a designated section of a clinic or emergency department, or even to set up a response center at a separate building. Designated internal sites should be chosen in advance and should be based on patient arrival sites; patterns of airflow and ventilation; accessibility of resources such as wall oxygen/suction; availability of adequate plumbing and waste disposal; and capacity to safely hold potentially large numbers of patients. Any triage or cohort site should have controlled entry to minimize the possibility of transmission.

Hand Hygiene

Either plain or antimicrobial-containing soaps may be used according to a facility's policy. Alcohol-based hand rubs are acceptable except when hands are visibly soiled or if the microorganisms contaminating the hands are hardy pathogens such as the spores of *Bacillus anthracis*.[1] Hands must be washed after touching any potentially contaminated materials and after removing gloves.

Personal Protective Equipment

Barriers such as gloves, gowns, and face protection should be worn using the guidelines outlined under Standard Precautions. Gloves must be worn when touching any potentially contaminated material. See Chapter 4 for additional information.

Isolation Precautions

Many of the agents likely to be used in a BT attack are not transmitted from person to person and re-aerosolization of these agents is unlikely.[4] All patients, including symptomatic patients with suspected or confirmed BT-related illnesses, should be managed utilizing Standard Precautions (see Chapter 6). For certain diseases or syndromes (e.g., smallpox and pneumonic plague) additional precautions will be needed to reduce the likelihood for transmission (see Table 23.2).

Laboratory

Any specimen sent to a clinical laboratory must have the agent under suspicion noted on the requisition slip. Double-bag the specimen, cleaning the outer bag carefully. Specimen packaging and transport must be coordinated with local and state health departments and the Federal Bureau of Investigation. There may be additional requirements for labelling or transporting these specimens as directed by local or federal law enforcement agencies.[1]

Transporting Patients

Most infections associated with BT agents cannot be transmitted from person to person. However, in general the transport and movement of patients with BT-related infections should be limited to movement that is essential to provide patient care, thus reducing any opportunity for transmission of microorganisms. If the patient requires Airborne Precautions (see Table 23.2), minimize dispersal of droplets by placing a surgical-type or N95 mask on the patient when transporting a patient to the hospital.

Waste Handling

Contaminated waste should be sorted and discarded in accordance with federal, state, and local regulations. Special precautions may be required for smallpox or viral hemorrhagic fever. See the APIC (http://www. apic.org/bioterror/) or CDC Web sites for guidance.

Disinfection and Sterilization

Decontamination of patients usually is not needed for aerosol exposures to BT agents. In patients with an acute exposure to a biological aerosol, infection has not yet developed. If there is visible contamination, wash the skin with soap and water. This will prevent the potential for aerosolization of the contaminant.[1,3,6] If the patient's clothing is contaminated, it should be removed and placed in a plastic bag.

Effective disinfection of potentially contaminated surfaces can be accomplished with diluted (1:10) bleach.[1] Rooms and bedside equipment of patients with BT-related infections should be cleaned using the same procedures that are used for all patients as a component of Standard Precautions, unless the infecting microorganism and the amount of environmental contamination indicate special cleaning. In addition to adequate cleaning, thorough disinfection of bedside equipment and environmental surfaces may be indicated for certain microorganisms that can survive in the inanimate environment for extended periods of time.

With the exception of linens used on patients with actual or suspected smallpox and viral hemorrhagic fever, linens should be handled in accordance with Standard Precautions. Although linens may be contaminated, the risk of disease transmission is negligible if it is handled, transported, and laundered in a manner that avoids transfer of microorganisms to other patients, personnel, and environments.

Occupational Health

Emergency department staff likely will be a first contact for patients with BT diseases, such as smallpox. Therefore, certain staff will need immunizations.[7] There are also some prophylactic measures that may be taken with certain BT agents, such as anthrax. It is important to know where to obtain the most current recommendations; check the CDC Web site for specific guidance.

Education

Appropriate education and training of staff ensure they will have a good understanding of the clinical presentation of BT agents, treatment options, and preventive

Table 23.2 Biological Agent Disease Resource[5]

Disease	Agent	Transmit Person to Person	Suspect Syndrome	Incubation Period	Duration of Illness	Infection Control Actions
Inhalation anthrax	*Bacillus anthracis*	No	Flu-like symptoms, abrupt onset of respiratory failure, widened mediastinum	1–7 days	3–5 days (usually fatal if untreated)	Standard Precautions
Pneumonic plague	*Yersinia pestis*	High (spread through droplets)	Fever, cough, chest pain, hemoptysis, rapid progression to dyspnea	1–4 days	1–6 days (usually fatal if untreated)	Airborne Precautions—for duration of illness
Tularemia	*Francisella tularensis*	No	Typhoidal—fever, headache, nonproductive cough	1–14 days (average 3–5)	≥2 weeks (30–60% fatal in untreated)	Standard Precautions
Smallpox	Variola virus	High (spread through droplets)	Fever, myalgias, rash prominent on face and extremities	7–19 days (average 12)	3 weeks (20–40% fatal in unvaccinated)	Airborne Precautions—until all crusts are shed
Viral hemorrhagic fevers	Marburg, Ebola, Lassa viruses	Moderate (spread through body fluids)	Fever, headache, malaise, myalgia, bleeding	3–21 days	7–16 days (usually fatal)	Standard Precautions
Botulism	*Clostridium botulinum*	No	Symmetric cranial neuropathies, blurred vision, symmetric descending weakness, respiratory dysfunction	1–2 days	Recovery takes months (5–10% fatal)	Standard Precautions
Brucellosis	*Brucella* species	No	Intermittent or irregular fever, headache, weakness, profuse sweating, chills, arthralgia, weight loss, and generalized aching	5–60 days	Variable	Standard Precautions
Q fever	*Coxiella burnetii*	Rare	Acute febrile illness, chills, retrobulbar headache, weakness, malaise, severe sweating	2–3 weeks	Variable	Standard Precautions
Melioidosis	*Burkholderia pseudomallei*	Rare	Ranges from asymptomatic illness to fatal septicemia	As short as 2 days to months	Variable	Standard Precautions

measures to stop spread. A survey of family practice physicians found that only 18% had previous training in BT preparations.[8] Objectives that might be included in training include:[9]

- Identify epidemiological factors that help differentiate between a natural epidemic and a BT attack.
- Match clinical syndromes to the BT agents.
- Describe chemotherapy and chemoprophylaxis for likely BT agents.
- Describe the role of vaccines in the treatment of patients exposed to BT agents.
- Identify appropriate personal protective measures for staff treating victims of BT.

Academic emergency departments and the CDC are collaborating on a surveillance system known as EMERGEncy ID NET (*http://www.cdc.gov/ncidod/osr/survsyss.htm*).[3] This system is designed to detect emerging infectious diseases. Another system to detect clusters of illness uses ambulatory care encounter records.[10] These systems can be used to help track disease syndromes that might represent BT.

Emergency management plans for the facility must include information on BT. Plans should provide information outlining contact information, including emergency telephone numbers for public health departments and law enforcement agencies. Annual disaster-preparedness drills should incorporate a BT scenario to test and refine BT-readiness plans at each individual facility. These plans should be developed in partnership with local health departments. See Appendix K for a sample policy and examples of educational materials. The possibility that biological weapons may be used is no longer unthinkable. Healthcare facilities must be prepared to meet this challenge.

References

1. *Bioterrorism Working Group Interim Bioterrorism Readiness Plan Suggestions.* Washington, DC: Association for Professionals in Infection Control and Epidemiology; April 2002, *http://www.apic.org/bioterror/default.cfm#Readiness%20Planning.*

2. Wetter, D. C., Daniell, W. E., and Treser, C. D. Hospital preparedness for victims of chemical or biological terrorism. *Am J Public Health.* 2001; 91:710–716.

3. Richards, C. F., Burstein, J. L., Waeckerle, J. F., and Hutson, H. R. Emergency physicians and biological terrorism. *Ann Emerg Med.* 1999; 34:183–190.

4. Simon, J. D. Biological terrorism. *JAMA.* 1997; 278:428–430.

5. *Control of Communicable Diseases Manual.* 17th Ed. Chin, J., ed. Washington, DC: American Public Health Association; 2000.

6. Keim, M., and Kaufmann, A. F. Principles for emergency response to bioterrorism. *Ann Emerg Med.* 1999; 34:177–182.

7. Smallpox Vaccination. Emergency Nurses Association Position Statements, 2002, *http://www.ena.org/about/position/Smallpox.asp.*

8. Chen, F. M., Hickner, J., Fink, K. S., Galliher, J. M., and Burstin, H. On the front lines: Family physicians' preparedness for bioterrorism. *J Fam Practice.* 2002; 51:745–750.

9. Younggren, B. N., and Lawrence, L. Emergency department preparedness in the event of bioterrorism. *Crit Decisions Emerg Med.* 1999; 14:1–10.

10. Lazarus, R., Kleinman, K., Dashevsky, I., Adams, C., Kludt, P., and DeMaria, A., et al. Use of automated ambulatory-care encounter records for detection of acute illness clusters, including potential bioterrorism events. *Emerg Infect Dis.* 2002; 8:753–760.

CHAPTER 24

Organizing for Infection Prevention, Surveillance, and Control

BACKGROUND

Each ambulatory care setting is unique; therefore, its specific needs must be considered to determine the appropriate structure of its infection prevention, surveillance, and control (IPSC) activities. The program must be appropriate to an organization's demographics, geography, volume of patient encounters, patient population served, clinical focus, and number of employees. Staff and data systems must be available to meet the needs of IPSC activities.[1–2]

There may be various groups or individuals responsible for the IPSC function; however, there should be one designated person with overall responsibility.[2] Benefits of a program coordinated under a specific individual include standardized patient care practices and education, evaluation of regulatory requirements, and improved surveillance activities.[3] Resources, both personnel and non-personnel, should be proportional to the size, case mix, and estimated infection risk of the population served.[2]

ORGANIZATIONAL STRUCTURE

The IPSC program must be under the responsibility and authority of one designated person. Depending on the needs of the organization, the designated person can be an individual with special training in infection prevention and control (i.e., an infection control professional [ICP]) or a staff member liaison with other responsibilities who is assigned the IPSC function.

Infection Control Professional

An ICP with specialized training can help ensure a safe working environment for patients and staff. Generally, ICPs provide ongoing surveillance, investigation, and evaluation of all IPSC practices and design policies and procedures, as well as educational training and on-the-job compliance procedures to ensure high-quality practices.[4–5] The ICP also helps the facility recognize potential risk management issues and keeps up to date on regulatory changes. A focus on epidemiological investigations and control activities is particularly useful for large ambulatory care sites, dialysis centers, and surgicenters.

Specific activities of an ICP include surveillance (especially for bloodstream and surgical site infections), along with tracking and trending of information; quality improvement; patient and staff education; development, review, and implementation of policies and procedures; product research; and evaluation of employee exposures and follow-up.[6] ICPs use their expertise in product evaluation to assist the institution in cost reduction and value analysis, and to contribute to cost avoidance in rejecting unnecessary items. In addition, they can demonstrate the financial impact of infections, and can develop and implement outcome measurement programs.[7] The ICP is also an important partner in patient safety activities.[8]

The ICP may act as a consultant to a staff member liaison, providing oversight for IPSC activities, or be assigned direct responsibility for the program. ICP consultants may be obtained through a formal contract or relationship with another facility, such as a hospital or health department.[2] A consultant ICP should be required to hold quarterly meetings with liaisons. These meetings can serve as a forum for troubleshooting problems related to maintaining compliance with IPSC policies.[4]

Staff Member Liaison

A staff member liaison often performs IPSC activities in addition to other assigned responsibilities. There may be a liaison assigned to each site of an institution or one person for the entire organization. Liaisons can be managers, staff nurses, lab technicians, or medical assistants. Many other functions interface with IPSC activities, including quality improvement, patient safety, customer satisfaction, safety, risk management, and staff development.[9] The staff member liaison may also be assigned one or more of these responsibilities. An ICP from a hospital or other facility may be contacted for consultation, as noted earlier. Staff member liaisons primarily help administer policies and procedures and are most useful in medical and dental offices.

This individual may also be responsible for dissemination of information to co-workers, collection of surveillance data, conduction of surveys, and provision of information on new policies and procedures.[3,9] A staff member liaison can be assigned primary responsibility for instituting all IPSC policies and procedures, educating staff, and serving as an infection prevention and control advocate.[4,10] These individuals may need to obtain authority from management to institute recommended changes or may be granted such authority.

Infection Control Committee

Regardless of which individual is assigned IPSC responsibilities, the scope of the program must be multidisciplinary to be successful. IPSC is a shared responsibility of the designated individual in partnership with clinical and support teams.[9] This team relationship may be formalized into an infection control committee (ICC). An ICC usually is charged with establishing guidelines to ensure a safe working environment in compliance with professional recommendations and regulations.[4] The multidisciplinary nature of the committee and administrative support help it ac-

complish its objectives. The ICP or staff member liaison provides support to the committee and carries out its goals.

RESOURCES

Another essential staff resource for the IPSC program is clerical support. Many activities in the IPSC program are clerical in nature, including tracking infection data, coordinating ICC agenda and minutes, and reporting information to health departments. One study noted that at least 21% of an ICP's time is spent on clerical functions.[6] Adequate clerical support will allow the ICP or staff member liaison to be more effective.

Other resources necessary to fulfill the responsibilities of the IPSC program include:[2]

1. Access to services of a physician trained in healthcare epidemiology;
2. Access to services of a trained ICP (if not one on site);
3. Computer support with Internet capability;
4. A budget for investigations; and
5. A budget for reference materials and continuing professional education.

To ensure access to the ongoing services of a person who is trained in IPSC, an ambulatory care facility may look to hospital-based infection control departments as a resource. In one study on the use of hospital-based ICPs, the majority of calls (51%) were infection prevention and control questions from personnel at other healthcare institutions.[11] These individuals are valuable resources who can be tapped by ambulatory care organizations.

TRAINING AND COMPETENCIES

Anyone who performs the activities of IPSC must be appropriately trained and able to demonstrate related competencies. This individual requires knowledge of microorganisms and appropriate laboratory tests, healthcare epidemiology, infectious diseases, and education techniques.[7,12] Standards are published, which include key criteria that can be used to evaluate both the competency of practice and individual performance in IPSC programs.

Professional standards[13] outline the general requirements for ICPs:

1. Professional accountability: The ICP is responsible for the development, evaluation, and improvement of his or her own practice in relation to the practice standards for infection control.
2. Qualifications: The ICP meets certain minimum qualifications to enter the profession.
3. Professional development: The ICP acquires and maintains current knowledge and skills in the areas of infection prevention and control and epidemiology.
4. Leadership: The ICP serves as a leader, mentor, and role model for the profession.
5. Ethics: The ICP makes decisions and performs activities in an ethical manner.

Practice standards[13] outline the elements of the IPSC program itself:

1. Infection prevention and control practice: The ISPC program consists of effective prevention and control activities that are specific to the practice setting, the population served, and the continuum of care.
2. Epidemiology: The ISPC program applies epidemiologic principles and statistical methods, including risk stratification, to identify target populations, analyze trends and risk factors, and design and evaluate prevention and control strategies.
3. Surveillance: The ISPC program uses a systematic approach to surveillance to monitor the effectiveness of prevention and control strategies that are consistent with the organization's goals and objectives.
4. Education: The ISPC program serves as an educational resource for infection prevention and control and healthcare epidemiology.
5. Consultation: The ISPC program provides expert knowledge and guidance in epidemiology and infection prevention and control-related issues.
6. Performance improvement: The ISPC program is an integral component of the plan for improvement of practice and patient outcomes.
7. Program management and evaluation: The ISPC program systematically evaluates the quality and effectiveness of the ISPC plan appropriate to the practice setting.
8. Fiscal responsibility: The ISPC program incorporates the principles of fiscal responsibility.
9. Research: The ISPC program applies relevant research findings to infection prevention and control practice.

ICPs can demonstrate this knowledge by passing an examination developed the Certification Board of Infection Control and Epidemiology (*http://www.cbic. org/*). Certification represents a commitment to continual improvement of infection prevention and control functions and their contribution to health care and patient safety.

The IPSC program represents an indicator of quality and safety that is important for patients and staff. To be successful, IPSC activities must be coordinated by knowledgeable individuals and supported by managers and supervisors. Well-designed, effective IPSC programs can limit the incidence of health care-associated infections and prevent potential legal claims and financial losses.[7]

References

1. *2000–2001 Standards for Ambulatory Care*. Oakbrook Terrace, IL: Joint Commission on Accreditation of Healthcare Organizations; 2000: 227–232.
2. Friedman, C., Barnette, M., Buck, A. S., Ham, R., Harris, J., and Hoffman, P., et al. Requirements for infrastructure and essential activities of infection control and epidemiology in out-of-hospital settings: A Consensus Panel report. *Am J Infect Control*. 1999; 27:418–430.
3. Nightingale, C. Clinic infection control. *Am J Infect Control*. 1998; 26:201, Abstract.
4. Hurt, N. The role of the infection control nurse in quality management in the ambulatory care setting. *J Healthcare Quality*. 1993; 15:43–44.
5. Jarvis, W. R. Infection control and changing health-care delivery systems. *Emerg Infect Dis*. 2001; 7:170–173.
6. Haim, L. Recommendations for optimizing an infection control practitioner's effectiveness in an ambulatory care setting. *J Healthcare Quality*. 1994; 16:31–34.
7. Rhinehart, E. Watching the bottom line. *Am J Infect Control*. 2000; 28;25–29.

8. Gerberding, J. L. Hospital-onset infections: A patient safety issue. *Ann Intern Med.* 2002; 137:665–670.

9. Jennings, J., Thibeault, M., Olmsted, R., and Craig, C. Ambulatory. In: *APIC Text of Infection Control and Epidemiology.* Washington, DC: Association for Professionals in Infection Control and Epidemiology; 2000: 38:1–29.

10. Ambulatory Care Settings. In: Jennings, J., and Wideman, J., eds., *APIC Handbook of Infection Control and Epidemiology.* 3rd Ed. Washington, DC: Association for Professionals in Infection Control and Epidemiology; 2002: 352.

11. Lavin, M. A., Wittrock, B., Zawacki, A., Ballinger, W., and Wurtz, R. Infection control "curbsides" from the community. *Am J Infect Control.* 1998; 26:83–84.

12. Goldrick, B. A., Dingle, D. A., Gilmore, G. K., Curchoe, R. M., Plackner, C. L., and Fabrey, L. J. Practice analysis for infection control and epidemiology in the new millennium. *Am J Infect Control.* 2002; 30:437–448.

13. Horan-Murphy, E., Barnard, B., Chenoweth, C., Friedman, C., Hazuka, B., and Russell, B., et al. APIC/CHICA–Canada infection control and epidemiology: Professional and practice standards. *Am J Infect Control.* 1999; 27:47–51.

Special Communication— Consensus Panel Report

Reprinted from Friedman C, Barnette M, Buck AS, Ham R, Harris J, Hoffman P, et al. Requirements for infrastructure and essential activities of infection control and epidemiology in out-of-hospital settings: A Consensus Panel report. Am J Infect Control. 1999;27:418-430. Used with permission of the Association for Professionals in Infection Control and Epidemiology, Inc.

SPECIAL COMMUNICATION

Requirements for infrastructure and essential activities of infection control and epidemiology in out-of-hospital settings: A Consensus Panel report

Candace Friedman, MPH, CIC
Marcie Barnette, MSN, RN
Alfred S. Buck, MD
Rosemary Ham, RN, MSN, CIC
Jo-Ann Harris, MD
Peggy Hoffman, RN
Debra Johnson, RN, CIC
Farrin Manian, MD
Lindsay Nicolle, MD
Michele L. Pearson, MD
Trish M. Perl, MD, MSc
Steven L. Solomon, MD

In 1997 the Association for Professionals in Infection Control and Epidemiology and the Society for Healthcare Epidemiology of America established a consensus panel to develop recommendations for optimal infrastructure and essential activities of infection control and epidemiology programs in out-of-hospital settings. The following report represents the Consensus Panel's best assessment of requirements for a healthy and effective out-of-hospital–based infection control and epidemiology program. The recommendations fall into 5 categories: managing critical data and information; developing and recommending policies and procedures; intervening directly to prevent infections; educating and training of health care workers, patients, and nonmedical caregivers; and resources. The Consensus Panel used an evidence-based approach and categorized recommendations according to modifications of the scheme developed by the Clinical Affairs Committee of the Infectious Diseases Society of America and the Centers for Disease Control and Prevention's Healthcare Infection Control Practices Advisory Committee.

INTRODUCTORY COMMENTARY

Central to the mission of health profession societies is a focus on the patient and a marshaling of the most current credible scientific evidence to provide the best and safest outcomes to preserve and restore the health of the patient. Quality health care requires teamwork and the ability to put into practice the processes necessary to ensure that quality. The following Consensus Panel report is the second in the series initiated by SHEA and APIC to establish recommendations designed to protect patients and health care workers from infections. The focus on the first report published in February 1998 was the acute care hospital. This report extends the scope of interest to extended care, selected ambulatory care, and home care settings. Both Consensus Panel reports have been collaborative and

From the Association for Professionals in Infection Control and Epidemiology (APIC) and the Society for Healthcare Epidemiology of America (SHEA) Consensus Panel. Candace Friedman, MPH, CIC, Panel Chair (APIC); Marcie Barnette, MSN, RN, National Association for Home Care (NAHC); Alfred S. Buck, MD, Joint Commission on Accreditation of Healthcare Organizations (JCAHO); Rosemary Ham, RN, MSN, CIC (APIC); Jo-Ann Harris, MD, Pediatric Infectious Diseases Society (PIDS); Peggy Hoffman, RN (NAHC); Debra Johnson, RN, CIC (APIC); Farrin Manian, MD (SHEA); Lindsay Nicolle, MD (SHEA); Michele L. Pearson, MD (SHEA); Trish M. Perl, MD, MSc (SHEA); Steven L. Solomon, MD, Centers for Disease Control and Prevention (CDC).

This report and the recommendations in it were formally

approved by the APIC and SHEA boards in 1999 and endorsed by the organizations represented by panel members: JCAHO, CDC, PIDS, and NAHC.

Reprint requests: APIC, 1275 K St NW, Washington, DC 20005-4006.

AJIC
Volume 27, Number 5

multidisciplinary. Professional societies, government agencies, and regulatory groups worked together to craft the most scientifically valid recommendations.

The first Consensus Panel concentrated on the acute care hospital because of the wealth of scientific information about control of nosocomial infections that developed in hospitals during the last 30 years. In the work of the current panel, the general framework and categories of recommendations from the first group turned out to be applicable in many ways to the out-of-hospital health care settings chosen. Of considerable interest is that almost all of the references used by the current Consensus Panel are from articles published and studies done in the 1990s. This fact alone helps confirm the validity of the 23 recommendations. However, this panel has clarified the many ways the patient populations differ in these out-of-hospital settings. Just as the care of the patient is now collaborative, so is the evolving structure of providing that care.

The focus of these recommendations is the "health care organization." This recognizes the continuing evolution of health care systems in the United States. The independent hospital and solo physician practices have been replaced by management, contractual, insurance, and other arrangements that have linked hospital, extended care facilities, ambulatory centers, and home health agencies together. The recommendations in this report and the recommendations in the one that preceded it give health care administrators, policy makers, and regulators a firm scientific basis for protecting patients and health care workers from a substantial number of infections.

The core of expertise in infection control is likely to reside within the acute care hospital infection control program. Health care organizations should draw on this expertise. It is the duty and responsibility of health care organizations to implement these recommendations.

William E. Scheckler, MD
SHEA, University of Wisconsin Medical School

During the past decade, health care delivery has undergone enormous changes; the nationwide growth in managed care organizations and the changing methods of provider reimbursement are restructuring the entire health care system. Diversification and integration strategies have blurred historical separations between the activities of hospitals, nursing homes, physicians, and other providers.[1] Services are being offered in, and in many cases, shifting to, less-costly settings, such as ambulatory clinics, work sites, and homes.

Factors that have contributed to the increasing trend of delivery of health care outside hospitals include the following: (1) economic forces resulting in earlier discharge of patients from hospitals, (2) advances in medical technology, and (3) the patient's desire to receive care outside the hospital. In addition, patients may be managed in their homes or in ambulatory care settings from the onset of illness rather than initiating care in the hospital. Such patient care settings (ie, home, ambulatory, and extended care) have increased markedly in recent years as has the complexity of care provided in these settings.

Infection prevention and control issues are important throughout this continuum of care. Infections in patients may lead to serious morbidity and mortality, readmission or admission to a hospital, increased use of antibiotics, and increased costs of care. Performing surgical procedures and invasive device insertions and managing and providing care for patients who are increasingly immunocompromised in these settings presents new infection control challenges.[2] Therefore, infection control practices must now encompass infections that patients may acquire as a result of their care or treatment

outside the acute care hospital as well as protect health care providers and caregivers in these settings.

Whereas there is an established body of information relating to the practice of infection control and epidemiology in inpatient settings,[3,4] there is no published consensus on how infection control programs should be structured and managed in settings outside the acute care hospital. The manner in which functional components of any health care organization (HCO)—including infection control—are administered and managed depends on various factors, including the size of the HCO, the types of patients for whom care is provided, the types of clinical activities performed, and whether the HCO is independently operated, is affiliated with a hospital, or is part of a larger network or health system. Therefore, infection control and epidemiology activities may be identified under various organizational labels or titles in out-of-hospital settings.

Concomitant with changes in the health care delivery system in the United States, changes have occurred in public health priorities that have an impact on infection control programs. The public health infrastructure has been the underlying foundation that supported the planning, delivery, and evaluation of public health activities and practices.[5] Among these activities has been cooperation with infection control programs in surveillance and support and assistance to infection control as needed. However, funding for public health has decreased in recent years, in some cases, with a change in activities by local and state agencies lessening their involvement in infection control. There are efforts to rebuild the US public health infrastructure to address infectious disease issues and provide tools and resources to facilitate interactions between HCOs and health departments.[5]

420 *Friedman et al*

AJIC
October 1999

Box 1. Settings referred to in this document

Health care settings addressed in document

Extended care
> Long-term care facility
> Rehabilitation facility
> Skilled nursing facility
> Hospice

Ambulatory care
> Outpatient surgery
> Dialysis center
> Infusion center

Home care
> Intravascular-related care
> Other device-related care

Health care settings *not* addressed in document*

Behavioral health
Out-of-home child care
Individual physician or practitioner office
Clinics
Respite care
Home hospice

---

*Except when discussed in the context of the settings addressed in the document

---

In 1998 a document entitled "Requirements for Infrastructure and Essential Activities of Infection Control and Epidemiology in Hospitals: A Consensus Panel Report"[6] was published. It outlined recommendations for infection control programs in the hospital. The purpose of the current document is to establish recommendations for the infrastructure and essential activities of infection control in relevant settings outside the hospital. The settings addressed and not addressed by this document are outlined in Box 1.

The health care settings not specifically addressed in this document must still implement appropriate infection control practices even though they may not have a formal infection control infrastructure. Health care providers in these settings should follow basic infection control practices and be prepared to identify and investigate problems. They also have a responsibility for ensuring communication with other health care settings on infectious disease issues. In time, they too may find it beneficial to affiliate with a more formal infection control program to provide services comprehensively across the continuum of care.

EXTENDED CARE SETTINGS

Currently, more than 1.5 million persons reside in nursing homes in the United States. This number is less than 10% of the US population that is currently older than 65 years; however, demographic trends suggest that at least 43% of the US population who turned 65 in

1990 will spend some time in an extended care facility.[7] There are many different types of extended care facilities, which vary considerably in the type of services they provide and the population they serve. These types include the following:

- Adult day care units
- Residential care facilities
- Rehabilitation facilities
- Long-term care facilities
- Nursing homes
- Chronic disease hospitals
- Veterans' Affairs nursing home care units

There are also residential facilities for persons who require both medical care and related psychosocial services. Young persons as well as elderly persons may reside in these facilities. However, the largest numbers of institutionalized persons reside in nursing homes, and more than 90% of these persons are elderly. Most information relating to infections in extended care facilities comes from nursing homes.[8]

The high frequency of infections in nursing home populations is well documented.[8] The 3 most common infection sites are respiratory tract, urinary tract, and skin and soft tissue. The reported overall incidence of infection has varied from 2.6 to 9.5 per 1000 resident-days, with respiratory infections accounting for 0.7 to 4.4 infections per 1000 resident-days, urinary tract infections, 0.1 to 2.4, and skin and soft tissue infections, 0.1 to 2.1. The differences in the reported rates of infection reflect a lack of uniform definitions used to identify infections, the use of different surveillance (case-finding) strategies, as well as differences in the types of populations studied, leading to wide variations in calculated risks of infection. In addition to high rates of endemic infections, outbreaks occur frequently.[8-12]

Many factors contribute to the frequency of infections in extended care facilities.[8] Recent changes in long-term institutional care, with increasing use and management of invasive devices, such as endotracheal or tracheostomy tubes, central intravascular lines, and percutaneous feeding tubes, have increased the likelihood of infection. For example, the prevalence of chronic indwelling urinary catheters in extended care facilities is universally associated with bacteruria.[13]

The extended care population presents unique problems in addressing issues related to infections. There is often uncertainty in making a specific clinical diagnosis of infection, as well as determining whether an infection is present in a patient or, if an infection is present, whether it is symptomatic.[14,15] Usual clinical diagnostic features are imprecise because of the complexity and chronicity of symptoms associated with comorbid illness. Bacteriologic diagnosis is problematic because of the very high prevalence of colonization of the upper respiratory tract and of

AJIC
Volume 27, Number 5

skin lesions with potentially pathogenic microorganisms.[8] The high frequency of infections, together with this diagnostic uncertainty, results in high intensity of antimicrobial use, much of which is empiric or provided for symptoms that may not be related to infection.[15]

There are substantial differences between acute and extended care institutions in patient characteristics, the type of care provided, the specific needs for increased social and personal contact, and staff resources. Recommendations for development of infection control programs in extended care have applied infection control practices to the extended care setting.[16] Nevertheless, there are no reported studies that evaluate the overall effectiveness of an infection control program in extended care facilities. However, there is ample evidence that implementation of infection control measures may control and limit the frequency and extent of outbreak situations.[17-21]

AMBULATORY CARE SETTINGS

The growth in managed care, with its attendant pressure to reduce the duration of or eliminate the inpatient stay, has resulted in a shift of many services previously delivered only in hospitals to that of ambulatory care settings. However, the delivery of health care in the outpatient setting is very different from that in the acute care facility. The patient mix and interactions are more varied; patients' clinical status may be well to acutely ill, requiring visits that may be brief or may last the entire day. Traditionally, infection control professionals have considered the risk for infection in the outpatient setting to be low. However, as more invasive procedures are performed in the ambulatory care setting, patients and health care workers alike are at risk for developing or transmitting infection. Goodman and Solomon[22] reviewed published articles and identified 53 reports of transmission of infection that occurred in the outpatient setting between 1961 and 1990. Their analysis revealed that most of the outbreaks were associated with nonadherence to infection control procedures.

Three areas of ambulatory care are especially important from an infection prevention and control perspective. These include the following:
- Ambulatory surgery setting: a setting in which surgical services are provided to patients not requiring hospitalization
- Ambulatory infusion setting: an out-of-home setting in which parenteral therapy is administered to patients who do not require hospitalization, including freestanding, physician office-based, or hospital-based centers
- Dialysis center setting: an out-of-hospital, out-of-home setting dedicated to the provision of dialysis services to patients with renal failure

Ambulatory care surgery settings

An increasing number of surgical procedures are performed in ambulatory care settings,[23] with a projected 75% of all surgical procedures in the United States being performed in such settings by the year 2000.[24] Moreover, an increasing number of "not-so-minor" surgical procedures are now performed in ambulatory care settings,[25,26] and patients with increasing levels of surgical risk are becoming candidates for outpatient surgery. Along with the provision of more complex ambulatory surgery procedures has come an increase in risk of developing procedure-related infections. For these reasons, it is essential to develop and implement an effective infection control program for ambulatory surgery.

Infusion center settings

It is estimated that 250,000 patients receive community-based parenteral therapies annually in the United States, with a projected growth rate of more than 10% per year.[27] Furthermore, it is estimated that 32% of antibiotic courses are currently administered at infusion centers.[28] Many other therapeutic products, such as chemotherapeutic agents, parenteral nutrition, blood components, and immunoglobulins, also are often administered in this setting.[29] A variety of locations are often used for administration of parenteral therapies, including physicians' offices, freestanding ambulatory infusion centers, and ambulatory care clinics.[30-32] As a result of the increasing frequency of parenteral therapies administered in infusion centers and the attendant risk of potentially serious bloodstream infections associated with such therapies, effective infection control programs must be developed and implemented in these centers.

Dialysis center settings

More than 180,000 patients undergo maintenance dialysis annually in the United States, with 85% receiving hemodialysis.[33] Most patients receive dialysis in centers that are affiliated with hospitals or are freestanding. Dialysis procedures and equipment are continually evolving, requiring ongoing education and training of personnel regarding proper infection control techniques. Bloodstream infections and pyrogenic reactions are not uncommon in dialysis centers.[33-38] Furthermore, numerous outbreaks of bloodstream infections and infections associated with arteriovenous fistulas, the peritoneal cavity, and exit sites of permanently placed long-term catheters have been associated with patient care in dialysis centers. These outbreaks are frequently a result of deficiencies in basic infection control practices.[33-37] Transmission of bloodborne pathogens (eg, hepatitis B virus, HIV, and hepatitis C virus) from

422 *Friedman et al*

AJIC
October 1999

patient-to-patient and patient-to-health care worker remain of particular concern in this setting.[39-42]

HOME CARE SETTINGS

The National Association for Home Care identified a total of more than 20,000 home care organizations in the United States as of 1996. This total represents an increase of approximately 89% over the past 10 years.[43]

Home care organizations are broadly defined as operational units that provide one or more home care programs to persons in their place of residence. Home care programs can include the following:

- Professional multidisciplinary services provided on an intermittent basis
- Private duty services provided on a hourly or shift basis
- Personal care and support services provided on part-time, intermittent, hourly, or shift basis
- Home infusion therapy that provides both pharmaceutical products and skilled nursing services
- Hospice care, which is an organized program of interdisciplinary services for terminally ill patients and their families to provide palliative medical care and supportive social, emotional, and spiritual services in the place of residence[44]

Durable medical equipment and supply companies, whereas not defined as home care organizations, are certainly ancillary to home care services and provide home care patients with products ranging from ventilators, wheelchairs, and walkers to catheters and wound care supplies.[45] Appropriate adherence to good infection control practice applies to these providers as well.

Home care organizations are caring for more acutely ill patients who often have a number of underlying medical conditions such as chronic obstructive pulmonary disease, cancer, AIDS, diabetes, renal failure, and decubitus ulcers. When combined with the use of invasive devices associated with home health treatment (feeding tubes, tracheostomies, vascular access devices, urinary catheters), these conditions significantly increase the patient's risk of infectious complications.[46,47]

There are limited data outlining the epidemiology of infections in home care. However, several outbreaks of bloodstream infections have been documented among persons receiving home infusion therapy.[48-50] Risk factors for bloodstream infection among patients receiving home infusion therapy include external central venous catheters,[48] multilumen central venous catheters,[51] and use of needleless infusion systems.[48-50,52]

Infection control implications are important not only for home care patients, but also for home care workers and informal caregivers. Patients with known or silent contagious diseases or conditions pose potential risks to home health professionals and other caregivers.

Because of these trends in home care, the patient, patient care providers, and home health workers are at risk for developing or transmitting infection.[50,53,54] Consequently, there is the need for prevention and control of home-acquired infections.[55,56] Surveillance and reporting are included in these activities because patients may develop infections after discharge from acute care or ambulatory care settings.

GOALS FOR INFECTION CONTROL AND EPIDEMIOLOGY

There are 3 principal goals for health care infection control and prevention programs, regardless of the setting:

- Protect the patient
- Protect the health care worker, visitors, and others in the health care environment
- Accomplish the previous 2 goals in a timely, efficient, and cost-effective manner, whenever possible

These goals are outlined completely in the first Consensus Panel report.[6] Achieving these goals is the driving force behind every recommendation and action of the infection control program. These goals are relevant to patient-care activities in any setting in which health care is provided, including skilled nursing facilities, acute care nursing homes, rehabilitation units, urgent care centers, same-day surgery facilities, ambulatory care centers, behavioral health facilities, and home care programs. However, this panel has chosen to focus on 3 major settings: extended care, ambulatory care, and home care. These areas were selected because we believe there is sufficient published information and expert experience to justify and support recommendations for these settings. However, we believe that the recommendations made are also appropriate, perhaps with minor modifications, for all other out-of-hospital settings. The goals, recommendations, and expected outcomes that follow represent a single standard of care for all health care settings outside of the hospital.

FUNCTIONS OF INFECTION CONTROL AND EPIDEMIOLOGY

The principal functions are:

1. To obtain and manage critical data and information, including surveillance for infections
2. To develop and recommend policies and procedures
3. To intervene directly to prevent infections
4. To educate and train health care workers, patients, and nonmedical caregivers

MANAGING CRITICAL DATA AND INFORMATION

The activities that comprise this function include developing and implementing surveillance plans, monitoring these plans, and internal and external reporting of infection information and data.

AJIC
Volume 27, Number 5

Surveillance systems for infections

The most important data management activity for all infection control programs is surveillance for infections and other adverse events in patients and staff. The type and method of surveillance must be tailored to the setting. It should be based on the types of infections most common to the care or services provided and the population served.[57-60] Persons performing infection surveillance must have access to all data and information vital to performing this activity; which will include access to computerized databases that are required for accurate and complete identification of infectious complications of health care.

Developing and implementing a surveillance plan

Documentation of the frequency, type, and associations of infections is an important component of the infection control program. Surveillance needs to be simple and pragmatic. The definitions used for surveillance of infection must be relevant to settings outside the acute care hospital.[15,47,61,62] These definitions should take into account the type of information routinely available in each setting.

Internal and external reporting of information and data

There are no nationally recognized benchmark data for infection rates outside the acute care hospital; therefore, each HCO should monitor its own data for trends. Attempts to compare infection rates among HCOs require careful evaluation of variations in patient characteristics in different facilities, access to and use of diagnostic tests, and the resources available in each setting to ensure the completeness and accuracy of surveillance. Efforts to develop external comparisons (eg, ORYX[63]) should be focused on infections that may be most readily identifiable and preventable and must take into account issues such as confidentiality, uniform definitions and data elements, infrastructures of data management, and data quality. Early priorities might include infections in persons with invasive devices, such as bloodstream infections in patients receiving infusion therapy, or diseases amenable to simple, effective interventions, such as vaccine-preventable diseases. Given their expertise, infection control professionals should be included in developing definitions for any national database.

It is important to develop procedures that facilitate communication of epidemiologically important information on infections regarding both patient and staff infections between and among HCOs.[46] This information needs to be shared effectively across all settings in the continuum of care to ensure feedback for completeness of surveillance in each setting and to permit appropriate infection control practices to be implemented as patient care requires. Fig 1 outlines a model for comprehensive surveillance of health care–associated infections illustrating the significance of sharing infection prevention and control information among all HCOs, settings, and public health departments to provide complete and useful surveillance data and other information. It is important to develop procedures to facilitate exchange of this information.

Complementary systems should be developed and maintained such that hospitals can report back to facilities and providers of extended care, home health care, or ambulatory care when their patients are hospitalized with an infection.[64] Similarly, persons in nonhospital settings must be able to notify hospital-based infection control professionals when extended care, home health care, or ambulatory care patients are found to have infections that were acquired in the hospital. In addition, infection control staff in out-of-hospital settings must be able to share such information among themselves. Local public health officials may be able to assist in this area (Fig 1).

Public health personnel are important collaborators in infection control. Public health agencies and infection control departments should be a focal point for prevention and control of infection by monitoring spread of microorganisms within the community, responding to infectious disease outbreaks, and coordinating communication and intervention across the continuum of care.

DEVELOPING AND RECOMMENDING POLICIES AND PROCEDURES

The activities that comprise this function include ensuring appropriateness and feasibility of policies, ensuring compliance with regulations, guidelines, and accreditation requirements, and employee health activities. To the greatest degree possible, HCOs should strive to ensure that policies and procedures are evidence-based and consistent with scientific knowledge and expert consensus.

Ensure appropriateness and feasibility

Written policies and procedures should address all elements of care. These elements will include environmental issues such as food handling, laundry handling, and cleaning, visitation policies, and direct patient care practices, including handwashing and immunization. The policies and procedures must be relevant to the setting, continually updated to remain current, and accessible to all staff.

424 *Friedman et al*

AJIC
October 1999

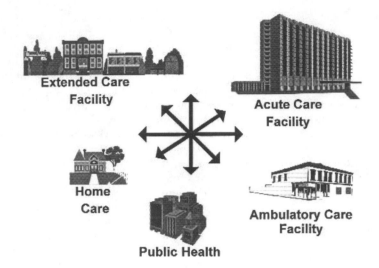

Fig 1. Outline of the significance of sharing infection prevention and control information among all HCOs and settings to provide complete and useful surveillance data and other information. Adapted from Jarvis W and Waller L, Centers for Disease Control and Prevention, 1998.

Sophisticated medical therapies are now increasingly performed outside the hospital and include intravascular infusion, dialysis, and mechanical ventilation.[65] Policies and procedures related to infection control practice in out-of-hospital settings might be patterned after current hospital standards and guidelines (eg, those issued by the Centers for Disease Control and Prevention's Healthcare Infection Control Practices Advisory Committee [HICPAC], APIC, and SHEA[66]). When establishing infection control policies and procedures, it is crucial that the means of implementing them be clearly outlined and consistent with evidence-based infection control and epidemiologic principles. The policies and procedures should describe what infection control measures are necessary to prevent transmission of infection.

Compliance with regulations, guidelines, and accreditation requirements

Regulations relevant to infection control in out-of-hospital settings occur at both the federal and state level. All HCOs are subject to regulation and oversight by various agencies, authorities, and government bodies. Some regulations may be specific to extended care, home health, or ambulatory care, whereas others are generally relevant to all health care facilities. Some nonlegislative standards may constitute required practices under certain conditions. For example, JCAHO standards may be incorporated into state licensing regulations as well as Medicare and Medicaid regulations.[67]

Employee health

Persons who work in health care settings are exposed more frequently to infectious diseases. They also may pose a risk to patients and other health care workers if they develop a communicable disease. Thus HCOs have the dual responsibility of preventing transmission of infections from patients to health care workers and limiting introduction of infections by staff members to interrupt spread both to patients and other staff. These objectives are achieved through an effective employee health program and policies.

The employee or occupational health program is a crucial component of the infection control program within an HCO. It is charged with developing and implementing systems for diagnosis, treatment, and prevention of infectious diseases in health care workers. It plays an important role in infection control within the HCO. The infection control program and the employee or occupational health program should have collaborative policies and procedures for health care personnel. These collaborative activities include placement evaluations, health and safety education, immunization programs, evaluation of potentially harmful infectious exposures and implementation of appropriate prevention measures, coordination of plans for managing outbreaks among personnel, provision of care to personnel for work-related illnesses or exposures, and maintenance of health records for all health care personnel.[68]

AJIC
Volume 27, Number 5

INTERVENING DIRECTLY TO PREVENT INFECTIONS

The activities that comprise this function include interruption of the transmission of infectious diseases, outbreak investigation and control, and performance improvement activities.

Endemic/epidemic disease

Epidemic disease may occur in any setting and can be associated with substantial morbidity and mortality.[8,16] Early intervention to prevent outbreaks or limit the spread of infections once an outbreak has been identified will interrupt transmission of disease, decreasing the impact on patients' health, patient care, and cost.[16-21]

The expertise and resources for infection control in a given HCO may be insufficient in an outbreak. Expertise related to outbreak management and infectious diseases may be obtained from state and local public health agencies, through linkages with other facilities, including acute care hospitals, or through a formal consultation arrangement with experts in infection control and health care epidemiology. The outbreak management team must have the authority to institute changes in practice or take other actions that are required to control the outbreak. As outbreaks may be anticipated to occur, plans to respond appropriately to such events should be developed before their occurrence.

Although the occurrence of outbreaks of infections often evokes considerable notice because they are easily identified and carry a connotation of danger, the morbidity and mortality that occurs as a result of endemic infections is greater than that associated with outbreaks.[69] Endemic cases represent the recurring health care–associated problems related to infectious disease in a particular setting. These endemic problems represent the baseline rate of infection among the population receiving care in that setting. The goal of infection control is to work consistently to decrease this baseline incidence; the management of these endemic infections encompasses techniques of epidemiology and quality improvement. Improvement in the endemic rate of infection within the HCO requires a review of processes that might lead to the development of the infection.[70]

Interrupting the transmission of infectious diseases

In-depth investigations must be conducted to obtain information once a problem or trend is identified.[34,35] Health care–associated infections may spread from person-to-person (eg, infections transferred from a staff member to a patient or from a patient to a staff member). Infections or microorganisms may also be spread from environmental sources (eg, from equipment or devices) to patients.

EDUCATING AND TRAINING HEALTH CARE WORKERS, PATIENTS, AND NONMEDICAL CAREGIVERS

The increasing complexity of care provided to patients and the increasing severity of illness of patients in out-of-hospital settings necessitates increasing awareness of appropriate measures of infection prevention and control. Staff, patients, and caregivers must receive ongoing training regarding proper infection control procedures.[55,56,71] In addition, it is essential that health care workers receive at least a rudimentary knowledge of the epidemiology of health care–associated infections specific to the setting in which they are employed. This knowledge will allow them to be better able to understand and comply with the practices and procedures necessary for the prevention and control of infections. The educational program should include education regarding surveillance, its uses, and the extent and nature of existing and potential problems related to infection in their organization.

RESOURCES

The resources for infection control and epidemiology should be proportional to the size, case mix, and estimated infectious risks of the populations served by the HCO. HCOs must comply with basic accreditation standards, federal regulations, and state and local licensing standards. Infection control functions are a critical component of quality health care, and adequate personnel and nonpersonnel resources are needed to ensure a quality program.

The infection control program must clearly be the responsibility of at least one designated person. In some HCOs, this person may also have other responsibilities (ie, infection control activities will be part time). In this situation, the expected number of hours per week that are devoted to infection control should be clearly stated.

Specific knowledge and training relevant to infection control and epidemiology makes this person more effective in overseeing an infection control program. Thus persons with this responsibility who are not specifically trained in infection control should have the opportunity to take courses and avail themselves of other educational opportunities that will increase their capacities in the field of infection control.

Some organizations will not be of a size or complexity sufficient to justify the resource commitment of full-time, on-site expertise in epidemiology and infectious diseases. If the person charged with the responsibility for infection control in the HCO is not specially trained or experienced in infection control, the HCO must ensure that oversight of the infection

AJIC
October 1999

Box 2. Recommendation categories

I. Strongly recommended
   Strongly recommended for implementation based on:
   • Evidence from at least one properly randomized, controlled trial, or
   • Evidence from at least one well-designed clinical trial without randomization, or
   • Evidence from cohort or case-control analytical studies (preferably from more than one center), or
   • Evidence from multiple time-series studies
II. Recommended
   Recommended for implementation based on:
   • Published clinical experience or descriptive studies, or
   • Reports of expert committees, or
   • Opinions of respected authorities
III. Recommended when required by governmental rules or regulations

---

control program is provided by an experienced person or group with such expertise. This augmentation, available on a contract basis or through a relationship with other facilities in an organization or outside the HCO (eg, a health department, private consultant, or other institution, as needed) ensures that the HCO has personnel trained in and familiar with basic infection control skills. Given the increasing emphasis on cost containment and the need to justify expenditures, a trained and experienced infection control professional can be especially helpful in evaluating the cost of the program and balancing these expenses against the benefits and requirements of the infection control program.[65]

One person should be charged with the infection control process and keep up-to-date on regulatory changes. Both the on-site staff responsible for infection control and any experts or consultants who participate in the program must be vested with the authority to carry out the components of the program and be supported throughout the organization by appropriate managerial and supervisory personnel. Within the management of the HCO, it is important to have a person(s) who facilitates and supports the infection control program.[72-74]

Persons who oversee infection control programs must have access to resources adequate to allow them to fulfill their responsibilities. In general, these resources include the following:
   • Personnel resources: infection control professionals, consultative services of a health care epidemiologist, and clerical support
   • Nonpersonnel support: access to office support, space, supplies, and equipment; computer support/Internet capability; microbiology laboratory support; reference laboratory testing; data manage-

ment and statistical support; clinical publications; budget to support outbreak or exposure investigations; and education

The Consensus Panel recommendations are as follows:

REQUIREMENTS FOR INFRASTRUCTURE AND ESSENTIAL ACTIVITIES OF INFECTION CONTROL AND EPIDEMIOLOGY IN OUT-OF-HOSPITAL SETTINGS

Whereas recommendations in this document are based on evidence for effectiveness whenever possible, limitations in information relevant to out-of-hospital settings means consensus of persons with expertise in these settings and infection control frequently must be accepted. Recommendations therefore are categorized in Box 2 by using a modification of the scheme developed by the Clinical Affairs Committee of the Infectious Diseases Society of America and the CDC HICPAC classification scheme.[75,76]

FUNCTIONS

Managing critical data and information, including surveillance for infections

Recommendation 1: Infection control personnel should develop policies and procedures for ongoing communication with other health care organizations (HCOs) to identify, prevent, manage, and control infections as patients move between HCOs throughout the continuum of care. *Category II.*
   • Report infectious complications and adverse events associated with medical and surgical procedures (eg, surgical site infections) to the HCO in which the procedure was performed or from which the patient was discharged
   • Report epidemiologically important infections to the HCO to which the patient will be transferred

Recommendation 2: Surveillance of health care–associated infections must be performed. *Category I*

Incorporate the following elements in the surveillance process:
   • Identification and description of the problem or event to be studied
   • Standard case definitions appropriate for the setting
   • Definition of the population at risk
   • Selection of the appropriate methods of measurement, including statistical tools and risk stratification
   • Identification and description of data sources and data collection
   • Definition of numerators and denominators
   • Preparation and distribution of reports to appropriate groups

AJIC
Volume 27, Number 5

Recommendation 3: Surveillance data must be appropriately analyzed and used to monitor and improve infection control and health care outcomes. *Category I*

Recommendation 4: Clinical performance and assessment indicators used to support external comparative measurements should meet the criteria previously delineated by APIC and SHEA for hospitalized patients.[77] *Category II*

Specifically, these indicators and their analyses must address:

- How process is related to outcome
- How to measure variation and quality
- That the numerators and denominators are defined
- That data collection is feasible, and the collected data are collected completely and reliably
- That the data are appropriately risk-adjusted when analyzed
- That data be adjusted for the populations' severity of illness and case-mix differences when analyzed before external comparison
- That personnel be trained regarding proper study and use of indicators
- That benchmarks be developed and used to compare the indicator's performance

Developing and recommending policies and procedures

Recommendation 5: Written infection prevention and control policies and procedures must be established, implemented, maintained, and updated periodically. *Both Categories II and III*

- The policies and procedures should be scientifically sound.
- The policies and procedures should lead to improved prevention of infections and other adverse events or improved patient and employee outcomes.
- The policies and procedures should be reviewed regularly to assess their practicality and cost-effectiveness.
- The policies and procedures should incorporate compliance with regulatory issues.

Recommendation 6: Policies and procedures should be monitored periodically for effectiveness, both to ensure that staff are able to comply fully with and fulfill organizational requirements and to ensure that the policies are having the desired result in preventing and controlling infections. *Both Categories II and III*

Compliance with regulations, guidelines, and accreditation requirements

Recommendation 7: HCOs should engage infection control personnel in maintaining compliance with relevant regulatory and accreditation requirements. *Both Categories II and III*

Recommendation 8: Infection control personnel should have appropriate access to medical or other relevant records, information in regard to the HCO's compliance with regulations, standards, etc, and to staff members who can provide information on the adequacy of the HCO's compliance with regard to regulations, standards, and guidelines. *Both Categories II and III*

Recommendation 9: The infection control program should collaborate with, and provide liaison to, appropriate local and state health departments for reporting of communicable diseases and related conditions and to assist with control of infectious diseases in the community. *Both Categories II and III*

Employee health

Recommendation 10: The infection control program personnel should work collaboratively with the HCO's employee health program personnel. *Category II*

- The HCO should have access to consultation and direction from a physician (or designee) with expertise in infectious disease and health care epidemiology.
- Infection control personnel should review and approve all employee health policies and procedures that relate to the transmission of communicable diseases in the HCO.

Recommendation 11: At the time of employment, all HCO personnel should be evaluated for conditions relating to communicable diseases. *Both Categories II and III*

The employment record should include the following:

- Medical history, including immunization status and assessment for conditions that may predispose personnel to acquiring or transmitting communicable diseases
- Tuberculosis screening
- Serologic screening for vaccine-preventable diseases, as deemed appropriate
- Such medical examinations as are indicated by the above

Recommendation 12: The HCO evaluates employees and other health care workers (eg, students, volunteers) for conditions related to infectious diseases that may have an impact on patient care, the employee, or other health care workers periodically. This evaluation should include a review of required immunizations and status of tuberculosis screening. *Both Categories II and III*

- Medical records of all health care workers must be kept confidential.
- The HCO should track employee immunization and tuberculosis screening status.

Recommendation 13: Employees must be offered immunizations based on regulatory requirements. HICPAC Personnel Guidelines and recommendations

428 *Friedman et al*

AJIC
October 1999

of the Centers for Disease Control and Prevention's Advisory Committee on Immunization Practices for health care workers should also be followed. *Both Categories I and III*

Recommendation 14: The HCO's employee health program should institute policies and procedures for the evaluation of exposed or infected health care workers. *Category I*

- Exposed health care workers should be evaluated for circumstances surrounding the exposure, evaluation of symptoms, need for postexposure prophylaxis, need for treatment, and work restrictions.
- Infected symptomatic and asymptomatic health care workers should be assessed for disease communicability, work restrictions, and treatment, as appropriate.

Intervening directly to prevent infections

Recommendation 15: Infection control personnel in HCOs must have the capacity to identify and implement measures to control endemic and epidemic infections and adverse events. *Category I*

- HCOs must have an ongoing system to obtain pertinent microbiologic data.
- Ongoing communication and consultation with clinical staff throughout the organization must be maintained to identify infectious and adverse events, to assist in maintenance and monitoring of infection control procedures, and to provide consultation.
- When an outbreak occurs, infection control personnel must have adequate resources and authority to ensure a comprehensive and timely investigation and the implementation of appropriate control measures.
- Institutional policies and procedures should be developed so that roles and responsibilities are outlined clearly.

Educating and training health care workers, patients, and nonmedical caregivers

Recommendation 16: HCOs must provide ongoing educational programs in infection prevention and control to health care workers. *Both Categories I and III*

- Infection control personnel knowledgeable regarding epidemiology and infectious diseases should be active participants in the planning and implementation of the educational programs.

Recommendation 17: Educational programs should be evaluated periodically for effectiveness. *Both Categories II and III*

- Educational programs should meet the needs of the group or department for which they are given and must provide learning experiences for persons with a wide range of educational backgrounds and work responsibilities.

- Participation of health care workers at educational programs should be documented.

Recommendation 18: The health care organization must have a mechanism to ensure that patients and caregivers receive appropriate information regarding infection prevention and control. *Category II*

Resources—personnel

Recommendation 19: The HCO must assure adequate personnel and supporting resources to fulfill the functions of the infection control program. *Category II*

Recommendation 20: All HCOs should have access to the ongoing services of a person who is trained in infection prevention and control (ie, an infection control professional [ICP]), who provides oversight for the infection control program. *Category II*

Recommendation 21: All HCOs should have access to continuing services of a physician trained in health care epidemiology. *Category II*

Recommendation 22: ICPs should be encouraged to obtain Certification in Infection Control. *Category II*

Other resources

Recommendation 23: Resources should be provided for continuing professional education of employees and infection control personnel who work directly for the organization. *Category II*

References

1. Marszalek-Gaucher E, Coffey RJ. Transforming healthcare organizations. San Francisco: Jossey-Bass; 1990. p. xi.
2. Jackson MM, Lynch P. Ambulatory care settings. In: Bennett JV, Brachman PS, editors. Hospital infections. 4th ed. Philadelphia: Lippincott-Raven; 1998.
3. Association for Professionals in Infection Control and Epidemiology. APIC infection control and applied epidemiology: principles and practice. St. Louis: Mosby; 1996.
4. A practical handbook for hospital epidemiologists. The Society for Healthcare Epidemiology of America. Herwaldt LA, Decker MD, editors. Thorofare (NJ): Slack; 1998.
5. Centers for Disease Control and Prevention. Preventing emerging infectious diseases: a strategy for the 21st century. Atlanta: US Department of Health and Human Services, Centers for Disease Control and Prevention; 1998.
6. Scheckler WE, Brimhall D, Buck AS, Farr BM, Friedman C, Garibaldi RA, et al. Requirements for infrastructure and essential activities of infection control and epidemiology in hospitals: a consensus panel report. AJIC Am J Infect Control 1998;26:47-60.
7. Kemper P, Murtaugh CM. Lifetime use of nursing home care. New Engl J Med 1991;324:595-600.
8. Nicolle LE, Strausbaugh LJ, Garibaldi RA. Infections and antibiotic resistance in nursing homes. Clin Microbiol Rev 1996;9:1-7.
9. Strausbaugh LJ, Crossley KB, Nurse BA, Thrupp LD. SHEA Long-Term Care Committee. Antimicrobial resistance in long-term care facilities. Infect Control Hosp Epidemiol 1996;17:129-40.
10. Outbreaks of pneumococcal pneumonia among unvaccinated residents in chronic-care facilities—Massachusetts, October 1995, Oklahoma, February 1996, and Maryland, May-June 1996. MMWR Morb Mortal Wkly Rep 1997;46:60-2.

AJIC
Volume 27, Number 5

Friedman et al **429**

11. Rice LB, Willey SH, Papanicolaou GA, Medeiros AA, Eliopoulos GM, Moellering RC Jr, et al. Outbreak of ceftazidime resistance caused by extended-spectrum beta-lactamases at a Massachusetts chronic-care facility. Antimicrob Agents Chemother 1990;34:2193-9.

12. Stevenson KB. Regional data set of infection rates for long-term care facilities: description of a valuable benchmarking tool. AJIC Am J Infect Control 1999;27:20-6.

13. Nicolle LE. Urinary tract infections in long term care facilities. Infect Control Hosp Epidemiol 1993;14:220-5.

14. Nicolle LE, Bentley D, Garibaldi R, Neuhaus E, Smith P, Antimicrobial use in long-term care facilities. Infect Control Hosp Epidemiol 1996;17:119-28.

15. McGeer A, Campbell B, Emori TG, Hierholzer WJ, Jackson MM, Nicolle LE, et al. Definitions of infection for surveillance in long-term care facilities. AJIC Am J Infect Control 1991;19:1-7.

16. Smith PW, Rusnak PG. Infection prevention and control in the long-term-care facility. SHEA Long-Term-Care Committee and APIC Guidelines Committee. AJIC Am J Infect Control 1997;25:488-512.

17. Auerbach SD, Schwartz B, Williams D, Fiorilli MG, Adimora AA, Breiman RF, et al. Outbreak of invasive group A streptococcal infections in a nursing home. Lessons on prevention and control. Arch Intern Med 1992;152:1017-22.

18. Arden NH, Patriarca PA, Fasano MB, Lui KJ, Harmon MW, Kendal AP, et al. The roles of vaccination and amantadine prophylaxis in controlling an outbreak of influenza A (H3N2) in a nursing home. Arch Intern Med 1988;148:865-8.

19. Layton MC, Calliste SG, Gomez TM, Patton C, Brooks S. A mixed foodborne outbreak with *Salmonella heidelberg* and *Campylobacter jejuni* in a nursing home. Infect Control Hosp Epidemiol 1997;18:115-21.

20. Yonkosky D, Ladia L, Gackenheimer L, Schultz MW. Scabies in nursing homes: an eradication program with permethrin 5% cream. J Am Acad Dermatol 1990;23:1133-6.

21. Nuorti JP, Butler JC, Crutcher JM, Guevara R, Welch D, Holder P, et al. An outbreak of multidrug-resistant pneumococcal pneumonia and bacteremia among unvaccinated nursing home residents. N Engl J Med 1998;338:1861-8.

22. Goodman RA, Solomon SL. Transmission of infectious diseases in outpatient health care settings. JAMA 1991;265:2377-81.

23. Manian FA. Surveillance of surgical site infections in alternative settings: exploring the current options. AJIC Am J Infect Control 1997;25:102-5.

24. Hecht AD. Creating greater efficiency in ambulatory surgery. J Clin Anesth 1995;7:581-4.

25. Davis JE. Ambulatory surgery...how far can we go? Med Clin North Am 1993;77:365-75.

26. Bookwalter JW 3rd, Busch MD, Nicely D. Ambulatory surgery is safe and effective in radicular disk disease. Spine 1994;19:526-30.

27. Williams DN, Rehm SJ, Tice AD, Bradley JS, Kind AD, Craig WA, et al. Practice guidelines for community-based parenteral anti-infective therapy. IDSA Practice Guidelines Committee. Clin Infect Dis 1997;25:787-801.

28. Kunkel MJ, Tice AD, Dalovisio JR, the Opivate OPAT Network. Patient registry for outpatient intravenous antimicrobial therapy [abstract]. Clin Infect Dis 1998;27:1050.

29. Liebert L, Bryant-Wimp J. Ambulatory infusion centers: hospital survival in an outpatient world. Infusion 1997;4(3):25-9.

30. Poretz DM. Outpatient parenteral antibiotic therapy. Management of serious infections. Part II: Amenable infections and models for delivery. Infusion center, office, and home. Hosp Pract 1993;28(Suppl 2):S40-S43.

31. Poretz DM. The infusion center: a model for outpatient parenteral antibiotic therapy. Rev Infect Dis 1991;13(Suppl 2):S142-S146.

32. Flores K. AIC: what's your role in the most talked about delivery model? Infusion 1998;4(11):35-8.

33. Favero MS, Alter MJ, Bland LA. Nosocomial infections associated with hemodialysis. In: Mayhall CG, editor. Hospital epidemiology and infection control. Volume 1. Baltimore: Williams & Wilkins; 1996. p.693-714.

34. Hindman SH, Favero MS, Carson LA, Petersen NJ, Schonberger LB, Solano JT. Pyrogenic reactions during haemodialysis caused by extramural endotoxin. Lancet 1975;2:732-4.

35. Gordon SM, Tipple M, Bland LA, Jarvis WR. Pyrogenic reactions associated with the reuse of disposable hollow-fiber hemodialyzers. JAMA 1988;260:2077-81.

36. Welbel SF, Schoendorf K, Bland LA, Arduino MJ, Groves C, Schable B, et al. An outbreak of gram-negative bloodstream infections in chronic hemodialysis patients. Am J Nephrol 1995;15:1-4.

37. Flaherty JP, Garcia-Houchins S, Chudy R, Arnow PM. An outbreak of gram-negative bacteremia traced to contaminated O-rings in reprocessed dialyzers. Ann Intern Med 1993;119:1072-8.

38. Lowry PW, Beck-Sague CM, Bland LA, Aguero SM, Arduino MJ, Minuth AN, et al. *Mycobacterium chelonae* infection among patients receiving high-flux dialysis in a hemodialysis clinic in California. J Infect Dis 1990;161:85-90.

39. Alter MJ, Favero MS, Maynard JE. Impact of infection control strategies on the incidence of dialysis-associated hepatitis in the United States. J Infect Dis 1986;153:1149-51.

40. Velandia M, Fridkin SK, Cardenas V, Boshell J, Ramirez G, Bland L, et al. Transmission of HIV in dialysis centre. Lancet 1995; 345:1417-22.

41. Tokars JI, Alter MJ, Favero MS, Moyer LA, Bland LA. National surveillance of dialysis associated diseases in the United States, 1991. ASAIO J 1993;39:966-75.

42. Almroth G, Ekermo B, Franzen L, Hed J. Antibody responses to hepatitis C virus and its modes of transmission in dialysis patients. Nephron 1991;59:232-5.

43. National Association for Home Care. Basic statistics about home care. Washington (DC): National Association for Home Care; 1997.

44. National Association for Home Care Uniform Data Set for Home Care and Hospice. Washington (DC): National Association for Home Care; 1998.

45. National Association for Home Care. How to choose a home care provider: a consumer's guide. Washington (DC): National Association for Home Care; 1997.

46. Smith PW. Forum: infection prevention in the home health setting. Asepsis 1994;16:9-11.

47. Rosenheimer L. Establishing a surveillance system for infections acquired in home healthcare. Home Healthc Nurse 1995;13(3):20-6.

48. Do AN, Ray BJ, Banerjee SN, Illian AF, Barnett BJ, Pham MH, et al. Bloodstream infection associated with needleless device use and the importance of infection-control practices in the home health setting. J Infect Dis 1999;179:442-8.

49. Kellerman S, Shay DK, Howard J, Goes C, Feusner J, Rosenberg J, et al. Bloodstream infections in home infusion patients: the influence of race and needleless intravascular access devices. J Pediatr 1996;129:711-7.

50. Danzig LE, Short LJ, Collins K, Mahoney M, Sepe S, Bland L, et al. Bloodstream infections associated with a needleless intravenous infusion system in patients receiving home infusion therapy. JAMA 1995;273:1862-4.

51. Tokars JI, Cookson ST, McArthur MA, Boyer CL, McGeer AJ, Jarvis WR. Prospective evaluation of risk factors for bloodstream infection in patients receiving home infusion therapy. Ann Intern Med In press 1999.

52. Chodoff A, Pettis AM, Schoonmaker D, Shelly MA. Polymicrobial gram-negative bacteremia associated with saline solution flush

AJIC
October 1999

430 *Friedman et al*

used with a needleless intravenous system. AJIC Am J Infect Control 1995;23:357-63.

53. Graham DR. Nosohusial infection: complications of home intravenous therapy. Infect Dis Clin Practice 1993;2:158-61.

54. Rosenheimer L, Embry FC, Sanford J, Silver SR. Infection surveillance in home care: device-related incidence rates. AJIC Am J Infect Control 1998;26:359-63.

55. Simmons B, Trusler M, Roccaforte J, Smith P, Scott R. Infection control for home health. Infect Control Hosp Epidemiol 1990;11:362-70.

56. Rhinehart E, Friedman MM. Infection control in home care. Gaithersburg (MD): Aspen Publishing; 1999.

57. Joint Commission on Accreditation of Healthcare Organizations. Comprehensive accreditation manual for home care: CAMHC/Joint Commission. Oakbrook Terrace (IL): Joint Commission on Accreditation of Healthcare Organizations; 1997.

58. Friedman MM. Designing an infection control program to meet JCAHO standards. Caring 1996;15:18-25.

59. Joint Commission on Accreditation of Healthcare Organizations. Comprehensive Accreditation Manual for Long Term Care: CAMLTC/Joint Commission. Oakbrook Terrace (IL): Joint Commission on Accreditation of Healthcare Organizations; 1997.

60. Joint Commission on Accreditation of Healthcare Organizations. Comprehensive Accreditation Manual for Ambulatory Care. Oakbrook Terrace (IL): Joint Commission on Accreditation of Healthcare Organizations; 1997.

61. Lorenzen AN, Itkin DJ. Surveillance of infection in home care. AJIC Am J Infect Control 1992;20:326-9.

62. Rhinehart E. Developing an infection surveillance system. Caring 1996;14:26-32.

63. ORYX. The next evolution in accreditation. Joint Commission on Accreditation of Healthcare Organizations. Nurs Manage 1997; 28:49-54.

64. White MC. Infections and infection risks in home care settings. Infect Control Hosp Epidemiol 1992;13:535-9.

65. Wade BH, Bush SE. Opportunities for extending infection control into the community. Infect Dis Clin Pract 1998;7:32-8.

66. Abrutyn E, Scheckler W, Goldmann DA, editors. Saunders infection control reference service. Philadelphia: WB Saunders; 1998.

67. Health care standards: official directory. Plymouth Meeting (PA): ECRI; 1990.

68. Bolyard EA, Tablan OC, Williams WW, Pearson ML, Shapiro CN, Deitchman SD, et al. Guideline for infection control in health care personnel, 1998. AJIC Am J Infect Control 1998;26:289-354.

69. Stamm WE, Weinstein RA, Dixon RE. Comparison of endemic and epidemic nosocomial infections. Am J Med 1981;70:393-7.

70. Friedman C, Chenoweth C. Infection control. In: Schmele JA, editor. Quality management. Albany (NY): Delmar Publishers; 1996.

71. Sheldon JE. 18 tips for infection control at home. Nursing 1995;25:32PP-32QQ.

72. Herrick S, Loos KM. Designing an infection control program. Home Care Provid 1996;1:153-6.

73. Bellen V. A model for a comprehensive infection control program in home healthcare. J Healthc Qual 1996;18:7-17.

74. Friedman MM. Joint Commission on Accreditation of Healthcare Organizations' infection control requirements: fact or fiction. Home Healthc Nurse 1997;15:236-8.

75. Gross PA, Barrett TL, Dellinger EP, Krause PJ, Martone WJ, McGowan JE Jr, et al. Purpose of quality standards for infectious diseases. Infectious Diseases Society of America. Clin Infect Dis 1994;18:421.

76. Pearson ML. Guideline for prevention of intravascular device-related infections. The Hospital Infection Control Practices Advisory Committee. AJIC Am J Infect Control 1996;24:262-93.

77. An approach to the evaluation of quality indicators of the outcome of care in hospitalized patients, with a focus on nosocomial infection indicators. The Quality Indicator Study Group. AJIC Am J Infect Control 1995;23:215-22.

APPENDIX B

Infection Control Program

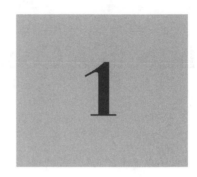

Infection Control Program

A. SOURCES OF PROGRAM DIRECTION

The first hospital infection prevention and control efforts in the United States began in the 1950s concurrently with the growth of intensive care and increasing staphylococcal infections.[1] Infection control (IC) programs extended into thousands of hospitals in the late 1960s and 1970s in response to urging from various organizations. The 1980s and 1990s brought changes to these programs from state and federal agencies, professional organizations, and scientific information published in journals. IC professionals need to be alert to these changing recommendations and information and make appropriate modifications to IC programs. In addition, local and state requirements must be followed. Specific agencies and organizations which have a major impact on programs include the:

CANDACE FRIEDMAN

1. American Hospital Association (AHA)

The AHA's Advisory Committee on Infections Within Hospitals published its first edition of *Infection Control in the Hospital* in 1968. The purpose of this manual was to describe the elements of an IC program that an AHA advisory committee "considers essential to the reduction and elimination of the human and economic wastage that results from our failure to prevent those nosocomial infections that are preventable . . . ." Three editions of the manual were printed, the last published in 1979.[2] The AHA impacted IC practice through educational programs and conferences, journals and other publications, briefings, and consultants. The AHA dissolved its infection control section in 1995 and began a collaboration with the Association for Professionals in Infection Control and Epidemiology (APIC) to meet the infection control needs of AHA members.

2. Association for Professionals in Infection Control and Epidemiology

a. The APIC was established in 1972 to provide education and science-based information to strengthen and improve the practice of infection prevention and control. Its purpose is to improve healthcare by serving the needs and aims common to all disciplines that are united by infection control and epidemiology activities.

b. APIC's major influences on IC practice are its guidelines and standards development, education and training programs, scientific journal, and governmental affairs activities. It established the Certification Board of Infection Control and Epidemiology in 1981 to administer an IC certification program. In 1993, the APIC Research Foundation was created to facilitate funding of priority-driven research projects. In 1997, the Center for Clinical Epidemiology was established to develop and disseminate information on adverse outcomes.

3. Centers for Disease Control and Prevention (CDC)

   a. In the 1960s the CDC began recommending that hospitals conduct surveillance of the occurrence of nosocomial infections.
   b. Training programs in IC surveillance were started at the CDC in the early 1970s. They stressed surveillance for infections, developing and implementing policies for prevention of infections, and reducing wasteful activities (e.g., environmental culturing). The CDC no longer offers these programs.
   c. The Hospital Infections Program (HIP) of the National Center for Infectious Diseases is the CDC's focus for information, surveillance, investigation, prevention, and control of nosocomial infections.
   d. In January 1970, the CDC began the National Nosocomial Infections Surveillance (NNIS) system as part of HIP's activities.
      1) One purpose of this program was to monitor trends in nosocomial infection rates, pathogens, and antibiotic susceptibility patterns in the United States.
      2) National surveillance of hospital nosocomial infections is coordinated and analyzed by NNIS.
      3) The NNIS program publishes hospital nosocomial infection rate data that many institutions use for comparison (i.e., benchmarking) and improvement efforts.[3]
   e. In 1974, the CDC initiated a study to determine the efficacy of infection control activities in reducing the risks of nosocomial infections in hospitals, the Study on the Efficacy of Nosocomial Infection Control (SENIC) project.
      1) The SENIC project defined an infection surveillance and control program as one containing three main elements:
         a) Epidemiologic surveillance for the occurrence of infections in patients within the hospital
         b) Formulation of policies and procedures to control infections based on data generated by surveillance and other sources
         c) Personnel specially trained in hospital epidemiology to collect the surveillance data and coordinate intervention activities
      2) The SENIC Project compared nosocomial infection rates that occurred in 1970 and

1976 in a stratified random sample of U.S. hospitals.[4]
      3) The project found that, in comparison with hospitals that had no program activities, those that established infection surveillance and control programs with a full-time–equivalent IC professional per 250 occupied beds, an effectual IC physician with special interest in infection control, and a program for reporting wound infection rates to surgeons, reduced their nosocomial infection rates by approximately 32%.[5]
   f. Hospital Infection Control Practices Advisory Committee (HICPAC)
      1) The HIP began a nosocomial infection guidelines and recommendation process in 1981. Several documents were developed for specific infection control practices. This process was discontinued in the mid-1980s.
      2) HICPAC was established in 1991 to provide advice and guidance to the CDC and others regarding the practice of hospital infection control and strategies for surveillance, prevention, and control of nosocomial infections.
      3) The committee influences IC programs through its periodic updating of guidelines and other policy statements regarding prevention of nosocomial infections.

4. Food and Drug Administration (FDA)

   a. The FDA is part of the Public Health Service. It is responsible for implementing, monitoring, and enforcing standards for the safety, efficacy and labeling of all drugs and biologics for human use.
   b. Of particular interest to the IC team are its activities related to food, blood, and antimicrobial products and chemical germicides used with medical devices.[1] (The Environmental Protection Agency is also involved in testing and use of hospital disinfectant products.)

5. Health Care Financing Administration (HCFA)

   a. As part of HCFA's required conditions for certification and participation in Medicare and Medicaid programs, healthcare facilities must comply with federal standards that include specific requirements for an active infection control program.[6]
   b. A program to investigate, control, and prevent infections in long-term care facilities accepting Medicare and Medicaid patients is mandated by HCFA.[7]

6. Joint Commission on Accreditation of Healthcare Organizations (JCAHO)

   a. Essentially, there were no governmental or private regulations or standards for IC programs until 1976 when IC programs became a requirement for accreditation by the Joint Commission.[1]

b. The JCAHO's standards for IC have been used by many institutions, including hospitals, long-term care facilities, behavioral-health facilities, and home-health agencies, to establish a framework for an infection prevention and control program.

c. These standards have undergone many revisions over the years. However, in general, the standards state that the goal of the surveillance, prevention, and control of infection function is for the healthcare organization to identify and reduce the risks of infections in patients and healthcare workers. There must be a functioning program, coordinating all activities related to the surveillance, prevention, and control of infections. The program should be doing the right things, doing these things well, be supported, and be focused toward improvement of processes and outcomes.[8,9]

d. As part of its Agenda for Change in 1987, the Joint Commission began a long-term project to develop quantitative indicators of patient care quality.[1] The goal is to have a continuous accreditation process that includes the use of both standards and performance measures to evaluate the performance of healthcare organizations.[10]

7. National Institute for Occupational Safety and Health (NIOSH)

a. NIOSH was established in 1970 and became part of the CDC in 1973. It is responsible for conducting laboratory and epidemiologic research on occupational hazards.[11]

b. Decisions regarding types of devices used for employee protection, eg, respirators, are part of NIOSH's mandate.

8. Occupational Safety and Health Administration (OSHA)

a. OSHA began its IC activities in 1987 with the draft publication of its blood-borne pathogens rules. These rules were finalized in 1991.[12]

b. In 1993, OSHA extended its activities to include prevention of tuberculosis in healthcare facilities.[13,14]

c. OSHA's standards focus on determining employees' health risks as the result of exposure to communicable diseases.

9. Society for Healthcare Epidemiology of America (SHEA)

a. SHEA was founded in 1980 to foster the development and application of the science of healthcare epidemiology.[15]

b. The organization provides educational programs, develops position papers, and produces two scientific journals. The society cosponsors

a training course in healthcare epidemiology with the CDC.

c. A multidisciplinary paper outlining the infrastructure for a hospital infection prevention and control program was coordinated by SHEA in 1997.[16]

B. OVERALL STRUCTURE AND FUNCTION

Each institution is unique and its specific needs must be considered when developing or reorganizing an IC program. Because of these differing needs, there may be various groups, individuals, and functions within the organization that are responsible for the IC program. The following information outlines various persons and activities related to an IC program.

1. Infection control team

a. Often the core of the IC program is the infection control professional, chair of the IC committee, and/or the healthcare epidemiologist. An individual responsible for employee health or administration may also be a part of the team.

b. The team is responsible for carrying out all aspects of the IC program.

c. Its members must be qualified and guided by sound principles and current information.

2. Infection Control Committee (ICC)

a. Authority: a facility may have an ICC to function as the central decision- and policy-making body for IC.

b. Reporting: the ICC chair reports either to the medical staff or administration.

c. Purpose: the ICC acts as the advocate for prevention and control of infections in the facility, formulates and monitors patient-care policies, educates staff, and provides political support that empowers the team.[17]

d. Meetings/membership: the ICC is multidisciplinary, composed of representatives from most departments; it meets regularly, often monthly. Representation typically includes members of administration and medical and nursing staff.

e. Decisions and dissemination of information.

1) Since infection problems and control measures often cross departmental lines, a multidisciplinary committee is important.

2) Often the ICC approves policies or procedures at meetings.

3) Dissemination of ICC information is crucial. Both surveillance data and policy decisions should be communicated throughout the organization. This may be accomplished through such mechanisms as routine reports to clinicians and/or department heads and through electronic methods. The ICC often ratifies the ideas of the infection control team; its members disseminate the information discussed in the meeting; and this com-

mittee gives political and administrative support to the infection control program.[18]

f. An ICC is not required by the JCAHO; some states do require an ICC. However, institutions may support a committee structure for the reasons outlined above. If a committee is not used, IC staff need to develop other mechanisms, eg, use of continuous quality improvement (CQI) models, to obtain multidisciplinary support for changes/actions.

   1) CQI models use a collaborative approach, including use of multidisciplinary teams. These teams meet regularly, often weekly.

   2) Teams are responsible for planning, policy development, and decision making. The team leader may be the IC professional.

   3) Dissemination of information: both surveillance data and policy decisions should be communicated throughout the organization. This may be accomplished, for example, through routine reports to clinicians and/or department heads and electronic methods.

   4) Monitoring, evaluation, and continuous improvement are overseen by top leadership.

3. IC professionals

   a. The role of IC professionals includes numerous responsibilities: collection and analysis of infection data; product/procedure evaluation; consultation on infection risk assessment, prevention, and control strategies; education efforts directed at interventions to reduce infection risks; implementation of changes mandated by regulatory and licensing agencies; application of epidemiologic principles to include activities directed at improving patient outcomes; provision of high-quality services in a cost-efficient manner; and participation in research projects.[16,19,20,21]

   b. Some IC professionals work less than full time on infection prevention and control. They may also be involved in such areas as employee health, quality management, and risk management. In a long-term care facility, IC professionals typically have multiple roles to fill and usually have only a few hours per week available to devote to IC activities, including surveillance.[22]

   c. Many training courses exist for IC professionals. Local and national APIC organizations, SHEA, state organizations, academic institutions, and private firms offer training courses for IC professionals. Various courses are available for both beginning and experienced professionals.

   d. An IC professional's time is split among surveillance, policy and procedure development, education, quality improvement, consulting, and investigating potential outbreaks. IC professionals may also take part in research activities.[21]

   e. Task and job analyses have been performed to specify what the IC professional's day-to-day work may entail.[23]

f. The IC professional may be involved in investigations related to adverse outcomes other than infections.

g. Certification for IC professionals is available through the Certification Board of Infection Control and Epidemiology.

h. There are two key IC professionals who are part of a program: the IC practitioner and the healthcare epidemiologist.

   1) IC practitioner (ICP)

      a) These professionals predominately have such backgrounds as nursing, medical technology, or microbiology.[24]

      b) Titles used by IC practitioners include infection control nurse, infection control coordinator, nurse epidemiologist, infection control officer, infection control practitioner.

      c) The ICP role involves the daily collaborative efforts within all facets of healthcare.[25]

      d) Typically functions as a consultant, educator, role model, researcher, and change agent. Responsibilities include education, surveillance, prevention and control, and quality improvement.[21]

   2) Healthcare epidemiologist

      a) May be the chair of the ICC or may occupy a separate position as either a technical advisor or a member of the committee.

      b) May be a physician with special training in healthcare epidemiology and infection prevention and control; often is an infectious diseases physician.

      c) Works closely with the medical staff.

      d) Specific training courses in healthcare epidemiology are offered throughout the United States cosponsored by SHEA and CDC.

4. Program reporting relationships

   a. Depending on the institution, IC professionals may report to administration, nursing or medical services, or quality-management departments. Other reporting relationships also exist.

   b. In some institutions, infection prevention and control is integrated with other departments (e.g., risk management, utilization management, and/or quality management).

5. Staffing

   a. On the basis of pilot studies in eight community hospitals in which different staffing levels were evaluated, the CDC recommended one full-time ICP for every 250 occupied beds.[26]

   b. The SENIC project strongly supported the 250-bed recommendation.[5]

   c. Because of increased demands on the IC professional's time for education and consultation, traditional staffing estimates are being evaluated.[27] One innovative method uses workload units.[28]

d. A point system for staffing was adopted by a working group of the Belgian Department of Health. The number of IC professionals is based on the number of points obtained by multiplying the number of beds of each patient-care unit by a factor that is specific for the patient population treated in the unit.[29]

e. Some innovative methods have been designed to extend the reach of an IC professional through computers,[30,31] nurse-advisors,[32] unit-based programs,[33] liaisons,[34] and clerical positions.[35]

6. Cost-benefit of IC programs

a. The SENIC project found that up to one-third of nosocomial infections could be prevented by effective IC programs.[5]

b. Part of a program's effectiveness is a reflection of the influence of IC professionals. They must be visible, provide a resource for staff, and use their scientific expertise when making specific recommendations. Effectiveness also depends on commitment to IC by administration.[36]

c. Decision analysis can be used to compare costs with outcomes.[37]

   1) Cost-effectiveness studies and cost-benefit studies are examples of decision analysis.

      a) Effectiveness refers to the outcome of care. It can be expressed as the number of cases of disease prevented, the number of lives saved, or the number of life-years saved.

      b) Cost-benefit analysis looks at outcome in terms of cost.

d. Various methods can be used to estimate how much healthcare related infections cost an institution.

   1) The cost of the program itself consists of such items as salaries, employee benefits, commodity expenses. Cost benefit estimates can be developed for both mortality and morbidity.[38]

   2) A crude estimate of cost can be obtained by multiplying the estimated numbers of nosocomial infections at various sites by the site-specific cost weights (cost per infection) derived from the SENIC project[39] adjusted for time.

   3) Other methods use actual cost weights or costs determined through prospective, randomized studies.[40]

   4) Prevalence surveys can also be used to assess the costs of nosocomial infections.[41]

7. Characteristics of the organization

a. The ability of the IC program to influence practices that affect quality patient care depends on certain characteristics of the patient population

and their risk of infection and characteristics of personnel.

b. These characteristics include number of beds, professional school affiliation, geographics, volume of patient encounters, patient population served, clinical focus, numbers of employees, and administrative philosophy.

c. It is important to understand these characteristics when developing a program to optimally meet the infection prevention and control needs of the organization and the patients it serves.

8. Influencing practice

a. There are internal and external characteristics of IC staff that are important in influencing and motivating patient-care providers.

   1) Internal characteristics include such factors as personal beliefs and motivation, inner energy and strength, and one's own perceptions about individual effectiveness in influencing the behavior of others.

   2) External characteristics include the visibility and availability of IC professionals, their assertiveness and diplomacy in managing conflict, their use of education and management strategies to bring about change, and their ability to work within the organization.

b. Written IC policies are often developed that relate to staff and patient-care practices, employee health, or sterilization/disinfection.

   1) General policies are applicable to staff in the whole facility. These policies may form the basis of an IC manual.

   2) Specific policies may be developed for each unit/area.

   3) These policies must be supported scientifically and address IC needs for the institution.

   4) The application of IC practices occurs primarily when providers of direct patient care consistently implement these policies to benefit patients and protect staff.

c. IC professionals usually attempt to affect patient-care outcomes by influencing the practices of patient-care providers.

   1) Teaching personnel to increase their knowledge and skills of patient-care practices is one method to influence patient care.

   2) Education of staff is crucial to the success of any IC program.

C. Administrative support

1. Administration

a. It is important that the administrative leaders of the organization approve and support the IC activities.

b. IC professionals should schedule regular meetings with the administrator to whom they are responsible. This helps to maintain liaison between the program and administration for forecasting and planning purposes and increases the awareness of the institution's leaders of the IC program's activities.

2. Support

   a. Every year goals and objectives for the IC program should be determined. These should be based on the institution's strategic goals.
   b. Staff and data systems needs should be defined by the specific requirements (goals and objectives) of the infection risk-reduction process of the organization.
   c. An annual evaluation of the IC program is important to outline achievements and activities of the program and describe support requirements. This annual review may also be helpful for the ICC and the IC department itself. The value of the IC program to the organization should be emphasized, as well as patient outcomes and cost savings. This evaluation report should be widely disseminated to leaders throughout the organization, in particular to the chief executive officer and board members.

D. Quality of an IC program

1. Vision/mission/values

   a. Decision makers need to be informed of the value of the IC program. One way to explain the importance of the program to others is through a mission statement and a description of the vision for the program.
   b. These governing ideas answer three critical questions: what? why? and how?
      1) *Vision* is the what?—the picture of the future the IC program seeks to create. Vision is long term.
      2) *Mission* is the why?—the answer to the question, 'Why does the IC program exist?' You need a vision to make the mission more concrete and tangible.
      3) *Core values* answer the question "How does the IC program want to act, consistent with our mission, along the path toward achieving our vision?" Values describe how the program functions on a day-to-day basis, while pursuing the vision.[42]
   c. Vision paints a picture of where the IC program wants the organization to go and what it wants it to be. What develops is a general picture. A vision needs to: (1) focus on strategic advantages—begun by identifying the IC program's strategic advantage in the organization—and (2) add value to others.[43]
   d. A mission statement defines the common purpose, focus, and context for all departmental activities. Mission statements enable a group to set boundaries for their activities, know what is and

isn't within their jurisdiction, and understand where they fit in the organization's overall improvement efforts.[44] The IC mission should support the overall institutional mission.

2. Customer identification

   a. A customer is anyone to whom the IC program provides service. Often the customer is the next person or group in a work process to receive the product, service, or information for the purposes of modifying or acting upon it. A customer is defined much more broadly than a patient; it includes the patient's family, physicians, nurses, and coworkers.
   b. Distinguish between external and internal customers. The distinction is based on the degree to which the IC professional can influence and negotiate customers' requirements. IC professionals are usually able to negotiate changes in requirements of internal customers if those requested are unrealistic. This is not ordinarily the case with external customers.[45]
      1) Internal customers of IC professionals may include nurses, physicians, administrators, technologists, and ancillary staff.
      2) External customers may include IC staff at other institutions and regulatory agency personnel.
   c. It is important that IC professionals know what is expected of them by the people they serve. Customer concerns must be given top priority. Every work process should be studied and constantly improved so that the final product or service exceeds customer expectations.[43] Quality has no meaning except as defined by the desires and needs of the customers.[46]

3. IC professional as supplier/customer

   For any transaction involving a product, service, or information, the person or organization being supplied something is the customer and the IC professional is the supplier. Supplier-customer roles switch for different transactions; every person is both a supplier and a customer at different times.[45] Figure 1-1 illustrates the

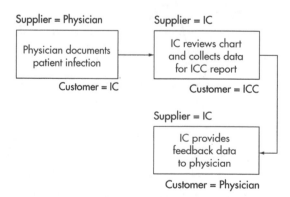

Figure 1-1 Two types of variation in processes.

APIC Text of Infection Control and Epidemiology

changing relationship of an IC professional with a physician after identification of a nosocomial infection and provision of data.

4. Multidisciplinary activities

   a. Major gains in quality and productivity most often result from collaborative teams—a group of people pooling their skills, talents, and knowledge to achieve a common goal. Teams identify processes or problems needing improvement and work together to find solutions.[44]

   b. Teams developed to work on IC issues should include individuals from multiple functional areas integral to the specific issue being studied.[47]

   c. Flowcharting the process at a macro level is one way to determine which areas should be involved in the team.

5. Epidemiologic method

   a. IC staff must be able to demonstrate their ability to apply the epidemiologic method. The staff must also be familiar with basic statistical techniques.

   b. Use of data to solve problems and evaluate processes is crucial. Using epidemiologic principles, data can be analyzed for trends and problems identified.

   c. The application of epidemiologic tools and principles to the problems of nosocomial infections is strongly connected to the continuous quality improvement concept of using dependable data to improve processes.[48]

6. Performance improvement

   a. Infection control staff have been active in various quality aspects of medical care for three decades.[49] The IC program is an essential component of quality patient care.[50]

   b. The IC program must be coordinated with the organization-wide process for assessing and improving organizational performance.[51,52]

   c. Quality assessment is an epidemiologic science. It provides the means for tracking and identifying clinical problems and providing information to clinicians that helps determine opportunities for improvement of patient care.[53]

   d. There should be ongoing study of ways to improve prevention and control processes to reduce nosocomial infection rates to the lowest possible levels.[54,55]

   e. Incorporate the principles of continuous quality improvement in the IC program.[56,57]

   f. Variation is inherent in hospital practices and outcomes. IC has routinely examined special causes; however, common causes must also be evaluated to reduce infection rates and eliminate variation.

      1) There are two types of variation in processes (see Fig. 1-2).[46] An unexpected, significant deviation outside predicted control limits is considered to represent a special cause of variation.

         a) Special causes tend to cluster by person, place, and time (i.e., epidemiologic).

         b) The cause of the problem is not part of the process; therefore, the problem only

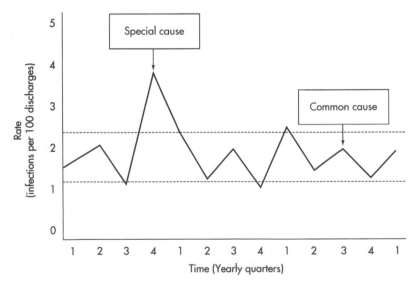

Figure 1-2 The changing relationship of an IC professional with a physician after identification of a nosocomial infection and provision of data.

occurs when the special cause is functioning.

   c) Special-cause variation represents changes that can be investigated and assigned to an identifiable source.[48]

2) Common-cause variation results from chance events that occur without a specific cause and from the inherent design of the process.

   a) Rates of specific processes and outcomes (e.g., nosocomial infections) fluctuate within statistically predictable bounds over time.

   b) The success of improvements can be ascertained by determining whether they improve the rate of a process or outcome significantly when compared with the predicted rate based on previous experience.[58]

f. Both outcomes and processes should be evaluated outcomes to understand the results, processes to understand what has been done to cause those results.[59-61]

1) Outcomes—performance measurement data can be used to improve care processes and to verify effectiveness of actions and improvement initiatives.[10]

2) Processes can be categorized as clinical, structural, or decision-making.[52]

   a) Clinical processes are those that directly influence patient care, such as skin care, intravascular practices.

   b) Structural processes involve the environment, such as needle disposal systems or regulated medical waste management.

   c) Decision-making processes involve various departments and issues, such as implementation of standard precautions.

g. Controlled trials to determine efficacy in reducing rates of infections are of interest to the IC team. An example of this type of study showed the efficacy of proper timing of perioperative antibiotics.[62]

7. Set priorities

a. Setting priorities allows better allocation of IC program resources.

b. Realistic strategies for surveillance and intervention should be developed.

c. Once annual program goals and objectives are stated, an action plan should be developed to outline the steps needed to accomplish each objective.[63,64]

d. The quality of the IC program should be assessed routinely by evaluating customer satisfaction,[65] appropriateness, efficacy, timeliness, availability, effectiveness, and efficiency.

REFERENCES

1. McDonald, LL. Health policy for infection control and epidemiology in critical care. *Crit Care Nurs Clin* 1995;7:727–732

2. American Hospital Association. *Infection Control in the Hospital.* Chicago, IL: American Hospital Association; 1969

3. National Nosocomial Infections Surveillance (NNIS) report: data summary from October 1986–April 1997, issued May 1997. *Am J Infect Control* 1997;25:477–487

4. Haley RW, Quade D, Freeman HE, et al. Study on the efficacy of nosocomial infection control (SENIC Project): summary of study design. *Am J Epidemiol* 1980;111:472–485

5. Hale RW, Culver DH, White JW, et al. The efficacy of infection surveillance and control programs in preventing nosocomial infections in US hospitals. *Am J Epid* 1985;121:182–205

6. Hospital conditions of participation: proposed rule, HCFA. *Fed Reg* 1997;62:66725–66763

7. US Department of Health and Human Services, Health Care Financing Administration. Medicare and Medicaid requirements for long–term care facilities. *Fed Reg* 1991;56:48826–48879

8. Joint Commission on Accreditation of Healthcare Organizations. Standards: surveillance, prevention and control of infection. In: JCAHO. *Accreditation Manual for Hospitals.* Chicago, IL: Joint Commission on Accreditation of Healthcare Organizations; 1998

9. Kobs A. Infection control. *Nurs Manage* 1997;28(8):17–19

10. Nadzam DM, Loeb, JM. Measuring and improving the performance of health care providers: accreditation in the 21st century. *Am J Infect Control* 1998;26:126–135

11. Request for comment on the proposed NIOSH document on guidelines for protecting the safety and health of health care workers. *Fed Reg* 1996;61:66281–66282

12. Department of Labor, Occupational Safety and Health Administration. Occupational exposure to bloodborne pathogens: final rule. *Fed Reg* 1991;56(235):64004–64182

13. Department of Labor, Occupational Safety and Health Administration. Occupational exposure to tuberculosis: proposed rule. *Fed Reg* 1997;62:54159–54309

14. Voelker R. New federal stances on TB control may be confusing to health care facilities. *JAMA* 1993;270:1903–1904

15. Larson E. A retrospective on infection control, Part 2: Twentieth Century—The flame burns. *Am J Infect Control* 1997;25:340–349

16. Scheckler WE, et al. Requirements for infrastructure and essential activities of infection control and epidemiology in hospitals: a consensus panel report. *Am J Infect Control* 1998;26:47–60

17. Wiblin RT, Wenzel RP. The infection control committee. *Infect Cont Hosp Epidemiol* 1996;17:44–46

18. Wenzel RP. Management principles and the infection control committee. In Wenzel RP, ed. *Prevention and Control of Nosocomial Infections.* 2nd ed. Baltimore, MD: Williams & Wilkins; 1993: 207–213

19. Schollenberger D. The infection control forum: where do we go from here? *Asepsis* 1990;12:11

20. Osguthorpe SG, Ormond L. Management constraints in infection control. *Crit Care Nurs Clin North Am* 1995;7:703–712

21. Practice and professional standards for infection control and epidemiology. *Can J Infect Control* 1998;13:7–9

22. Smith PW, Rusnak PG. Infection prevention and control in the long–term care facility. *Am J Infect Control* 1997;25:488–512

23. Bjerke NB, Fabrey LJ, Johnson CB, et al. Job analysis 1992: infection control practitioner, *Am J Infect Control* 1993;21:51–57

24. Jackson MM, Soule BM, Tweeten SS. APIC strategic planning member survey, 1997. *Am J Infect Control* 1998;26:113–125

25. The role of the infection control practitioner. *Can J Infect Control* 1996;11:36–37

26. Eickhoff TC, Brachman PS, Bennett JV, et al. Surveillance of nosocomial infections in community hospitals, I: surveillance methods, effectiveness, and initial results. *J Infect Dis* 1969;120:305–317

27. Friedman C, Chenoweth C. A survey of infection control professionals staffing patterns at University HealthSystem Consortium institutions. *Am J Infect Control* 1998;26:239–244

28. Kuwaki–Chuman I, Becker L, Hardy MJ, et al. Development and application of infection control workload unit tool to determine staffing needs. *Am J Infect Control* 1993;22:117

29. Reybrouck G. Scoring system suggested to determine staffing level. *Am J Infect Control* 1986;14:148

30. Wenzel RP, Streed SA. Surveillance and use of computers in hospital infection control. *J Hosp Infect* 1989;13:217–229

31. Gransden WR. Information, computers and infection control. *J Hosp Infect* 1990;15:1–5

32. Amundsen J, Drennan DP. An infection control nurse–advisor program. *Am J Infect Control* 1983;11:20–23

33. Colletti MA, Kasey C, Fellencer C. Unit–based infection control: it makes a difference. *Am J Infect Control* 1987;15:32A–34A

34. Ross KA. A program for infection surveillance utilizing an infection control liaison nurse. *Am J Infect Control* 1982;10:24–28

35. Haim L, Booth JH, Greaney K. Recommendations for optimizing an infection control practitioner's effectiveness in an ambulatory care setting. *J Health Care Q* 1994;16:31–34

36. Mehtar, S. Infection control programmes – are they cost-effective? *J Hosp Infect* 1995;30(S):26–34

37. Nettleman, MD. Cost-effectiveness and cost-benefit analysis in infection control. In: Wenzel RP, ed. *Prevention and Control of Nosocomial Infections* 3rd ed. Baltimore, MD: Williams & Wilkins; 1997:19–32

38. Wenzel RP. The economics of nosocomial infections. *J Hosp Infect* 1995;31:79–87

39. Haley RW. *Managing Hospital Infection Control for Cost-effectiveness.* Chicago, IL: American Hospital Association; 1986

40. Wakefield DS, Pfaller MA, Hammons GT, et al. Use of the appropriate evaluation protocol for estimating the incremental costs associated with nosocomial infections. *Med Care* 1987;25:481–488

41. French GL, Cheng AFB. Measurement of the costs of hospital infection by prevalence surveys. *J Hosp Infect* 1991;18(suppl A): 65–72

42. Senge PM. *The Fifth Discipline: The Art & Practice of the Learning Organization.* New York, NY: Doubleday; 1990:223–235

43. Belasco JA. *Teaching the Elephant to Dance: The Manager's Guide to Empowering Change.* New York, NY: Crown Publishers; 1990: 99–103

44. Scholtes PR. *The Team Handbook: How To Use Teams To Improve Quality.* Madison, WI: Joiner Associates; 1988

45. Marszalek-Gaucher E, Coffey RJ. *Transforming Healthcare Organizations: How To Achieve and Sustain Organizational Excellence.* San Francisco, CA: Jossey-Bass; 1990:85

46. Gabor A. *The Man Who Discovered Quality.* New York, NY: Random House; 1990:82

47. Vander Hyde K, Friedman C. Using a quality improvement team for determining strategies to reduce body substance exposures. *Am J Infect Control* 1994;22:108

48. Brewer JH, Gasser CS. The affinity between continuous quality improvement and epidemic surveillance. *Inf Cont Hosp Epidemiol* 1993;14:95

49. Nyström B. The role of hospital infection control in the quality system of hospitals. *J Hosp Infect* 1992;21:169–177

50. Post BA, Kreutzer-Baraglia L. Infection control. In: Spicer JG, Robinson MA. eds. *Managing the Environment in Critical Care Nursing.* Baltimore, MD: Williams & Wilkins; 1990:42

51. Johnson J, Bonadonna L, Webster B. Integrating infection control practices into unit-based quality improvement. *Am J Infect Control* 1993;21:106

52. Atkins PM. Reducing risks through quality improvement, infection control, and risk management. *Crit Care Nurs Clin* 1995;7:733–741

53. Donabedian A. Contributions of epidemiology to quality assessment and monitoring, *Inf Cont Hosp Epidemiol* 1990;11:117–121

54. Karanfil L, Josephson A, Alonzo H. An infection control quality improvement (QI) approach to nosocomial bacteremia in neonates. *Am J Infect Control* 1991;19:108

55. Kelleghan S, Salemi C, Padilla S, et al. An effective quality improvement program for prevention of nosocomial ventilator pneumonia. *Am J Infect Control* 1991;19:122

56. McKenzie M, Taylor G. Infection control in an environment of continuous quality improvement. *Am J Infect Control* 1992;20:96

57. Cook JD, Lewis L, Thomassen K. Using total quality management to achieve proper isolation. *Am J Infect Control* 1994;22:123

58. Kritchevsky SB, Simmons BP. Continuous quality improvement. *JAMA* 1991;266:1817–1823

59. Joint Commission on Accreditation of Healthcare Organizations. Standards: performance improvement. In: JCAHO. *Accreditation Manual for Hospitals.* Chicago, IL: Joint Commission on Accreditation of Healthcare Organizations; 1998

60. Friedman C, Richter D, Skylis T, Brown D. Process surveillance: auditing infection control policies and procedures. *Am J Infect Control* 1984;12:228–232

61. Baker OG. Process surveillance: an epidemiologic challenge for all health care organizations. *Am J Infect Control* 1997;25:96–101

62. Classen DC, Evans RS, Pestotnik SL, et al. The timing of prophylactic administration of antibiotics and the risk of surgical-wound infection. *New Engl J Med* 1992;326:281–286

63. Bennett G, Baker O. Developing an integrated quality improvement program. *Am J Infect Control* 1990;18:118–125

64. Haley RW. Surveillance by objective: a new priority-directed approach to the control of nosocomial infections. *Am J Infect Control* 1985;13:78–89

65. Friedman C, Baker CA, Mowry-Hanley, et al. Use of the total quality process in an infection control program: a surprising customer-needs assessment, *Am J Infect Control* 1993;21:155–159.

SUGGESTED READINGS

Chaudhuri AK. Infection control in hospitals: has its quality-enhancing and cost-effective role been appreciated? *J Hosp Infect* 1993;25: 1–6

Farr BM. Organization of infection control programs. In: Abrutyn E. ed. *Saunders Infection Control Reference Service.* Philadelphia, PA: WB Saunders Co; 1998:13–15

Friedman C, Chenoweth C. Infection control. In: Schmele JA. ed. *Quality Management in Nursing and Health Care.* Albany, NY: Delmar Publishers; 1996:507–519

Haley RW. The development of infection surveillance and control programs. In: Bennett JV, Brachman PS. eds. *Hospital Infections.* 4th ed. Philadelphia, PA:1998, Lippincott–Raven; 1998:53–64

Hoffman KK. The modern infection control practitioner. In: Wenzel RP. ed. *Prevention and Control of Nosocomial Infections.* 3rd ed. Baltimore, MD: Williams & Wilkins; 1997:33–45

Jackson MM. Infection prevention and control in the managed care era: dinosaur, dragon, or dark horse? *Am J Infect Control* 1997;25:38–43

Mehtar S. *Hospital Infection Control: Setting Up with Minimal Resources.* London, England: Oxford University Press; 1992.

Mehtar S. How to cost and fund an infection control programme. *J Hosp Infect* 1993; 25:57–69

Pugliese G, Kroc KA. Development and implementation of infection control policies and procedures. In: Mayhall CG. ed. *Hospital Epidemiology and Infection Control.* Baltimore, MD: Williams & Wilkins; 1996:1068–1079

Selwyn S. Hospital infection: the first 2500 years. *J Hosp Infect* 1991; 18(suppl A):5–64, 1991.

Wenzel RP, Pfaller MA. Feasible and desirable future targets for reducing the costs of hospital infections. *J Hosp Infect* 1991;18(suppl A): 94–98.

Triage Screening Tools

Sample Triage Policy

Sample Triage Screening Protocol

Tuberculosis Screening Tool

Figure C.1a   Sample Triage Policy   (Front of Form)

> **Guideline: Triage for Infection Prevention in Ambulatory Care**
>
> For suspected chicken pox, measles, rubella, or other airborne infections and unidentified rashes:
>
> The nurse will triage the patient phone call and will discuss with the physician or assigned clinician whether the patient must be seen, whether the visit can be rescheduled, or whether the case can be handled over the telephone.
> If the patient will be seen:
>
> 1. Advise the patient to come to an alternate door and not the main entrance, when available.
> 2. Determine the immune status of the staff. Recommend that only staff members who are immune care for the patient. All non-immune staff who must care for the patient must wear masks.
> 3. At the time of entry to the facility, have the patient wear a mask (surgical or isolation).
> 4. Place the patient in an exam room immediately to avoid time in the waiting room.
> 5. Keep the exam room door closed.
> 6. When the patient leaves, clean surfaces contaminated with blood or body fluid as for any patient, using Standard Precautions.
>
> Patients with suspected active, pulmonary TB must be handled according to Airborne Precautions. The patient is to be moved to a facility with negative pressure isolation rooms, such as _____ Hospital, as soon as possible or sent home with appropriate instructions.
>
> If possible exposure occurs, contact _____ or _____.
> (Infection Control)   (Employee Health)

Figure C1.b   Part of the Intake Form   (Back of Form)

> Pediatric Outpatient Note   Patient Stamp:
>
>
> Exposures: (circle one)
>   Chicken pox   Y or N   Date _____
>   Measles   Y or N   Date _____
>   Rash   Y or N

Figure C.2   Sample Triage Screening Protocol

Diseases Screened	Where Screening Occurs: Check-In Desk, Triage Area, Waiting Room, or Treatment Room	Actions
Bacterial meningitis	Triage area	
Chicken pox	Check-in desk	Place in negative pressure room
Measles	Check-in desk	Place in negative pressure room
Mumps	Check-in desk	Place in negative pressure room
Pertussis	Check-in desk	Place in negative pressure room
Respiratory syncytial virus	Check-in desk	Cohort patients
Tuberculosis	Treatment room	Place in negative pressure room

Figure C.3   Tuberculosis Screening Tool—Emergency Department

For all patients presenting with a respiratory complaint, ask: "Do you have a productive cough (producing sputum)?"

If NO: Continue with normal screening procedure.

If YES: Ask patient if he/she has any of the following:

Blood in sputum

Fevers

Night sweats

Unexplained weight loss

Past history of TB

Previous positive TB test

Recent exposure to someone who is sick with TB

Risk factors for HIV infection

If the patient, or patient representative, answers YES to at least one of the questions above and the patient does not require critical care intervention, immediately put the patient in a room designated for isolation. Hang a sign indicating "Airborne Precautions" on the door and keep the door closed. Anyone entering the room must wear a mask. The patient must remain in this room with the door closed.

If the patient, or patient representative, answers YES to at least one of the questions above and the patient requires close monitoring, do the following:

1. Place a mask on the patient. If the patient cannot wear a mask, place an oxygen mask on the patient;
2. Place the patient in a bay furthest away from other patients and concentrated staff areas, and;
3. Instruct staff working in the same bay with the patient to wear a mask.

If the patient will be admitted, transfer the patient to an isolation room set at negative pressure as soon as patient safety permits.

APPENDIX D

Isolation Tools

Contact Precautions Sign

Droplet Precautions Sign

Airborne Precautions Signs

Isolation Precautions Table

CONTACT PRECAUTIONS

1. **Gloves:** Wear for any patient contact and contact with any item that touched the patient. Remove gloves before leaving the room.

2. **Hands:** Wash upon exiting the room.

3. **Face Protection:** No, except as for Standard Precautions.

4. **Gowns:** Wear for any patient contact or contact with items close to the patient.

STANDARD PRECAUTIONS at all times!

Figure D.1   Contact Precautions Sign

DROPLET PRECAUTIONS

1. **Gloves:** Wear for any patient contact. Remove before touching environmental surfaces. Wash hands after removing gloves.

2. **Hands:** Wash upon exiting the room and after contact with the patient.

3. **Face Protection** (e.g., mask/goggle combination): Wear if the patient is coughing *and* if coming within 2 to 3 feet of the patient.

4. **Gowns/Barriers** (diaper, towel, or blanket): Wear if your body will be contacting the patient, exam room bed, or immediate surrounding area.

STANDARD PRECAUTIONS at all times!

Figure D.2 Droplet Precautions Sign

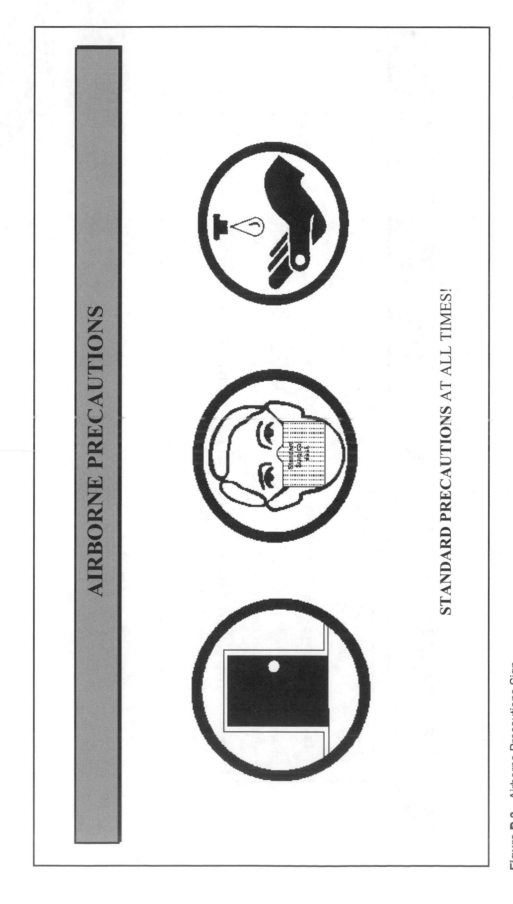

Figure D.3 Airborne Precautions Sign

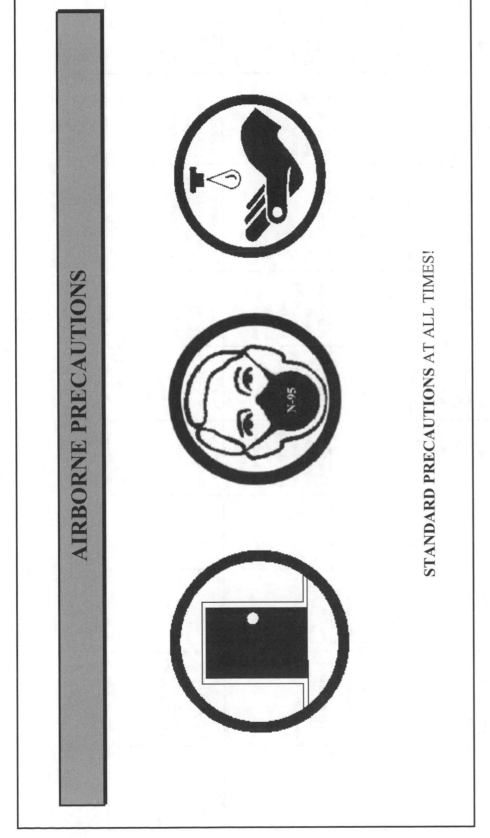

Figure D.4   Airborne Precautions Sign—Use for Tuberculosis

Table D.1   Isolation Precautions

	Principle	Diseases	Room	Gloves	Mask	Gown	Eye Protection (facemask/goggles)	Handwashing	Equipment Handling
Standard Precautions (SP)	Precautions used for *all* patients to prevent exposure to diseases spread through moist body substances.	Not focused on any specific disease; focuses on interactions and practices with all patients.		When handling moist body substances or items soiled with moist body substances.	If face is likely to be splattered with moist body substance. Always worn with eye protection.	If clothes are likely to be splattered with moist body substance.	If face is likely to be splashed with moist body substance.	Wash after removing gloves or having any contact with moist body substance or nonintact skin.	Clean immediately if soiled with body substances.
Airborne Precautions	Precautions used to prevent exposure to diseases spread through the air.	Examples: Chicken pox, disseminated Herpes zoster (shingles), tuberculosis	Isolation room set at negative pressure.	No (except as per SP)	Mask required unless immune.	No (except as per SP)	No (except as per SP)	According to SP	According to SP
Contact Precautions	Precautions used to prevent illness spread by contact.	Examples: Scabies, RSV, VRE, VRSA		Wear for any patient contact and contact with any item that touched patient.	No (except as per SP)	Wear for any patient contact or if working close to patient.	No (except as per SP)	Wash after touching potentially contaminated articles and before leaving room.	Wipe with disinfectant prior to removal from room.
Droplet Precautions	Precautions used to prevent spread of microbes through large particle droplets.	Examples: Influenza, pertussis, rubella		No (except as per SP)	Wear if patient is coughing *and if* coming within 2–3 feet of patient.	Wear for any activity involving patient contact or if working close to patient.	Wear if patient is coughing *and if* coming within 2–3 feet of patient.	Wash after patient contact and upon exiting room.	Wipe with disinfectant prior to removal from room.

Education Tools

Antibiotic Resistance Precautions—A Patient's Guide

Sample Handout for Patients in Isolation/Precautions

Figure E.1   Antibiotic Resistance Precautions—A Patient's Guide

What are antibiotic-resistant bacteria?

You have had a positive culture for a bacterium that cannot be treated easily with antibiotics. This type of bacteria is commonly known as **antibiotic-resistant bacteria**. Antibiotic-resistant bacteria will not make you any sicker than more common bacteria and are sometimes treatable with a combination of antibiotics and/or with newer kinds of medications.

In many cases, the body's own immune system is able to attack antibiotic-resistant bacteria to either rid them from the body or to keep them "in check" by not allowing them to grow to numbers that might lead to illness.

Healthy people are in no danger of becoming sick from antibiotic-resistant bacteria because their bodies are very good at fighting off *any bacteria* that are not common to their own bodies. People with chronic conditions, weakened immune systems (decreased ability to fight off disease), on long-term antibiotics, or who have many or lengthy hospitalizations are at risk for becoming sick with *any* of the bacteria that are typically in their surroundings.

Antibiotic Resistance Precautions

Extra precautions are taken to prevent antibiotic-resistant bacteria from spreading to other patients. These precautions are called **contact precautions** and are practiced *in addition to* the usual precautions we use for *all* patients to prevent the spread of *any* kind of microorganism (bacteria and other germs).

When initiating precautions, a sign will be placed on your exam room door outlining the extra precautions the staff will need to take when providing your care. They include:

- Hands will be washed whenever exiting the room.
- A long-sleeved gown will be worn if contact will be made with you or the immediate area around you.
- Gloves will be used for any contact with you.

Answers to Some Common Questions

Do I need to worry about taking this bacteria home to my family?

In most cases you do not need to use special precautions at home because most people have defenses that will not allow this bacteria to "take hold." If someone in your home has been on antibiotics for many weeks and also is immune-compromised, tell your nurse or doctor, and he or she will tell you what you can do to prevent exposing this person to the resistant organism.

What precautions should family caregivers take for infected persons in their homes?

Outside of healthcare settings, there is little risk of spreading these bacteria to others; therefore, healthy people are at low risk of getting infected. In the home, the following precautions should be followed:

- Caregivers should wash their hands with soap and water after physical contact with the infected or colonized person.
- Towels used for drying hands after contact should be used only once.
- Disposable gloves should be worn if contact with body fluids is expected, and hands should be washed after removing the gloves.

What are enterococci?

Enterococci are bacteria that live in the bowel. Enterococci can go to other parts of the body and cause an infection. Vancomycin is an antibiotic used to treat infection caused by enterococci. If bacteria are resistant to vancomycin it means that vancomycin will not treat the infection. When this happens it is called "vancomycin-resistant enterococci" or VRE.

Will I ever be rid of VRE?

Over time your normal bowel organisms may take the place of VRE. You may no longer be isolated when stool or rectal swabs are negative for VRE.

What is Staphylococcus aureus?

Staphylococcus aureus, or *S. aureus*, is a bacteria usually found on a person's skin and mucous membranes. It may cause infections on broken skin or wounds. Methicillin and Vancomycin are antibiotics used to treat infections caused by *S. aureus*. If *S. aureus* is resistant to Methicillin, it is called MRSA. If *S. aureus* is resistant to Vancomycin, it is called VRSA. This means that the infection may be more difficult to treat. If someone has a VRSA or MRSA infection, other antibiotics may be used.

Will I ever get rid of MRSA or VRSA?

Over time your normal skin organisms may take the place of MRSA or VRSA and you will no longer be placed in precautions.

Figure E.2   Sample Handout for Patients in Isolation/Precautions

ANSWERS TO YOUR QUESTIONS:
AIRBORNE PRECAUTIONS

What is Airborne Precautions?

Airborne Precautions is a way to protect other patients, visitors, and staff from breathing in the microbes that are breathed out from a person with certain diseases. You will be in a room with a special air system that provides fresh air to the room and prevents the room's air from going to the rest of the building. The door to your room must stay closed. There will be a sign on your door that states "Airborne Precautions."

Why are people wearing masks?

Most staff entering your room will wear a mask to protect themselves.

Can I leave the room?

It is important that you stay in the room until we have completed our evaluation. If you need to leave your room for any reason, check with a nurse. If you must leave, you will be given a mask to wear. If you cough or sneeze, please cover your mouth — even if you are wearing a mask.

Disinfection/Sterilization Tools

Sample Procedure for Disinfection

Sample Procedure for Sterilization

Steam Autoclave Spore Test Log

Endoscopy Competency

Autoclave Competency

High-Level Disinfection Competency

Temperature Log for Medication Refrigerator

Patient Food Refrigerator/Freezer Log

Sample Procedure for Disinfection

Name of instrument: _____

Performed by (underline): medical assistant   nurse   other _____

Personal protective equipment needed (underline):   gloves   gowns
                                                             face shield   mask/goggles

Disassembly instructions, if applicable:

Disinfectant used:

Procedure: After each use:

1. Immediately immerse instrument into water or soapy water to avoid drying of secretions or body fluid.
2. Clean with enzymatic instrument detergent. Special equipment needed (underline):
   brushes   cleaning cloths   ultrasonic cleaner
3. Rinse with tap water.
4. Drip dry (to avoid diluting the disinfectant chemical).
5. Completely immerse in disinfectant.
6. Soak for _____ minutes at room temperature.
7. Rinse with running tap water, or use a clean basin (not the same basin as used for the initial rinsing) filled with fresh water.
8. Dry.
9. Storage location, to prevent contamination: _____ .

Figure F.1   Sample Procedure for Disinfection

Sample Procedure for Sterilization

Name of instrument: _____

Performed by (underline): medical assistant   nurse   other _____

Personal protective equipment needed (underline):   gloves   gowns

face shield   mask/goggles

Disassembly instructions, if applicable:

Procedure. After each use:

1. Immediately immerse instrument into water or soapy water to avoid drying of secretions or body fluids.
2. Clean with instrument detergent. Special equipment/procedures needed (circle):
   brushes or cleaning cloths   ultrasonic cleaner
3. Rinse with tap water.
4. Dry.
5. Wrap. Indicate type of wrap (e.g., peel pouch, surgical wrap): _____ .
6. If not part of the wrap, include internal and external chemical indicators.
7. Label with date of sterilization and load number if more than one sterilizer load is run per day.
8. Place in autoclave.
9. Remove when cycle is finished and packs are completely dry.
10. Specify storage location in closed cabinet or drawer to avoid contamination: _____
    _____ .

Figure F.2   Sample Procedure for Sterilization

STEAM AUTOCLAVE SPORE TEST LOG

Location of Sterilizer: _____

If the sterilizer is used at least once a week, a spore test must be run weekly. If it is used less than once a week, a spore test must be run with each load. Run a control with every test.

For any positive results and for questions on sterilizer monitoring policies, contact Infection Control, email or phone number _____.

For autoclave malfunction, contact Maintenance, email or phone number _____.

Maintain records for ___ years.

Date of Test/Control	Date of Results	Test Result (positive or negative)	Control Result (positive or negative)	Operator's Initials	Contents of Load—General Description	Follow-up, if Positive

Figure F.3 Steam Autoclave Spore Test Log

ENDOSCOPY COMPETENCY

Instructions for RN: Place check mark next to each critical behavior. Sign your name and date. Note: Staff must demonstrate all Critical Behaviors for each demonstration before considered to be competent.

Staff name _____ Circle: MA, RN, LPN, other_____

RN Signature _____ Date _____

File completed form in employee's folder.

Competency: Cleans and disinfects endoscopes in the absence of an automatic endoscope reprocessor.

Critical Behaviors	Preceptor Initial/Date		Recommended Resources	Evaluation
	Met	Needs improvement		
1. Demonstrates use of personal protective equipment during endoscope reprocessing: a. Gloves must be worn. b. Gowns and face protection (goggles and mask, or face shield) must be used if splashing is likely to occur.			Standard Precautions Infection Control Disinfection Guidelines	To demonstrate competence, the staff person must perform the following:
2. Demonstrates precleaning (removal of gross contamination immediately following use): a. Wipes insertion tube with enzymatic detergent solution. b. Suctions detergent solution through each channel of the endoscope. c. Clears air and water channels according to manufacturer's instructions.			Infection Control Policy—Endoscopy: High-Level Disinfection SGNA self-study module: "Endoscope Cleaning and High-Level Disinfection"	1. Observe a competent staff person clean and disinfect an endoscope. and 2. Perform a satisfactory return demonstration of the cleaning and disinfecting of an endoscope with observation by and feedback from a competent staff person.
3. Demonstrates leak testing according to endoscope manufacturer's instructions.				
4. Demonstrates the process of cleaning in enzymatic detergent: a. Detaches all removable parts—see 10c. b. Immerses and thoroughly cleans the exterior of the endoscope. c. Brushes entire suction/biopsy channel system. Repeats brushing until no debris is visible on the brush. d. Attaches cleaning (all-channel) adapter, or uses suction or syringes. e. Rinses scope under running water to remove residual detergent. f. Flushes all channels with water.			SGNA video: "Endoscope Cleaning and High-Level Disinfection" Product label instructions for enzymatic detergent and disinfectant Endoscope manufacturer's instructions	

(continues)

Figure F.4 Endoscopy Competency

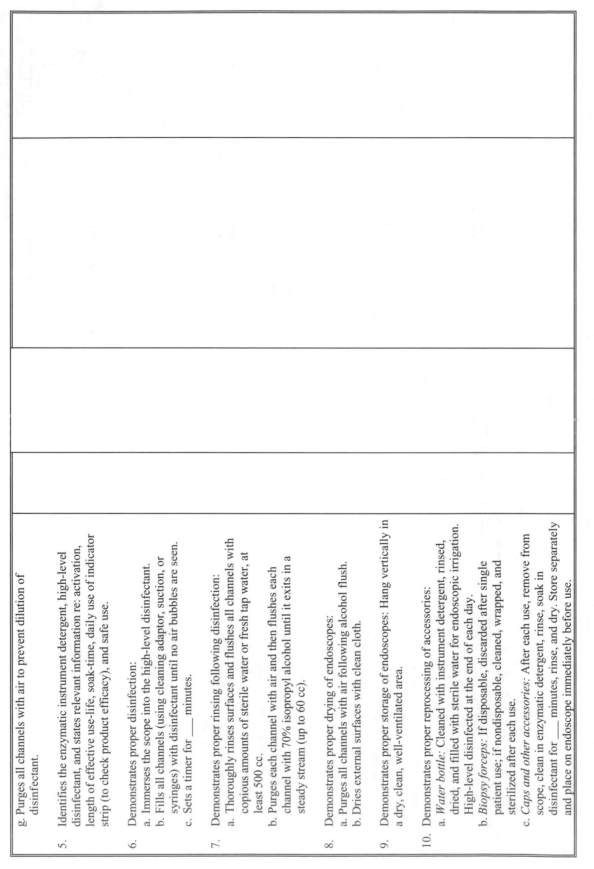

g. Purges all channels with air to prevent dilution of disinfectant.

5. Identifies the enzymatic instrument detergent, high-level disinfectant, and states relevant information re: activation, length of effective use-life, soak-time, daily use of indicator strip (to check product efficacy), and safe use.

6. Demonstrates proper disinfection:
   a. Immerses the scope into the high-level disinfectant.
   b. Fills all channels (using cleaning adaptor, suction, or syringes) with disinfectant until no air bubbles are seen.
   c. Sets a timer for ___ minutes.

7. Demonstrates proper rinsing following disinfection:
   a. Thoroughly rinses surfaces and flushes all channels with copious amounts of sterile water or fresh tap water, at least 500 cc.
   b. Purges each channel with air and then flushes each channel with 70% isopropyl alcohol until it exits in a steady stream (up to 60 cc).

8. Demonstrates proper drying of endoscopes:
   a. Purges all channels with air following alcohol flush.
   b. Dries external surfaces with clean cloth.

9. Demonstrates proper storage of endoscopes: Hang vertically in a dry, clean, well-ventilated area.

10. Demonstrates proper reprocessing of accessories:
   a. *Water bottle:* Cleaned with instrument detergent, rinsed, dried, and filled with sterile water for endoscopic irrigation. High-level disinfected at the end of each day.
   b. *Biopsy forceps:* If disposable, discarded after single patient use; if nondisposable, cleaned, wrapped, and sterilized after each use.
   c. *Caps and other accessories:* After each use, remove from scope, clean in enzymatic detergent, rinse, soak in disinfectant for ___ minutes, rinse, and dry. Store separately and place on endoscope immediately before use.

Figure F.4 Endoscopy Competency (continued)

AUTOCLAVE COMPETENCY

Instructions for RN: Place check mark next to each critical behavior. Sign your name and date. Note: Staff must demonstrate all Critical Behaviors for each demonstration before considered to be competent.

Staff name _____   Circle: MA, RN, LPN, other _____

RN Signature _____   Date _____

File completed form in employee's folder.

Competency: Cleans and sterilizes reusable devices using an autoclave.

Critical Behaviors	Preceptor Initial/Date		Recommended Resources	Evaluation
	Met	Needs Improvement		
1. States criteria for determining when a device requires sterilization between patient uses: a. Contact with vascular or normally sterile tissue, and b. Labeled for reuse versus single-use (in accordance with FDA single-use device law).			Written procedures for each item to be sterilized Infection Control Policies for Sterilization Monitoring	To demonstrate competence, the staff person must perform the following:
2. Verbalizes the importance of performing sterilization consistently for each item that meets the above criteria, regardless of the diagnosis of the patient.			Operator's manual for autoclave	1. Observe a competent staff person clean and sterilize equipment (e.g., surgical pack), perform preventive maintenance on the autoclave, and perform the BI test.
3. Locates and refers to written procedures for device reprocessing and Infection Control Policies for Sterilization Monitoring.				
4. Locates and refers to operator's manual for autoclave, as appropriate.				and
5. Describes the process for ensuring that a device moves from soiled to clean/decontaminated, to sterilized, to storage without contamination.				2. Perform a satisfactory return demonstration of the cleaning and sterilizing of equipment,
6. Demonstrates the following when preparing items for sterilization: a. Wears gloves. Other personal protective equipment is worn if splashing is anticipated. b. Cleans device with specified instrument enzymatic detergent, rinses with tap water, and dries.				

Figure F.5   Autoclave Competency

(continues)

preventive maintenance of the autoclave and the BI test, with observation by and feedback from a competent staff person.

c. Wraps device in peel pouch or approved autoclave wrap.
d. Includes internal sterilization indicator (if not included as part of the pouch).
e. If using autoclave wrap, tapes with autoclave-sensitive tape.
f. Labels each item with the date of sterilization.

7. Explains the term event-related sterility, including the necessity of checking indicator tape, external and internal monitors, sterilization parameters, package integrity, and biological indicator (spore test) results to ensure sterility of package contents.

8. Demonstrates loading and operation of the autoclave in accordance with the operator's manual:
   a. If needed, adds distilled or deionized water.
   b. Places packs or peel pouches in autoclave tray with no pack touching side of autoclave or loads cassette.
   c. Closes and locks autoclave door.
   d. Chooses cycle appropriate to the load and starts cycle.
   e. At end of cycle, carefully opens door slightly to allow for drying and to prevent steam burns.
   f. Does not touch or handle packs or peel pouches until cool and dry to prevent contamination of item.
   g. When cooled and dry, places sterilized packs or peel pouches on shelves in designated clean storage room or in closed cupboards/drawers of other rooms to prevent contamination.

9. States steps involved in preventive maintenance (PM) as specified in owner's manual:
   a. Cleans inside of autoclave and gasket at regular intervals.
   b. Checks gasket and interior surfaces for damage and removes any debris at regular intervals.
   c. Drains water, flushes, and fills with distilled or deionized water at regular intervals.
   d. Checks any other items specified in the autoclave manual.
   e. Calls Maintenance with any questions or problems with autoclave function.

Figure F.5   Autoclave Competency (continued)

Competency: Biological Indicator (BI) to test and document autoclave performance

1. Verbalizes the frequency with which to perform BI:
   a. Weekly, or
   b. With every load, if autoclave is used less than once per week.

2. States the need to perform a "control run" with each test run and demonstrates the method for doing so.

3. Demonstrates the following when performing BI test:
   a. Verifies that expiration date has not been exceeded.
   b. Places BI into peel pouch or wrap.
   c. Places test pack in the autoclave with a normal load and into the most difficult area to sterilize, generally near the drain or door.
   d. Performs the sterilization cycle.
   e. After the cycle is complete and packs are dry and cool, removes the BI.
   f. Opens the peel pouch or wrap and removes BI.
   g. Prepares BI for incubation.
   h. Describes length of incubation period.
   i. Describes expected color of control versus color result of test, and which colors correspond to positive and negative.
   j. Locates and appropriately documents control and test results in the BI log.

4. States what "positive results" are and steps to take for a positive result:
   a. Run the autoclave again with another BI test.
   b. If the repeat is positive, call Maintenance and Infection Control.
   c. Institute recall procedure.

Figure F.5 Autoclave Competency (continued)

HIGH-LEVEL DISINFECTION COMPETENCY

Instructions for RN: Place check mark next to each critical behavior. Sign your name and date. Note: Staff must demonstrate all Critical Behavoirs for each demonstration before considered to be competent.

Staff name _____   Circle: MA, RN, LPN, other_____

RN Signature _____   Date _____

File completed form in employee's folder.

Competency: Performs high-level disinfection safely and effectively.

Critical Behaviors	Preceptor Initial/Date		Recommended Resources	Evaluation
	Met	Needs Improvement		
1. States criteria for determining when a device requires high-level disinfection between patient contacts: a. Contact with mucous membranes or non-intact skin, and b. Labeled for reuse versus single use (in accordance with FDA single-use device law).			Written procedures for each item to be disinfected Infection Control Policies for High-Level Disinfection	To demonstrate competence, the staff person must perform the following:
2. Verbalizes the importance of performing high-level disinfection consistently for each item that meets the above criteria, regardless of the diagnosis of the patient.			Product label instructions for enzymatic detergent and disinfectant	1. Observe a competent staff person clean and disinfect a device (e.g., vaginal speculum).
3. Locates and refers to written procedures for device reprocessing and Infection Control policies for High-Level Disinfection.			Material Safety Data Sheets (MSDS) for detergent and disinfectant	and
4. Identifies the enzymatic instrument detergent, high-level disinfectant, and states relevant information re: dilution or activation, length of effective use-life, soak-time, daily use of indicator strip (to check product efficacy), and safe use.				2. Perform a satisfactory return demonstration of the cleaning and disinfecting of a device, with observation by and feedback from a competent staff person.
5. Identifies the steps involved in the safe and effective use of a high-level disinfectant: a. References MSDS. b. Activates product according to label. c. Covers container. d. Labels container with expiration date. e. Labels container with product name, health, and physical hazards.				

(continues)

Figure F.6 High-Level Disinfection Competency

f. Uses gloves for contact.

g. Checks product efficacy each day of use with indicator strip.

h. Calls Safety Management Services or Industrial Hygienist for chemical exposure and safety issues.

6. Describes the process for ensuring that a device moves from soiled, to clean/decontaminated, to disinfected, to storage without contamination.

7. Demonstrates the following when performing high-level disinfection:

a. Wears gloves. Other personal protective equipment is worn if splashing is anticipated.

b. Cleans device with specified instrument detergent, rinses with tap water, and dries (to avoid diluting disinfectant).

c. If same sink will be used for final rinse, wipes sink with disinfectant cleaner.

d. Immerses device completely into the disinfectant.

e. Sets timer for minutes (if watch or clock is used, the time must be posted).

f. Removes device from disinfectant and rinses thoroughly in either a basin of fresh water or under running water.

g. Dries and stores device in a covered location to prevent contamination.

Figure F.6 High-Level Disinfection Competency (continued)

TEMPERATURE LOG FOR MEDICATION REFRIGERATOR

SITE: _____

LOCATION: _____

MONTH: _____

Temp °F	Temp °C	Date:	1	2	3	4	5	6	7	8	9	10	11	12	13	14	15	16	17	18	19	20	21	22	23	24	25	26	27	28	29	30	31
		Time/initials																																
50°F	10°C																																	
49	9.4																																	
48	8.9																																	
47	8.3																																	
46	7.8																																	
45	7.2																																	
44	6.7																																	
43	6.1																																	
42	5.5																																	
41	5																																	
40	4.4																																	
39	3.9																																	
38	3.3																																	
37	2.8																																	
36	2.2																																	
35	1.7																																	
34	1.1																																	
33	0.5																																	
32	0																																	
31	-0.5																																	
30	-1.1																																	

Please place an "X" in the box of the observed temperature. Record time and your initials, above. Record "C" on each day the unit is closed.

If out of range (in the gray area), contact Pharmacy. Adjust the thermostat. In one hour, reread and record the new temperature. If still out of range, report to Supervisor. Move medications to a working refrigerator until the temperature is within range. Supervisor should contact Maintenance to report problem and request urgent repair.

Corrective Actions	Date	Name	Corrective Actions	Date	Name
_____	_____	_____	_____	_____	_____
_____	_____	_____	_____	_____	_____
_____	_____	_____	_____	_____	_____

Turn in completed log to manager.

Figure F.7 Temperature Log for Medication Refrigerator

Patient Food Refrigerator/Freezer Log

Room: _____ Year: _____

1. Read and record temperatures daily (M-F, if area is not open on weekends). Initial.
2. Circle any temperature out of standard. Document corrective action on back of form.
3. Maintain logs for 3 years.
4. Defrost freezer if ice builds up.

	1	2	3	4	5	6	7	8	9	10	11	12	13	14	15	16	17	18	19	20	21	22	23	24	25	26	27	28	29	30	31
Jan Refrig. ≤41°F or ≤5°C																															
Freezer ≤0°F or ≤−17.8°C																															
Initials																															
Feb Refrig. ≤41°F or ≤5°C																															
Freezer ≤0°F or ≤−17.8°C																															
Initials																															
March Refrig. ≤41°F or ≤5°C																															
Freezer ≤0°F or ≤−17.8°C																															
Initials																															
April Refrig. ≤41°F or ≤5°C																															
Freezer ≤0°F or ≤−17.8°C																															
Initials																															
May Refrig. ≤41°F or ≤5°C																															
Freezer ≤0°F or ≤−17.8°C																															
Initials																															
June Refrig. ≤41°F or ≤5°C																															
Freezer ≤0°F or ≤−17.8°C																															
Initials																															
July Refrig. ≤41°F or ≤5°C																															
Freezer ≤0°F or ≤−17.8°C																															
Initials																															
August Refrig. ≤41°F or ≤5°C																															
Freezer ≤0°F or ≤−17.8°C																															
Initials																															
Sept Refrig. ≤41°F or ≤5°C																															
Freezer ≤0°F or ≤−17.8°C																															
Initials																															
Oct Refrig. ≤41°F or ≤5°C																															
Freezer ≤0°F or ≤−17.8°C																															
Initials																															
Nov Refrig. ≤41°F or ≤5°C																															
Freezer ≤0°F or ≤−17.8°C																															
Initials																															
Dec Refrig. ≤41°F or ≤5°C																															
Freezer ≤0°F or ≤−17.8°C																															
Initials																															

Figure F.8   Patient Food Refrigerator/Freezer Log (front)

Corrective Action Procedure and Documentation for Food Refrigerators and Freezers

1. Circle any temperature out of standard (refrigerator ≥ 41°F / 5°C; freezer ≥ 0°F / –17.8°C).

2. For **refrigerators** less than 45°F or 4.9°C, do nothing and check the refrigerator the next day.
   If on the next day the refrigerator is still above normal but less than 45°F/4.9°C, adjust the temperature gauge down and recheck in a couple of hours.
   If adjustments to temperatures do not resolve the problem, discard food and call Maintenance.

3. For **freezers** less than 10°F or –16.8°C, do nothing and check the freezer the next day.
   If on the next day the freezer is still above normal but less than 10°F /–16.8°C, adjust the temperature gauge down and recheck in a couple of hours.
   If adjustments to temperatures do not resolve the problem, discard food and call Maintenance.

Date	Temperature	Corrective Action	Result	Signature

Figure F.8   Patient Food Refrigerator/Freezer Log (back)

Surveillance Tools

Sample Surveillance Plan 1

Sample Surveillance Plan 2

Data Analysis

Forms

Sample Surveillance Plan 1

Scope of services: Infusion therapy
Case mix (patient population): Patients have cancer and are being treated with chemotherapy
Patient volume: The ambulatory care site has approximately 100 visits per month.
Types of invasive procedures: None
Types of medical procedures: Infusion
Types of equipment used: Intravascular (IV) therapy equipment

Infection prevention and control staff performs continuous, priority-directed, targeted surveillance. This method of surveillance was chosen to focus on those areas or services with a potential for prevention–infusion therapy.

Specific Surveillance Indicators:

Blood:
Purpose: To check for bloodstream infection (BSI) resulting from IV-access procedure.

- If center visit within past 48 hours *and* clinical information consistent with BSI.

IV site:
Purpose: To check for intravascular-site infections resulting from IV access.

- If center visit within past 48 hours *and* clinical information consistent with IV-site infection.

Data are collected using microbiology laboratory reports to identify positive cultures that might indicate infected patients. The IV sites are evaluated during each visit. Patients are also requested to provide information on infections. The CDC's National Nosocomial Infections Surveillance System definitions for nosocomial infections are followed.

Data are presented routinely to the Infusion Center Quality Improvement Team and the Infection Control Committee in the form of rates. Any problem areas are also brought to the attention of the infusion center staff. Data are used in studies for improving patient care.

If a cluster of infections or an outbreak is identified, an investigation is performed to identify root causes. Control measures are recommended at various stages prior to, during, and after the investigation. Surveillance is continued to ensure control of the problem. Sustained improvement is evaluated routinely through surveillance and review of microbiology laboratory culture results.

Sample Surveillance Plan 2

Scope of services: Eye surgery
Case mix (patient population): Patients who require eye surgery
Patient volume: There are approximately 500 visits per month.
Types of invasive procedures: Eye surgery
Types of medical procedures: None
Types of equipment used: Surgical instruments

Infection control (IC) staff performs continuous, priority-directed, targeted surveillance. This method of surveillance was chosen to enable IC staff to focus on the population at risk (e.g., those areas where frequent infectious complications are found—surgery).

Specific Surveillance Indicators:

Wounds:

Purpose: Surveillance for post-discharge surgical-site infection (SSI), surveillance for SSI resulting from outpatient procedure.

- If patient had surgery within past 30 days (one year if implant), check clinical information for signs/diagnosis of SSI.
- If patient had outpatient surgery within applicable timeframe *and* clinical information indicates SSI or possible SSI.

Eye:

Purpose: Surveillance for specific infections of past importance or reported importance in IC literature.

- Eye: If patient had eye exam within seven days of wound culture. *Specific purpose:* To detect outbreak/cluster of EKC (adenovirus causing epidemic keratoconjunctivitis).

Data are collected using microbiology laboratory reports to identify positive cultures that might indicate infected patients. In addition, a reporting system is used to identify patients with potential post-surgical or eye infections. Health care-associated infections are identified through ongoing concurrent medical record review. The CDC's National Nosocomial Infections Surveillance System definitions for nosocomial infections are followed.

Data are used in studies for improving patient care. IC staff works with the quality assurance staff on improvement projects. Studies are performed as needed to evaluate accuracy and completeness of case finding.

Data are presented routinely to the Infection Control Committee in the form of rates. Any problem areas are also brought to the attention of the nurse manager and the medical director. At completion of problem follow-up, an epidemiologic formal report is written. Recommendations are made related to the problem in order to decrease infectious complications and improve patient care.

If a cluster of infections or an outbreak is identified, an investigation is performed to identify root causes. A casecontrol or cohort study may be performed. One area of review is adequate staffing. Control measures are recommended at various stages prior to, during, and after the investigation. Surveillance is continued to ensure control of the problem. In general, epidemiologic methods are used to evaluate results, investigate problems, and determine measures for improvements. Sustained improvement is evaluated routinely through surveillance and review of microbiology laboratory culture results.

DATA ANALYSIS

Line Listing

Name	Reg No.	Insertion Date	Type of CVC	Symptom Date	Site	Microbes
Murphy C	247799	06/11/2001	tunneled	08/12/2001	BSI	CPS
Ward M	295154	06/02/2001	tunneled	09/27/2001	BSI	ENT
Alexander C	234545	09/01/2001	tunneled	09/05/2001	BSI	KP
Regina T	234546	09/15/2001	tunneled	10/20/2001	BSI	CNS
Spink A	272355	11/11/2000	tunneled	10/25/2001	BSI	CNS
Leah H	235644	06/11/2000	tunneled	11/11/2001	BSI	PA
White F	235689	10/13/2001	PICC	12/24/2001	BSI	CNS

Rates

Outcome Measures

Surgical site infection (SSI) rate

    Numerator: Number of SSIs

    Denominator: Number of operations

    Rate (%): Number of SSI ÷ Number of operations × 100

Dialysis-related infection rate

    Numerator: Number of access site infections

    Denominator: Number of dialysis months (total cumulative months all patients received dialysis during a specific time period [e.g., one month])

    Rate per 1000 dialysis-months: Number of access site infections ÷ Number of dialysis months × 1000

Process Measures

Immunization rate

    Numerator: Number of persons immunized for influenza

    Denominator: Number of persons eligible for influenza vaccine

    Immunization Rate (%): Number of persons immunized for influenza ÷ Number of persons eligible for influenza vaccine × 100

Biological Indicator Failures

    Numerator: Number of positive biological indicators

    Denominator: Number of sterilizers tested with biological indicators

    Rate (%): Number of positive biological indicators ÷ Number of sterilizers tested with biological indicators × 100

Tables, Graphs, and Charts

Table

A table is a set of data arranged in rows and columns; it can note comparisons.

Use: To present the frequency an event (e.g., infection) occurs.

Catheter-Related Bloodstream Infections

    Numerator: Number of bloodstream infections

    Denominator: Number of catheter days

	Infusion Area 1	Infusion Area 2	Infusion Area 3
2000	10.0**	4.0	5.3
2001	7.9	3.0	11.9
Benchmark*	6.8	6.8	6.8

*From the literature

**Rate per 1000 catheter-days

Graph

A graph is a method of showing data using a system of coordinates; it is very visual.

Use: Can aid in understanding and interpreting data.

Types: Line, bar, histogram

Bloodstream Infections in Infusion Patients

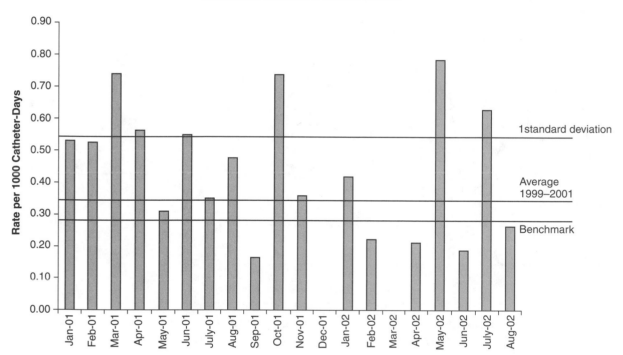

Run Chart

A run chart is a line or bar graph.

Use: To study observed data for trends or patterns over time.

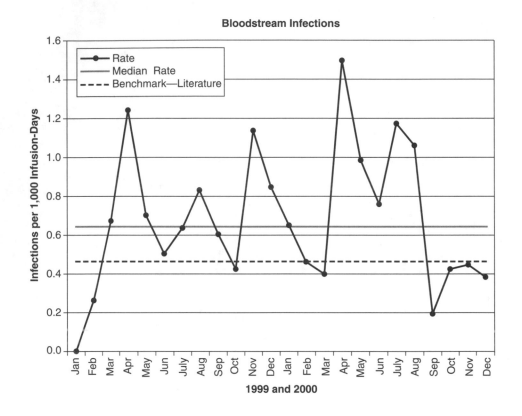

Bloodstream Infections

Chart

A chart is a method of illustrating information using only one coordinate.

Use: To compare magnitudes of different events; to compare parts of an entire picture.

Types: Run, Pareto, geographic, pie

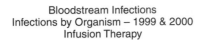

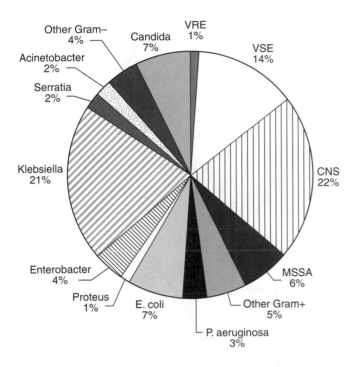

Control Chart

A control chart is a graph of data to help display the type of variation in processes; it is a line graph plus statistical control limits used as reference lines. A control chart identifies trends and special causes.

> *Special cause:* An unexpected, significant deviation outside what is predicted. Special causes tend to cluster by person, place, and time. Special cause variation represents changes that can be investigated and assigned to an identifiable source.
>
> *Common cause:* Variation that results from chance events that occur without a specific cause and from the inherent design of the system. As a result of this common cause variation, rates of specific processes and outcomes fluctuate over time.

Use: Focuses attention on detecting and monitoring variation over time; distinguishes special from common causes of variation; helps focus direction on improving a process.

Types: The type of data determines the chart used; for infection prevention and control purposes, u and p charts are used.

> *u chart:* Uses attribute data (discrete events, e.g., infections) and has a variable sample size.
>
> *p chart:* Uses attribute data (discrete events, e.g., tests) and a sample size greater than 50.

Tip: The p and u charts create changing control limits if the sample sizes vary in each group.

Example (u):

A violation of the upper control limit is noted in April 1999. A cause is sought, and it is discovered that a new type of IV administration set was instituted that month, allowing cross-contamination. Once the problem is corrected and this special cause is eliminated, the rate declines. Apart from that deviation, the monthly rate fluctuates within the control limits. The month-to-month variations represent chance events, not correctable sources of variation.

Long-term, the processes underlying the development of bloodstream infections may be investigated to reduce the mean overall and, therefore, establish new control limits.

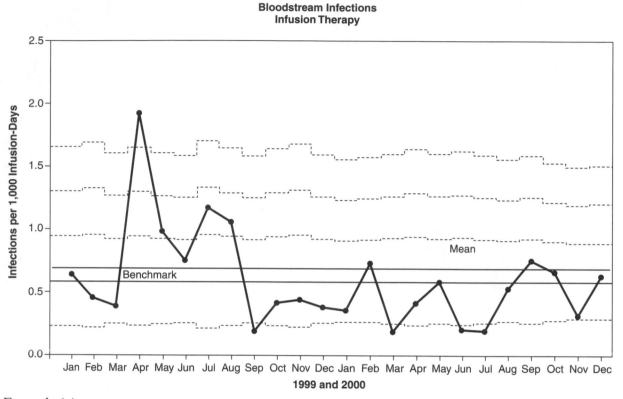

**Bloodstream Infections
Infusion Therapy**

Example (p):

Tuberculin tests are administered annually to employees during their anniversary month. Improvement in employee compliance can be seen starting in late 1998 after specific measures are put into place. Control charts assist in identification of improvement in these rates.

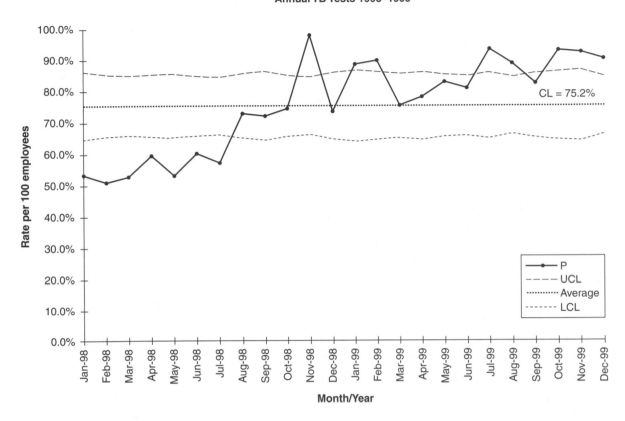

Annual TB Tests 1998–1999

Statistical Techniques

The following statistical techniques may be performed using Microsoft Excel or Epi Info (obtained from *http://www.cdc.gov/epiinfo/*).

Descriptive Statistics

These numbers organize, describe, and summarize data in a concise manner.

Mean: Sum of observations divided by the number of observations; the mathematical average.

Example:
observations = 7, 16, 3, 12, 8, 3   number of observations = 6
mean = $(7+16+3+12+8+3) \div 6 = 49 \div 6 = 8.2$

Other measures include median, ratio, rate, and standard deviation.

Inferential Statistics

This is a process by which we can draw conclusions regarding a population from results observed in a sample. These procedures rely on probability. Conclusions drawn depend on whether the test results are statistically significant; that is, it is unlikely that the results could occur by chance.

Chi Square Test (2×2 Table): Used to test differences between two samples.

Contingency table for test:

	Disease	
Factor	**Y**	**N**
Y	a	b
N	c	d

Formula: $X^2 = \dfrac{n(|ad - bc|)^2}{(a+b)(c+d)(a+c)(b+d)}$

The p-value is obtained by looking up the value obtained in a X^2 table. However, there are Web sites that will compute the p-value easily, such as *http://members.aol.com/johnp71/ctab2x2.html*.

Example:

	Disease	
Factor	**BSI**	**no BSI**
TPN	21	79
No TPN	5	95

Formula: $X^2 = \dfrac{200(|1995 - 395|)^2}{(26)(174)(100)(100)} = 9.95$

Looking up the value in a X^2 table results in a p-value of 0.002.

Fisher's Exact Test: Used to test differences between two samples for small sample size tables.

Formula: $p = \dfrac{(a+c)!(b+d)!(c+d)!(a+b)!}{n!a!b!c!d!}$

There are Web sites that will compute the p-value easily, such as *www.matforsk.no/ola/fisher.htm*.

t-test: Evaluates the difference between two samples.

Comparing the mean of a sample (number of observations ≤ 30) with a known standard. Want to know if the mean is statistically different from a known number, e.g., a NNIS rate.

Formula: sample of n observations with mean $\bar{x}$ and a standard deviation of s.

$t = \dfrac{\bar{x} - \mu}{s / \sqrt{n}}$

Look up calculated t-value on a Student's t-table for n − 1 degrees of freedom to obtain p-value.

Example: You have 24 months of data for bloodstream infections in your infusion therapy center. The mean is 6.8 and the standard deviation is 1.2. The benchmark 50th percentile is 4.5.

$$t = \frac{6.8 - 4.5}{1.2 / \sqrt{24}} = \frac{2.3}{0.25} = 9.3 \quad \text{degrees of freedom} = 24 - 1 = 23$$

The t-test value for p = 0.005 is 2.807 and for p = 0.0005 is 3.768; therefore, since the t value in the example is 9.3, the p-value is <0.0005.

Forms

Ambulatory Surgery Form (front)

Dr. _____

Below is a list of your patients for the time period _____ to _____.

Please indicate whether any of these patients developed a post-operative infection. All

information is confidential.

| | | Infection? | |
Date of Surgery	Patient Name/Medical Record Number	Yes (Note date of infection)	No

Ambulatory Surgery Form (back)

Infection Criteria:

Superficial Incision—Surgical Site Infection

Infection occurs within 30 days after the operation *and* infection involves only skin or subcutaneous tissue of the incision *and* at least *one* of the following:
1. Purulent drainage, with or without laboratory confirmation, from the superficial incision.
2. Organisms isolated from an aseptically obtained culture of fluid or tissue from the superficial incision.
3. At least one of the following signs or symptoms of infection: pain or tenderness, localized swelling, redness, or heat *and* superficial incision is deliberately opened by surgeon, *unless* incision is culture-negative.
4. Diagnosis of superficial incisional SSI by the surgeon or attending physician.

Deep Incision—Surgical Site Infection

Infection occurs within 30 days after the operation if no implant is left in place or within one year if implant is in place and the infection appears to be related to the operation *and* infection involves deep soft tissues (e.g., fascial and muscle layers) of the incision *and* at least *one* of the following:

1. Purulent drainage from the deep incision but not from the organ/space component of the surgical site.
2. A deep incision spontaneously separates or is deliberately opened by a surgeon when the patient has at least one of the following signs or symptoms: fever (>38°C), localized pain, or tenderness, unless site is culture-negative.
3. An abscess or other evidence of infection involving the deep incision is found on direct examination, during reoperation, or by histopathologic or radiologic examination.
4. Diagnosis of a deep incisional SSI by a surgeon or attending physician.

Please return this form to: _____ by (date) _____.

Thank you.

Confidential document information

From University of Michigan Hospitals and Health Centers

Site Review Form (1 of 4)

Infection Control—Site Review Form

Site: Medical Director:
Address: Administrator:
Phone: Nursing Manager:
Office Manager: Reviewer:
                                               Date of Visit:

	Yes	No	N/A	Recommendations, References, or Comments
Manager Interview				
Do you notify the health department of reportable diseases?				
Have all eligible staff received TB skin test within the past year?				
Do you have competencies in place for staff who reprocess endoscopes or other instruments, or use the autoclave?				
Do you have a triage process in place to identify and separate patients with airborne infections, including TB?				
Bloodborne Pathogen Standards				
Have all staff received IC training within the past year?				
Is approved disinfectant available for blood spill clean-up?				
Are eating and drinking observed where specimens and blood are handled?				
Is the process for reporting body substance exposures known to staff?				
Can staff locate the Exposure Control Plan?				
Employee Interview (sample #___)				
Do you know what to do if you have a body substance exposure (e.g., needlestick)?				
Can assigned staff verbalize the toy cleaning procedure or policy?				
Waiting Room				
Is the area clean?				
Are the toys clean?				
Can clerical staff verbalize triaging of possibly infectious (airborne) cases?				

Site Review Form (2 of 4)

Infection Control—Clinic Site Review Form				page 2
	Yes	No	N/A	Recommendations, References, or Comments
Exam/treatment room assessment				
Are exam gloves available?				
Are face protection (goggles, masks or faceshields) and gowns available?				
Are sharps containers < 3/4 full?				
Are soap dispensers disposable, or if not, are they cleaned when empty (not topped off)?				
Is antimicrobial soap or alcohol-based hand rub available?				
Is antiseptic agent available for patient skin prep prior to minor surgery, peripheral IV placement, and blood draw?				
Are any patient-care items under sink?				
Are any multidose vials (MDVs) outdated?				
Is room clean, including exam table?				
Is disinfectant cleaner available?				
Are soiled and clean linen separated?				
Are clean, sterile supplies stored in closed cabinets, drawers, or so as to avoid contamination?				
Are clean, sterile supplies away from splash zone of sink?				
Are sterile supplies set up immediately before use on individual patients?				
Are irrigation solutions (500, liter bottles) labeled, discarded w/in 24 hours of opening?				
Is soiled equipment transported safely to utility room?				
Clean storage room or area				
Are patient care items off the floor?				
Are sterile packs rotated "first in first out"?				
Is "event-related" sterility used?				
Is linen stored covered (if on shelving in hall) and off the floor?				
Refrigerators				
Are separate refrigerators available for specimens, medications, and patient food?				
Are temperature logs in use and up-to-date (temps logged daily)?				
Does the specimen refrigerator have a biohazard label?				
Are any food or medications in the specimen refrigerator?				
Are medications past expiration date, including multi-dose vials (MDVs)?				

Site Review Form (3 of 4)

Infection Control—Clinic Site Review Form				page 3
	Yes	No	N/A	Recommendations, References, or Comments
Utility room				
Are sharps containers, red bags, and biohazard buckets located where needed?				
Do red bags or biohazard buckets contain only/mostly regulated medical waste?				
Are clean storage and soiled utility rooms separated?				
If in the same room, are areas labeled or well marked/delineated?				
If utility room is used for storage, are cabinets and shelves closed so as prevent contamination of patient ready items?				
If glutaraldehyde is used, is ventilation adequate?				
Process Observation				
Equipment Reprocessing Are single use devices used once, then discarded?				
Are gloves, gowns, and face protection available?				
Are written procedures available for each device reprocessed?				
Are devices that contact mucous membrane, non-intact skin high level disinfected?				
Are devices that contact sterile or vascular tissue sterilized?				
Does workflow proceed from soiled to decontaminated to disinfected/sterilized to storage?				
Are devices soaked immediately after use?				
Are devices cleaned with enzymatic instrument detergent and rinsed with running or in basin of fresh water?				
If needed, are ultrasonic cleaners used?				
Are devices dried after cleaning?				
Disinfectant safely, effectively used: Are containers: completely covered? • Labeled with chemical name? • Labeled with expiration date? • Checked each day of use for effectiveness?				
Are devices completely immersed in disinfectant?				
Is soak time according to product label?				
Is timer used to measure soak time?				
Are devices rinsed thoroughly after use?				
If used, are endoscopes reprocessed according to policy and strict procedures?				

Site Review Form (4 of 4)

Infection Control—Clinic Site Review Form				page 4
	Yes	No	N/A	Recommendations, References, or Comments
Autoclave				
Is biological indicator performed weekly or with every load if run less often?				
Is log up to date?				
If test is positive, are staff aware of follow-up procedure?				
Is preventive maintenance program in place (including cleaning and draining of autoclave)?				
If items are autoclaved unwrapped, is indicator used in each load?				
Are items labeled with date of sterilization?				
Are packs labeled with external and internal indicators and/or are peel pouches with these labels as part of the wrap used?				
Are packs placed in autoclave according to autoclave manual?				

General Comments

From University of Michigan Hospitals and Health Centers

Infection Control Surveillance Data Entry Form

Patient ID# _____

Patient Name _____

Visit Date ____/____/_____   Age _____   Sex _____

Service _____

Operation Y / N   Procedure _____

Date ____/____/_____   Duration: Hrs _____ Min _____

Surgeon _____

General Anes Y / N   ASA _____   Wound Class _____

Emergency Y / N   Trauma Y / N   Implant Y / N

Room #_____

Endoscopic Approach Y / N   Multiple Procedures Y / N

Infection Date ____/____/_____

Site _____

48 hrs Preceding Infection

BSI: Central line Y / N   TPN Y / N

Tunneled line Y / N

PNEU: CXR Confirmed Y / N

Ventilator Y / N

Other information:

Invasive procedures/devices Y / N

2° Bloodstream Infection Y / N

DX _____

Prophylactic antibiotics

Surg. Prophy abx (Type & Route)	Incision Time	Time Admin.

Notes

Culture

Date	Source	Results	Comments

SIGNS/SYMPTOMS WITHIN 24 HOURS OF VISIT/PROCEDURE
(Circle all that may be considered related to suspected infection.)

Circle and indicate dates

fever (38°C/100.4°F) chills   leukocytosis (>10k)   hypotension (systolic <90)   oliguria   mental confusion
apnea   tachypnea   decreased O_2 sat.   respiratory distress   bradycardia   hyperglycemia

Resp: rales   dullness to percussion   wheezing cough   change in character of sputum   mental confusion
              increased production of respiratory secretions   new onset of purulent sputum
LRI   rhonchi   lung abscess   empyema
URI   erythema of pharynx   sore throat   cough   hoarseness   purulent exudate   abscess   rhinnorhea
Vascular: pain, erythema, or heat at vascular site   purulent drainage at vascular site
Skin   pain/tenderness   localized swelling   erythema   heat   purulent drainage   abscess
/Wound   pustules   vesicles   boils   change in burn wound appearance
Eye   purulent exudate from (circle one or more): conjunctiva, eyelid, cornea, meibomian glands, lacrimal glands
              eye pain   visual disturbance   hypopyon   conjunctivitis
GI   diarrhea (acute onset?)   nausea   vomiting abdominal pain/tenderness   jaundice   gross blood in stools
              anorexia   purulent material from intraabdomial space   abscess   abdominal distension   prefeeding residuals
Urinary: (circle one or >) urgency frequency, dysuria, suprapubic tenderness   pyuria (≥10wbc/mm³)
Bone/Joint   drainage from suspected site   bone pain   joint pain   effusion or limited motion   vertebral disc pain

APPENDIX H

Outbreak Investigation Tools

Protocol and Example

Definition of Terms

Information of Epi Info

OUTBREAK INVESTIGATION PROTOCOL AND EXAMPLE: MT. SINAI EYE CENTER

1. Confirm that an outbreak exists.
   a. Case finding (Need to develop criteria/case definition): Look for additional cases. Use laboratory database to help with case finding, determine historical information. Get special report from microbiology, if necessary.

   b. Compare current situation with historical data or information in the literature.
   c. Report to health department, if reportable disease or if health department requires reporting of outbreaks.
   d. Have specimens held, as appropriate (for further testing).
   e. Verify the diagnosis of cases; identify the agent.
      a. Characterize signs and symptoms.
      b. Check susceptibilities to compare microbes.
      c. Obtain additional specimens, as appropriate.
   f. Communicate initial information to appropriate staff.
   g. Search for additional cases; collect critical data and specimens.
      a. Perform routine surveillance.
      b. Discussions with staff (request that you be informed if they notice patients with signs/symptoms of case definition).
      c. Use data collection tool (develop one with required data elements).
2. Characterize the cases by person, place and time.
   a. Develop line list of cases.
   b. Develop chronological graph and/or placement map, as appropriate.
   c. Develop epidemic curve, as appropriate.
   d. Evaluate patient characteristics (e.g., underlying disease).
   e. Calculate rates.
   f. Review data and determine whether a problem exists.
3. Formulate tentative hypotheses (best guess as to root causes).
   a. Look for a potential carrier issue.
   b. Identify if contaminated solutions, equipment.

A case patient was defined as any Center patient [with EKC] examined at the Center during the month preceding the onset of disease. EKC = epidemic keratoconjunctivitis.
Case patients were identified by review of infection control reports and patient records during July.
Historical data revealed that in the pre-outbreak period there were only three cases of EKC from January to June.

All cases cultured Adenovirus (the causative agent). Symptoms included ocular redness, swelling, tearing, photophobia, and ocular discomfort.

The medical director and administrator of the Center were informed on July 20.
Data were collected onto standardized forms and analyzed by EpiInfo software. Staff was interviewed to determine practices during examinations (e.g., technique for administration of eye drops/dye, processing of equipment between patients, and hand hygiene). Observations were made of infection prevention and control practices.

See Table 21.1 and Figure 21.1. In the outbreak period there were 19 cases of EKC in 1800 visits to the Center (attack rate of 1.1%). The mean incubation period was 6.3 days (range 5–10 days). All patients had pneumotonometry performed during their examination. Because there was a dramatic increase in the number of EKC patients with a peak on July 17, this appeared to be a common source outbreak.

Hypothesis: The infections are associated with tonometer use or eye manipulation (e.g., drops, dye, etc.). Staff interviews identified that tonometers were wiped with a clean tissue between patients.

   c. Evaluate if person-to-person spread and what
      cause might be (e.g., staffing issues, cleaning
      issues, etc.).

   d. Communicate tentative findings.

      a. nurse manager, medical director/chief of
         service

      b. appropriate leaders

Findings were verbally discussed with the medical director on July 21. Use of tonometers was stopped.

4. Test hypotheses.

   a. May not need to do this; descriptive epidemiology (as in 2) may be enough to identify problem.

Environmental cultures of surfaces, equipment, and solutions were obtained. All were negative.

   b. Perform cultures of equipment, environment.

   c. Observe practices.

   d. Discuss with staff.

   e. Case-control or cohort study.

   f. Review staffing of area.

5. Institute appropriate control measures.

6. Evaluate efficacy of control measures.

   a. Perform intensive surveillance looking for additional cases. Amount of time depends on type of outbreak and its epidemiology.

Control measures instituted July 23:

1. All suspected cases were sent to a separate waiting area and were seen in one specific exam room.
2. Gloves were worn during examinations.
3. Surfaces were cleaned with approved disinfectant cleaner between patients.
4. Tonometer tips were removed and disinfected with bleach solution between patients.

7. Communicate findings.

   a. To nurse manager/medical director.

   b. Interim reports.

      a. If cluster continuing despite control measures, write an interim report outlining measures and any issues that are outstanding regarding recommendations made. Continue to go back to step 5.

Reports written and sent to medical director and administrator.

   c. Write final report.

      a. For unit-based problems—to nurse manager, medical director/chief of service, other areas, as appropriate.

      b. For patient-to-patient transmission—to nurse manager, medical director/chief of service

   d. Communicate with health department, if appropriate.

No additional cases were identified after control measures were instituted.

DEFINITION OF TERMS

The following list includes important epidemiologic terms used in outbreak investigations.

Attack rate: An incidence rate calculated for a short time period, as in an epidemic.

Case: A patient having the particular disease or condition under study.

Case definition: Parameters that determine which patients should be included as cases.

Case-control study: A study that includes cases of disease and a suitable reference group for comparison. Data on selected attributes or risk factors are collected from both groups using similar methods, and then the frequencies are compared between the two groups using statistical analyses.

Cohort study: A method of comparing the future disease experience of a group or population. The population is characterized by exposures that may be important in causing a certain disease. The incidence over time of that disease is tracked for the population, and disease rates for exposed and unexposed persons are then compared.

Common-source outbreak: Involves patient exposures to a single contaminated source (e.g., a contaminated solution or device).

Cluster of infections: Defined by geographic and temporal grouping.

Endemic: Expected frequency of infections; the typical level of disease.

Epidemic: Disease in excess of the normal frequency.

Epidemic curve: A graph (histogram) showing cases of the disease during the outbreak by time, with time on the X-axis and the number of cases on the Y-axis.

Incidence rate: The number of new cases of an infection or disease during a defined period of time divided by the population at risk during that time.

Incubation period: The time from initial exposure to an infection to the onset of the first sign or symptom associated with the infection.

Outbreak or **epidemic of health care-associated infections:** When the expected frequency of infections is exceeded. A single episode of a rare infection or isolation of an unusual pathogen also can be considered an outbreak if the occurrence of cases is not expected (e.g., one case of legionellosis, one surgical site infection caused by group A streptococcus).

Pseudoinfection: Isolation of a microorganism by stain or culture from a patient who does not have signs or symptoms characteristic of infection with that microbe.

Pseudo-outbreak or **pseudoepidemic:** Involves a cluster of patients from whom the same microorganism is isolated but who do not have signs or symptoms suggestive of infection (e.g., a cluster of pseudoinfections). Often, pseudo-outbreaks involve false-positive cultures of clinical specimens from patients. They may be associated with:

- Contamination of materials used in diagnostic specimen collection (e.g., contaminated blood culture bottle tops)
- Specimen collection contamination
- Laboratory contamination
- Contamination of equipment used in diagnostic procedures
- Improper blood-drawing technique
- Contamination of antiseptic solutions used for skin preparation

INFORMATION ON EPI INFO

Epi Info and Epi Map are public domain software packages designed for the global community of public health practitioners and researchers. Both provide for easy form and database construction, data entry, and analysis with epidemiologic statistics, maps, and graphs. Although "Epi Info" is a CDC trademark, the programs, documentation, and teaching materials are in the public domain and may be freely copied, distributed, and translated.

With Epi Info 2000 and a personal computer, epidemiologists and other public health and medical professionals can rapidly develop a questionnaire or form, customize the data entry process, and enter and analyze data. Epidemiologic statistics, tables, graphs, and maps are produced with simple commands such as READ, FREQ, LIST, TABLES, GRAPH, and MAP. Epi Map 2000 displays geographic maps with data from Epi Info 2000.

Key Features of Epi Info 2000

- Maximum compatibility with industry standards, including:
  - Microsoft Access and other SQL and ODBC databases
  - Visual Basic, Version 6
  - World Wide Web browsers and HTML
- Extensibility, so that organizations outside the CDC can produce additional modules
- Epi Map, an ArcView®-compatible GIS
- NutStat, a nutrition anthropometry program that calculates percentiles and z-scores using either the 2000 CDC or the 1978 CDC/WHO growth reference
- Logistic regression and Kaplan-Meier survival analysis
- Teaching exercises
- Microsoft Windows 95, 98, NT, and 2000 compatible
- Allows analysis and import of other file types

System Requirements

- Windows 95, 98, NT, or 2000 required
- 32 MB of random access memory. More RAM (64 MB minimum) recommended for Win NT
- 200 megahertz processor recommended
- At least 50 megabytes of free hard disk space
- Download from *http://www.cdc.gov/epiinfo/*

APPENDIX I

Exposure Control Plan

Bloodborne Pathogens Exposure Control Plan Example

BLOODBORNE PATHOGENS EXPOSURE CONTROL PLAN: MT. SINAI INFUSION CENTER

Prepared July 1, 2002

In accordance with the OSHA Bloodborne Pathogens standard (*http://www.osha-slc.gov/SLTC/bloodbornepathogens/index.html*) the following exposure control plan has been developed.

Exposure Determination

The following employees are determined to be at risk from occupational exposure to bloodborne pathogens. The exposure determination was made without regard to the use of personal protective equipment. At this facility the following job classifications are in this category:

- Nurses
- Physicians
- Medical Assistants

The tasks/procedures that might result in exposure to blood or other potentially infectious material (OPIM) are as follows:

- Blood drawing (phlebotomy)
- Changing visibly soiled beds
- Cleanup of surfaces contaminated by blood/body substances
- Emptying drainage receptacles, including urine receptacles, bed pans, and emesis basins
- Intravascular (IV) catheters: initiation, termination
- Reprocessing of medical instruments

Schedule and Method of Implementation

Compliance with the Bloodborne Pathogens Standard became mandatory when this facility opened in December 2000.

Methods of Compliance

All staff use Standard Precautions in order to prevent contact with blood and other potentially infectious materials. All blood/OPIM is considered potentially infectious regardless of the perceived status of the patient.

Engineering and work practice controls are used to reduce or eliminate potential employee exposures to blood and body fluids. Engineering controls are reviewed and updated on a yearly schedule to ensure their effectiveness. New safety-engineered devices are evaluated annually. The following engineering controls are used: ·

- Safety (needle-less) IV administration sets
- Safety IV catheters
- Safety butterfly needles
- Blunt medication fill needles
- Sharps containers

Readily accessible handwashing facilities and alcohol-based hand rub are provided to employees near patient care areas. Supervisors will ensure that employees wash their hands immediately or as soon as feasible after removal of gloves or other personal protective equipment.

Contaminated needles and other contaminated sharps will not be bent or recapped. Shearing or breaking of contaminated needles is prohibited. Immediately, or as soon as possible after use, contaminated reusable sharps are placed in appropriate containers until properly reprocessed. Containers are located at each patient cubicle.

Eating, drinking, smoking, applying cosmetics or lip balm, and handling contact lenses are prohibited in work areas. Food and drink are not kept in refrigerators, freezers, shelves, cabinets, or on countertops where blood or OPIM are present. All procedures involving blood or OPIM are performed in such a manner as to minimize splashing, spraying, spattering, and generation of droplets of these substances.

Personal Protective Equipment

Where occupational exposure remains after institution of these controls, personal protective equipment (PPE) will also be used. Employees are provided, at no cost, with appropriate PPE. Supervisors ensure that employees use appropriate PPE and that equipment in the appropriate sizes and types is readily accessible.

Cleaning, laundering, and disposal of PPE are provided by the Center at no cost to the employees. If blood or OPIM penetrate a garment, the garment is removed immediately or as soon as feasible.

All PPE is removed prior to leaving the work area. When PPE is removed it is placed in an appropriately designated container. Gloves are worn when it can be reasonably anticipated that there may be hand contact with blood, OPIM, mucous membranes, or non-intact skin, and when handling or touching contaminated items or surfaces. Disposable (single-use) gloves are replaced as soon as practical when contaminated or as soon as feasible if they are torn, punctured, or when their ability to function as a barrier is compromised. Disposable gloves are not washed or decontaminated for re-use. Masks, in combination with eye protection devices such as goggles or glasses with solid side shields, or chin-length face shields, are worn whenever splashes, spray, spatter, or droplets of blood or OPIM may be generated.

Appropriate protective clothing, such as gowns, lab coats, or clinic jackets, is worn in occupational exposure situations.

Specimens of blood or OPIM are placed in a container that prevents leakage during collection, handling, processing, storage, transport, or shipping. If outside contamination of the primary container occurs, the primary container is placed within a plastic bag that is properly labeled as containing biohazardous materials. If the specimen could puncture the primary container, the container is placed within a second container that is puncture-resistant in addition to the above characteristics.

Equipment that may become contaminated with blood or OPIM is examined prior to servicing or shipping and will be decontaminated as necessary. A label containing the biohazard logo and the word "biohazard" is attached to the equipment, stating which portions remain contaminated if cleaning is not feasible.

Housekeeping and Waste Disposal

The Center ensures that the work site is maintained in a clean and sanitary condition. Management determines and implements an appropriate written schedule for cleaning and method of decontamination.

All equipment and environmental and working surfaces are cleaned and decontaminated after contact with blood or OPIM. Contaminated work surfaces are decontaminated with Cleanex after completion of procedures; immediately or as soon as feasible when surfaces are overtly contaminated, or after any spill of blood or OPIM; and at the end of the work shift if the surface may have become contaminated since the last cleaning.

Broken glassware that may be contaminated is not to be picked up directly with the hands. It is cleaned up using a brush and dustpan. Reusable sharps that are contaminated with blood or OPIM are not stored or processed in a manner that requires employees to reach into the containers with their hands.

When moving containers of contaminated sharps or waste from the area of use, the containers are closed prior to removal and placed in a secondary container if

Personal Protective Equipment for Patient Care Activities

	Handwashing following Activity	Gloves	Gown/Plastic Apron	Face Protection
Blood drawing (phlebotomy)	X	X		
Changing visibly soiled beds	X	X	P	
Cleanup of surfaces contaminated by blood/body substances	X	X	P	
Emptying drainage receptacles, including urine receptacles, bed pans, emesis basins	X	X	P	P
Intravascular catheters: initiation, termination	X	X		
Reprocessing medical instruments	X	X	P	P
Resuscitation*	X	X		

X = Always

P = If there is a potential for soiling or splattering

*Use of mouth-to-mask device

leakage is possible. The secondary container is closable and labeled as biohazardous.

Communication of Hazards to Employees

The workplace risks associated with blood and OPIM are communicated to at-risk employees.

Labels and Signs

Warning labels must be affixed to or printed on containers and bags of biohazardous waste, refrigerators and freezers containing blood or OPIM, and other containers used to store or transport blood or OPIM. Labels include the biohazard logo and the word "biohazard."

Information and Training

The Center ensures that all employees with occupational exposure participate in a training program that is provided during working hours. The training is provided at the time of initial assignment and at least annually thereafter. The Center ensures that additional training is provided when changes such as modification of tasks or institution of new procedures affect employees' occupational exposure.

The bloodborne pathogens training program covers basic risks and prudent practices to avoid occupational exposure:

- Bloodborne Pathogens Standard purpose, policy, and responsibilities
- Modes of transmission, epidemiology, and symptomatology of bloodborne diseases
- Exposure Control Plan—means by which the employee may obtain a copy of the document
  - Tasks and other activities that may involve exposure to blood and OPIM
  - Methods that will prevent or reduce exposure, including appropriate engineering controls, work practices, and personal protective equipment
  - Personal protective equipment—types, selection, proper use, storage location, removal, handling, decontamination, and disposal
- Hepatitis B immunization program, including information on the efficacy, safety, administration,

and benefits of the vaccine and that the vaccine will be offered at no cost to the employees
- Appropriate actions to take and persons to contact in an emergency; procedure to follow if an exposure incident occurs, including the method of reporting the incident and the medical follow-up that will be made available
- Post-exposure evaluation and follow-up that the department is required to provide for the employee following an exposure incident
- Labels, signs, and color-coding pertaining to biohazards required by departmental policy
- Opportunity for interactive questions and answers

Hepatitis B Immunization Program

The hepatitis immunization series is provided, free of charge, to all employees determined to be at-risk. The immunization program is conducted through Mt. Sinai Hospital. Employee participation in the immunization program is on a completely voluntary basis. If an employee chooses not to participate in the immunization program, he/she is required to document the declination with a special form. (See Appendix J.) A copy of this form will be retained for the duration of the employee's tenure.

Post-Exposure Evaluation and Follow-Up

In the event an employee sustains an occupational exposure to blood or body substances, evaluation, follow-up, and counseling is provided free of charge.

If necessary, first aid is administered immediately for any cuts or punctures, and any exposed skin is washed with soap and water. The employee reports the injury to the supervisor as soon as possible. The supervisor assesses the situation and determines whether the incident constitutes an occupational exposure. The supervisor then completes any necessary accident forms and refers the employee to Mt. Sinai Hospital. A sharps injury log is maintained.

The employee will report to the Hospital as soon as possible, report the occupational injury as a potentially infectious nature, and provide an injury report form that the supervisor issued. The employee provides the following details on the injury:

- the type of injury the employee received

- the type of biohazardous material to which the employee was exposed
- circumstances under which the exposure occurred
- the hepatitis B immunization status of the employee

The physician will provide the employee with a confidential medical evaluation and follow-up of the incident:

- evaluation of the exposure risk of the incident based on the exposure source
- a written list of recommended options for testing
- preventive treatment
- explanation to the employee of the rationale and benefits of these tests and treatments

Recordkeeping

Employee records concerning training, exposures, and medical surveillance are maintained by the Center's manager.

Training Records

Training records for training in Bloodborne Pathogens are maintained for a period of three years by the Center's manager. It will include:

- the dates of the training
- the contents or a summary of the training
- the names of persons conducting the training
- the names and job titles of all persons attending the training sessions

Vaccination/Declination Records

The supervisor maintains vaccination records and declination forms for an employee's tenure at the Center.

Annual Review and Update

This Exposure Control Plan is carefully reviewed and updated annually by the Center's manager.

Occupational Health Tools

Latex Questionnaire for Heath Care Workers

	Yes	No
1. Have you ever been told by a physician that you are allergic to rubber?	____	____
2. Have you ever been tested for latex allergy and had a positive reaction?	____	____
3. Have you ever experienced an unexplained reaction, such as a drop in blood pressure, hives, or wheezing, during a medical, dental, or surgical procedure?	____	____
4. Have you ever experienced swelling or itching in the mouth or throat associated with dental procedures?	____	____
5. Have you ever experienced a rash or persistent itching while wearing rubber gloves?	____	____
6. Have you ever experienced hives, swollen mouth, runny nose, eye irritation, swollen throat, or wheezing after blowing up a balloon or contact with a rubber product?	____	____
7. Have you experienced itching or hives after using a latex condom or diaphragm, or after a rectal or vaginal examination?	____	____
8. Does your mouth or throat itch when you eat bananas, chestnuts, or avocados?	____	____
9. Did you have multiple surgeries during infancy or childhood?	____	____
10. Do you have allergies, asthma, or eczema?	____	____

HIV Post-Exposure Prophylaxis (PEP) Algorithm

Step 1: Source Material
❑ Blood
❑ Bloody fluid
❑ Other infectious materials (semen/vaginal, CSF; synovial, pleural, peritoneal, pericardial, or amniotic fluid; tissue)

If any of the above are checked, go to Step 2:

❑ Other than above (urine, stool, non-bloody saliva): NO PEP NEEDED

Step 2: Source HIV Class
❑ Class 1: (asymptomatic/high CD4 count, viral load less than 1,500 copies/ml)
❑ Class 2: (CD4 count low, AIDS, high viral load)

Step 3: Type of Exposure
❑ Intact skin→NO PEP NEEDED
❑ Percutaneous exposure (laceration or needlestick)
    ❑ Less severe (solid needle, superficial scratch)
        ❑ Class 1 source→Basic 2 drug regimen
        ❑ Class 2 source→Expanded 3 drug regimen
    ❑ More severe (large bore hollow needle, deep puncture, visible blood on device or device used in artery/vein)
        ❑ Class 1 source→Expanded 3 drug regimen
        ❑ Class 2 source→Expanded 3 drug regimen
❑ Mucous membrane/non-intact (dermatitis, abrasion, open wound) skin
    ❑ Small volume (few drops, short duration of exposure)
        ❑ Class 1 source→*Consider* basic 2 drug regimen
        ❑ Class 2 source→Basic 2 drug regimen
    ❑ Large volume (major splash or long duration of contact)
        ❑ Class 1 source→Basic 2 drug regimen
        ❑ Class 2 source→Expanded 3 drug regimen

Step 4: PEP Recommendation
❑ NONE
❑ Basic 2 drug regimen: combination zidovudine and lamivudine—1 pill 2 times daily for 4 weeks.
❑ Expanded 3 drug regimen: combination zidovudine and lamivudine—1 pill 2 times daily plus a protease inhibitor (250 mg.) 3 pills 3 times daily for 4 weeks.

If employee accepts PEP, perform pregnancy test, obtain consent for PEP, and provide medication instructions sheets; follow-up in EHS at 1 week for med/sx review/follow-up at 2 and 4 weeks for medication labs; follow-up at 6 weeks, 3 months, and 6 months for AHIV.

Special Considerations:
• Unknown source: Generally, PEP not warranted unless likelihood of HIV infection in source is high.
• Source unable to be tested: PEP generally not warranted unless source has risk factors for HIV.
• Source patient with anti-HIV drug resistance, pregnant employee: Consult with Infectious Disease consultant regarding appropriate regimen.

Source: Updated U.S. Public Health Service Guidelines for the Management of Occupational Exposures to HBV, HCV, and HIV and Recommendations for Postexposure Prophylaxis. *MMWR.* 2001; 50(RR-11):1–42.

Immunization Inventory

PART I—TO BE COMPLETED BY THE APPLICANT

Name _____

Last   First   M.I.

Date of Birth ___/___/___   Job Title _____

Department _____   Supervisor _____

PART II—TO BE COMPLETED AND SIGNED BY A LICENSED HEALTH CARE PROVIDER
(Dates must include month and year.)

1. RUBELLA
   - ❑ Rubella (or MMR) vaccine   Month/Year: _____/_____
   - ❑ Rubella Titer Month/Year: _____   Result: _____
2. MUMPS
   - ❑ Mumps (or MMR) vaccine   Month/Year: _____/_____
   - ❑ Mumps Titer Month/Year:_____   Result: _____
3. RUBEOLA (Measles)
   - ❑ Rubeola or MMR Vaccine (2 doses):

Dose 1: Month/Year _____/_____   Dose 2: Month/Year _____/_____
   - ❑ Rubeola Titer: Month/Year: _____/_____   Result: _____
4. CHICKENPOX (Varicella)
   - ❑ Had disease
   - ❑ Varicella vaccine Dose 1: Month/Year _____/_____ Dose 2: Month/Year _____/_____
   - ❑ Varicella Titer: Date: _____/_____   Result: _____
5. HEPATITIS B VACCINATION
   - ❑ Dose 1: Month/Year ___/___ Dose 2: Month/Year ___/___ Dose 3: Month/Year ___/___
   - ❑ Antibody Titer: Month/Year _____/_____   Result: _____
6. DIPHTHERIA/TETANUS
   - ❑ Had primary Series
   - ❑ Last booster: Month/Year _____/_____
7. TUBERCULOSIS SKIN TESTING

Most recent Mantoux PPD test: Month/Year _____/_____ ❑ positive ❑ negative

_____ mm *If positive, chest x-ray required (attach copy of report).*

   (If PPD done within past 12 months, it will be used for first step of two-step testing.)

HEALTH CARE PROVIDER COMPLETING THIS FORM:

Name: _____   Address: _____

(Printed)

Signature: _____   Date: _____   Phone: (___)_____

* *

EMPLOYEE HEALTH SERVICE REVIEW: _____

_____

Signature: _____   Date: _____

DOCUMENT ALL VACCINATIONS AND TB SKIN TESTS GIVEN ON EMPLOYEE HEALTH RECORD.

Hepatitis B Vaccine Declination Form

I understand that due to my occupational exposure to blood or other potentially infectious materials I may be at risk of acquiring hepatitis B virus (HBV) infection. I have been given the opportunity to be vaccinated with hepatitis B vaccine, at no charge to myself. However, I decline hepatitis B vaccination at this time. I understand that by declining this vaccine, I continue to be at risk of acquiring hepatitis B, a serious disease. If in the future I continue to have occupational exposure to blood or other potentially infectious materials and I want to be vaccinated with hepatitis B vaccine, I can receive the vaccination series at no charge to me at that time.

Employee Name _____

Employee Signature & Date _____

Supervisor Name _____

Supervisor Signature & Date _____

Bioterrorism Tools

Sample Bioterrorism Policy

Educational Material

SAMPLE BIOTERRORISM POLICY

Policy

The Health Center will develop responses to the medical needs of patients and staff who have or may have been exposed to a source of biological contamination. The response should minimize the risk of secondary infection by exposure of staff members and other patients while providing the highest level of patient care.

Purpose

The purpose of this policy is to assign responsibility, define treatment sites, and outline the Center's response to an internal or external biological contamination exposure or suspected related infection.

Definitions

Biological agent: A rare microorganism (may be highly contagious) that poses serious immediate health risks to the individual and potentially to others who come in contact with an infected individual (examples: plague, anthrax, smallpox)
Cohort: Place together in one area
HD: Health Department

Policy Standards

A. All patients are managed using Standard Precautions because biological agents are generally not spread from person to person through aerosolization.
B. Airborne Precautions, including use of an isolation room, is used for any patient with suspected smallpox or pneumonic plague.
C. Patients with similar signs and symptoms may be cohorted in a designated area.

Procedure Actions

Follow the appropriate scenario:

1. Patient potentially exposed to biological agent calls to ask what to do.
2. Patient(s) potentially exposed to biological agent comes to Health Center.
3. Patient comes to Health Center with disease suspected to be caused by biological agent.

Scenario 1: Patient potentially exposed to biological agent calls to ask what to do.

Call to Health Center. Staff asks questions: Performs medical triage—if person asymptomatic, follow this scenario; if person has symptoms, tell the person to go to the nearest emergency department.

> First: Ask if caller called police.
> If yes, police will follow up with person.
> If no, ask caller to call police.
> *Note:* Police will contact County Hazardous Material Department.

Scenario 2: Patient(s) potentially exposed to biological agent comes to Health Center.

Patient goes to isolation or private room. Ask patient(s) to remove clothing and place it in a plastic bag. Label bag with patient's name and seal the bag. Have patient wash with soap and water if there was skin exposure. Provide patient with gown. Provide biological plan patient information sheet(s). Screen patients for the presence and extent of bodily injury. Screen patient(s) for degree and location of biological agent exposure. Contact County Office of Emergency Management and HD. Decontaminate all equipment and space used in the Health Center before release for routine use. Help patients and families cope with emotional distress resulting from the incident. Keep family informed of patient's condition. Call the health department to determine the necessity of obtaining vaccines and/or pharmaceuticals (e.g., antibiotics). Determine necessity of prophylaxis or vaccination of personnel.

Scenario 3: Patient comes to Health Center with disease suspected to be caused by biological agent.

Provide immediate care. Review information on isolation protocol and treatment regimen. Place mask on patient if smallpox or plague suspected. Call EMS to transport patient to Emergency Department. Alert Emergency Department that patient is en route. Keep family informed.

Provide educational materials to patient/family. Contact County Office of Emergency Management and HD. Decontaminate all equipment and space used in the Health Center before release for routine use. Call the health department to determine the necessity of obtaining vaccines and/or pharmaceuticals (e.g., antibiotics). Determine necessity of prophylaxis or vaccination of personnel.

EDUCATIONAL MATERIAL

Anthrax

You may have been in contact with *Anthrax*. Here is an outline that will help you decide what to do.

What is anthrax?

Anthrax is an acute infection caused by the bacterium *Bacillus anthracis*. Anthrax most often occurs in warm-blooded animals (e.g., cattle, goats, and sheep). These animals pick up the anthrax spores from direct contact with contaminated soil. Humans often pick up the spores through contact with anthrax from these animals or their products (e.g., goat hair). Person-to-person spread has not been found. You may have been exposed by drinking the bacteria from contaminated water or breathing bacteria spread through the air or ventilation systems.

What are the symptoms of anthrax?

The symptoms will depend on how a person is exposed to the disease. The first symptoms (look for them during the next one to six days) may seem like a common cold. After a few days, the symptoms may progress to severe breathing problems and shock. The type of anthrax people get from breathing in the bacteria can result in death one to two days after the start of symptoms.

When anthrax gets into a person's skin, it is called cutaneous anthrax. People who already have cuts or scratches are more likely to get the illness. Areas of uncovered skin, such as arms, hands, face, and neck, are most often at risk.

What are cleaning protocols?

Because you may have been in contact with anthrax through your skin or clothing, you should remove your clothing. Place all clothing and any potentially contaminated items carefully in plastic bags and then shower using lots of soap and water. Use a bleach solution (one part household bleach to 10 parts water) to clean contaminated items. This would include objects such as letters or the surface in direct contact with the item. Wash your hands with soap and water after touching these items.

Any person in direct contact with the contaminated item or substance should receive an antibiotic. This should be taken until the substance is proved not to be anthrax.

How is anthrax spread?

Breathing in anthrax bacteria that are released into the air causes the most grave form of human anthrax, and chance of death may be high even with the correct treatment. The chance of getting anthrax through intact skin is low even after being in contact with anthrax spores.

Can anthrax be spread from person to person?

Direct person-to-person spread of anthrax does not occur often through breathing. Contact with contaminated items may spread the illness through the skin.

What is the treatment for anthrax?

Drugs called antibiotics are used to treat anthrax. The first antibiotic of choice is penicillin. Other drugs used are erythromycin, tetracycline, or chloramphenicol. To get rid of anthrax, treatment should begin early. If not treated, a person with anthrax can die from the illness.

Who should I contact?

If you show any of the symptoms above, contact your doctor as soon as you can.

What if I have other questions?

If you have questions, contact your local health department's communicable disease section or review this Web site: *http://www.cdc.gov/ncidod/dbmd/disease-info/anthrax_g.htm*.

Smallpox

You may have been exposed to *Smallpox*. Here is an outline that will help you decide what to do.

What is smallpox?

Smallpox is an illness caused by a virus called variola. This virus causes an infection known by a certain type of skin rash. The last known case of widespread smallpox was in October 1977. The last known case of smallpox that was caused by working with smallpox in a lab was in 1978. Most people in the United States are no longer immune to smallpox. You may have been exposed by breathing the virus in from the air.

What are the symptoms of smallpox?

Symptoms of smallpox are flu-like symptoms. These include fever (102–105°F), headache, tiredness, weakness, backache, and overall muscle aches. Other symptoms are generalized illness, vomiting, stomach pain, and rash often on face, arms, and legs. Look for symptoms during the next seven to 17 days.

What are cleaning protocols?

You should remove your clothing and other items on your person. Place all items in plastic bags. Shower using a lot of soap and water. Further cleansing of people who have had direct contact with smallpox is not needed. Wash your hands well after coming in contact with any item soiled with discharge from a person with smallpox.

How is smallpox spread?

Smallpox germs are spread through the air and when coming in contact with skin sores. You can catch the virus during all stages of the disease. It is easy to catch until the sores scab (in about three weeks).

Can smallpox be spread from person to person?

Yes, it can be spread very easily from person to person.

What is the treatment for smallpox?

There is no treatment for smallpox. Vaccination can prevent the illness. In the year 2003, however, smallpox is almost gone all over the world. The risk of getting smallpox from vaccination, although very small, is now greater than the risk of smallpox disease itself. Thus, smallpox vaccination is only recommended for lab workers who work with smallpox or related viruses, military personnel, and some health care workers. This may change in the future.

Who should I contact?

If you have any of the symptoms listed above, contact your doctor as soon as you can.

What if I have other questions?

If you have questions, contact your local health department's communicable disease section or review this website: *http://www.bt.cdc.gov/agent/smallpox/overview/disease-facts.asp*.

Viral Hemorrhagic Fever

You may have been exposed to *viral hemorrhagic fever*. Here is an outline to help you decide what to do.

What is viral hemorrhagic fever?

The term viral hemorrhagic fever (VHF) refers to a group of illnesses that are caused by many different viruses. These viruses can cause mild illness, but many of them cause severe illness and death.

What are the symptoms of VHF?

Certain signs and symptoms vary by type of virus, but the first signs and symptoms often include fever, feeling dizzy and tired, muscle aches, and weakness. People with severe cases of VHF often show signs of bleeding under the skin, in body organs, or from body parts such as the mouth, eyes, or ears. Very ill cases may also develop shock, nervous system problems, coma, and seizures. Some types of VHF are linked with kidney failure. Look for symptoms during the next 4 to 21 days.

What are cleaning protocols?

No special cleaning of clothing or skin is needed. Wash your hands after coming in contact with any soiled item.

Can VHF be spread from person to person?

With some viruses, humans can spread the virus to one another. This type of spread of the virus can occur through close contact with infected people or their body fluids.

What is the treatment for VHF?

Patients receive supportive care, but most often there is no cure. There is no vaccine for VHF.

Who should I contact?

If you have any of the symptoms outlined above, contact your doctor as soon as you can.

What if I have other questions?

If you have questions, contact your local health department's communicable disease section or review this Web site: *http://www.cdc.gov/ncidod/diseases/virlfvr/virlfvr.htm.*

Index

Note: Italicized page locators indicate tables/figures.